TEXTBOOK OF

Urinalysis and Body Fluids

TEXTBOOK OF
Urinalysis and Body Fluids

Doris L. Ross, Ph.D., M.T. (ASCP), C.L.S.
Professor, Medical Technology
Associate Dean, School of Allied Health Sciences
Assistant Professor, Department of Pathology and Laboratory Medicine,
 Medical School
The University of Texas Health Science Center at Houston

Ann E. Neely, M.Ed., M.T. (ASCP)
Instructional Materials Specialist, Department of Medicine,
 Section of Hematology/Oncology
Medical College of Georgia
Augusta, Georgia

 ACC APPLETON-CENTURY-CROFTS/Norwalk, Connecticut

83 84 85 86 87 / 10 9 8 7 6 5 4 3 2 1

Prentice-Hall International, Inc., London
Prentice-Hall of Australia, Pty. Ltd., Sydney
Prentice-Hall of India Private Limited, New Delhi
Prentice-Hall of Japan, Inc., Tokyo
Prentice-Hall of Southeast Asia (Pte.) Ltd., Singapore
Whitehall Books Ltd., Wellington, New Zealand

Library of Congress Cataloging in Publication Data

Ross, Doris L.
    Textbook of urinalysis and body fluids.

    Includes bibliographical references and index.
    1. Urine—Analysis.   2. Urine—Examination.
3. Body fluids—Analysis.   I. Neely, Ann E.   II. Title.
[DNLM: 1. Urine—Analysis.   2. Body fluids—Analysis.
QY 185 T355]
RB53.R6 1982   616.07′56   82-11572
ISBN 0-8385-8913-8

Design: Jean M. Sabato

This textbook is dedicated to:

Violet Keiller, M.D., Martha Gregg, M.T. (ASCP),
and Twila McIntire, M.T. (ASCP),
who first taught me urinalysis.
Doris Ross

And to:

The authors' families
Ann E. Neely
Kathryn Kilpatrick Cheek

CONTRIBUTORS

Kathleen Becan-McBride, Ed.D., M.T. (ASCP), C.L.S.
Program Director and Associate Professor
Program in Medical Technology
School of Allied Health Sciences
Assistant Professor in Pathology and Laboratory Medicine
The Medical School
The University of Texas Health Science Center
at Houston

Darlean Brown, B.S., M.T. (ASCP)
Supervisor
Hematology Laboratories
Hermann Hospital
Department of Pathology and Laboratory Medicine
The Medical School
Clinical Instructor
Program in Medical Technology
School of Allied Health Sciences
The University of Texas Health Science Center
at Houston

Kathryn Kilpatrick Cheek, M.D., M.H.Ed., M.T. (ASCP)
Formerly Instructor, School of Medical Technology
Medical College of Georgia
Augusta, Georgia

Linda P. Crum, M.A., M.T. (ASCP), C.L.S.
Formerly Education Coordinator
Program in Medical Technology
School of Allied Health Sciences
The University of Texas Health Science Center
at Houston

Diana Garza, M.S., M.T. (ASCP), C.L.S.
Senior Education Coordinator and Instructor
Program in Medical Technology
School of Allied Health Sciences
The University of Texas Health Science Center
at Houston

Karen Lorimor, B.S., M.T. (ASCP), C.L.S.
Quality Control Coordinator
Hermann Hospital Clinical Laboratories
Department of Pathology and Laboratory Medicine
The Medical School
Clinical Instructor
Program in Medical Technology
School of Allied Health Sciences
The University of Texas Health Science Center
at Houston

Barbara Smith Michael, B.S., M.T. (ASCP), R.T.-HI (CSLT), C.L.S.
Instructor and Educational Resources Coordinator
Program in Medical Technology
School of Allied Health Sciences
The University of Texas Health Science Center
at Houston

CONTENTS

PREFACE

ALTHOUGH SEVERAL good books on urinalysis are available to the clinical laboratory scientist, none covers exclusively urinalysis and body fluids in one volume. This separation makes it difficult for the student of clinical laboratory sciences to recognize the common factors responsible for the abnormalities in these fluids. Our textbook is designed to place these related areas together and thus assist in the recognition of the relationships that exist. This relationship is already recognized in programs of medical technology where both subjects are taught by the same instructor in one course.

Much could be written about any one of the topics covered in this book. It has been a challenge to the authors to select information and present it in a way that is most appropriate for an understanding of the practice of urinalysis and the examination of body fluids. One of the most profound rewards of our efforts is the increased respect for writers to whom we refer. It has been our earnest desire that no information has been misread or misinterpreted in the organization of the material and that we have cited the most appropriate source when several were available.

The need for clinically relevant information in the examination of body fluid specimens is clearly evident from the increasing number of specimens submitted to the clinical laboratory. There is currently no one book available that considers the examination and the clinical interpretations related to all the body fluids covered here. The authors of this portion of the book have written the procedures and the clinical interpretations of the body fluids as a ready source for practice and for teaching. Since no other book filled this need the methods of performance of these tests have been included.

The detailed procedures for the performance of the tests on urine, including some of the special tests, have been adequately covered in previous publications on the subject. The urinalysis portion of the book provides the reader with the pathophysiological concepts of the formation of urine as well as the principles and problems encountered in the examination of urine in the clinical laboratory. Some of the information may not be required for the performance of the routine examination of urine; however, these concepts are included for those students who want to learn more than the methods. The authors understand that the time available and the course's particular objectives must determine how the content of this book can be used. Accordingly, the information within the chapters has been arranged so that certain units may be disregarded without confusing the student. Objectives, review questions, and case studies are included to make the study of urinalysis and body fluids interesting and memorable for students in medical technology, medical laboratory sciences, and laboratory medicine.

Appreciation is expressed to the following

for their contribution to the urinalysis part of the book: Dr. Donald C. Cannon, who encouraged this endeavor; Dr. Ruth Bulger and Dr. Regina Verani for their critique and assistance; Mr. David Payne and Mr. Brad Perkins for the art work and photography; and the secretarial staff, all of whom are representative of the support given by the Department of Pathology and Laboratory Medicine of the Medical School; and Dr. Alton Hodges, Dean, and the staff of the School of Allied Health Sciences of the University of Texas Health Science Center at Houston for their support.

Appreciation is also extended to Dr. Jose M. Trujillo, Director, and Ms. Phyllis Sedgewick of the Department of Laboratory Medicine, and Mr. John Kuykendall of The University of Texas M.D. Anderson and Tumor Institute of Houston for the photographs of urinary sediment. For their contributions to the body fluids portion of the book, we are indebted to the following: Ms. Bonnie Szymik and Ms. Betty Blisset for selecting and providing specimens, Dr. Jonathan Kraus for assistance in interpretations of specimens, Dr. David Lehmiller and Dr. Dee McFarland for their initial inspiration, and Ms. Barbara Edwards, all of the Department of Pathology; Ms. Ann Anderson, School of Medical Technology; Dr. Larry Lutcher and Ms. Betty Williams, Department of Medicine, for their assistance and encouragement. Also, Dr. Frank Winekoff for his contribution in organizing material about malignant cell characteristics and guidance in comparative studies of Wright stained and Hematoxylin-Eosin stained specimens; Ms. Leslie Laurens for the illustrations; Mr. Roosevelt Brown, Medical Illustration Services; and Ms. Theresia Renick, Ms. Jenny Moore and Ms. Peggy Salter for typing the manuscript.

We hope that this book will contribute to a better understanding of the examination of urine and body fluids.

TEXTBOOK OF
Urinalysis and Body Fluids

Doris L. Ross

CHAPTER 1

Fluid Formation in the Body

Objectives

It is expected that the information presented in this chapter will enable the reader to:

1. Identify the forces involved in ultrafiltration from the capillary.
2. Utilize data about Starling's forces to determine the resulting ultrafiltration or reabsorption.
3. Define the term "interstitial fluid."
4. Calculate the ion distribution at equilibrium of solutions on either side of a membrane, one side of which contains nondiffusible protein.
5. Identify the relative water composition of the body spaces.
6. Compare the water content and osmolality of interstitial and intracellular fluid.
7. Explain the difference in ion content between interstitial fluid and blood plasma.
8. Evaluate substances used to determine extracellular water.
9. Distinguish normal from abnormal anionic and cationic composition of extracellular and intracellular fluid.
10. Correlate the body cavity containing the fluid with the appropriate term applied to that effusion.
11. Determine the relationship between conditions of edema and dehydration and the laboratory results that may be anticipated in each case.

The molecular activities of the cells in the human body occur in an aqueous environment. The ebb and flow of this sea within and the alteration of its composition influence and, in turn, are influenced by the metabolic processes that are life sustaining.

Fluid enters the body by ingestion and absorption through the intestinal tract. Some of the body fluid is derived from the oxidation within the tissues. The average individual ingestion of water in the form of liquids and solid foods is about 2.2 L/day. Other sources and ways in which water is lost from the body are shown in Table 1.1.

Once the fluid is absorbed, it becomes a part of the circulating blood plasma. Fluid distribution in the body is determined by blood flow as well as certain forces and cellular functions that occur in the capillaries of the body.

DIFFUSION

The formation of interstitial fluid begins with the process of transudation or ultrafiltration across the endothelial cells of the capillary wall. Ultrafiltration occurs by passage of water, small molecules, and ions through pores at intercellular spaces between the adjacent endothelial cells, through vesicles, or through fenestrae in the cells of the capillary wall. The surface area of capillaries of voluntary and heart muscle in the adult has been estimated to be about 465 m² (5,000 sq ft), about 1 sq m (10 to 11 sq ft) of which is lateral spaces between adjacent endothelial cells. These gaps (4 to 6 nm) allow the passage of horseradish peroxidase (40,000 daltons) and

limited passage of albumin (65,000 daltons). Some solutes and water may also be actively transported across the capillary endothelial cells. The magnitude of the entire process is such that a volume of fluid equivalent to the entire plasma volume crosses the capillaries in 60 seconds.

One of the forces involved in this process is that described by the Gibbs-Donnan effect. The Gibbs-Donnan rule states that the product of the number of charges of diffusible anions and cations on one side of a permeable membrane will equal the product of the same ions on the other side of the membrane at equilibrium. Therefore, if a nondiffusible anion, e.g., protein (Pr^-) at physiologic pH, is on one side of such a membrane, the diffusible ions will not be distributed equally on either side of the membrane at equilibrium. However, the total cations will equal the total anions within each compartment. An example of this effect is shown in Figure 1.1. It can be seen that the total number of particles on the side containing the protein will be greater, and therefore a greater osmolality will exist on that side.

The osmolalities of the interstitial fluid and intracellular fluid have been determined to be similar. The total concentrations of sodium, potassium, and other solutes will not necessarily be identical in both fluids because osmolality is a colligative property and, thus, is a function of the number of particles in solution. The number of ionic charges has no effect on the osmolality.

Even though the osmolality of the blood plasma is greater than that of interstitial fluid, the size of each compartment is constant in the steady state. A consideration of the forces

TABLE 1.1. WATER IN AND OUT OF THE BODY

Source			Loss		
Fluids of diet	1,200 ml	48%	Lungs	500 ml	20%
Food	1,000 ml	40%	Skin	500 ml	20%
Oxidation in			Urine	1,400 ml	56%
tissues	300 ml	12%	Feces	100 ml	4%

From Hawk PB, Oser BL, Summerson WH: Practical Physiological Chemistry, 13th ed, 1954, p 1080. Courtesy of McGraw-Hill Book Co.

Initial		Equilibrium	
5 Pr⁻	10 Cl⁻	5 Pr⁻	
5 Na⁺	10 Na⁺	4 Cl⁻	6 Cl⁻
		9 Na⁺	6 Na⁺
A	**B**	**A**	**B**

Figure 1.1. The Gibbs-Donnan effect of ion distribution. (Modified from Pitts RF: Physiology of the Kidney and Body Fluids, 3rd ed, 1974. © 1974 Year Book Medical Publishers, Inc., Chicago.)

that play a role in this constant distribution of water between interstitial tissues and the circulating blood plasma led Starling, in 1896, to propose the now classic Starling hypothesis.[1] According to the hypothesis, blood is filtered out of the capillary at the arteriolar end and is returned to the capillary from the interstitial tissue at the venular end (Fig. 1.2). The forces promoting ultrafiltration from the capillary are the hydrostatic pressure due to blood pressure that decreases in the direction of the venule and the interstitial oncotic pressure due to the small concentration of protein in that fluid. The opposing forces are the plasma oncotic pressure and the pressure from the turgidity of the interstitial tissue. The net pressure of approximately 1.4 kilopascal (kPa) at the arteriolar end of the capillary favors ultrafiltration, whereas at the venular end the net pressure of less than 0 favors reabsorption. The excess of the ultra-

filtrate enters the lymphatic circulation. Other important factors in the maintenance of plasma and interstitial volume are the activity of the precapillary sphincters in the regulation of hydrostatic pressure, the total surface area, and the permeability of the capillaries.

DISTRIBUTION OF BODY WATER

Water represents 50 to 70 percent of the body weight. Thirty to forty percent of this water is located in the tissue cells, about 16 percent in the interstitial fluid, and about 4.5 percent in the blood plasma (Fig. 1.3). One to three percent is located in the transcellular water of the cerebrospinal, digestive, pleural, synovial, intraocular, and peritoneal fluids.[2] The transcellular fluid is separated from the

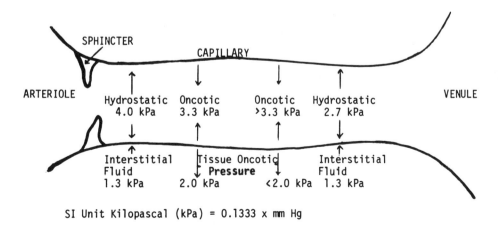

Figure 1.2. Starling hypothesis of forces governing ultrafiltration.

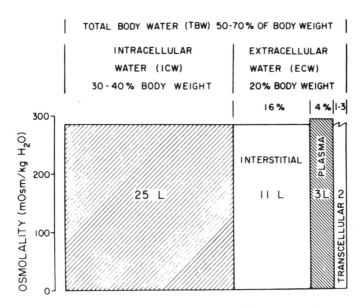

Figure 1.3. Distribution of body water. Approximate sizes of the major body fluid compartments, expressed as percentage of body weight and in mean absolute values for an adult human being who weighs 70 kg (154 pounds). The ranges of normal among individuals are considerable, and thus no one value should be taken too rigidly. The plasma has a slightly higher osmolality than the intracellular and interstitial compartments. This small difference can be ignored when dealing with problems of fluid balance. (From Valtin H: Renal Function: Mechanisms Preserving Fluid and Solute Balance in Health, 1973, p 16. Courtesy of Little, Brown, and Company. Copyright 1973.)

blood by epithelial cells in addition to the capillary endothelial barrier of the other interstitial fluid compartments.

The water content of plasma is 94 percent, and that of intracellular fluid is 75 to 80 percent. For the entire body, the water content is measured by administering a substance that will become distributed throughout all compartments of body fluids. Such substances are antipyrine and deuterated or tritiated water. The dilution of the substance is measured by spectrophotometry or by its radioactivity in the blood plasma after time for equilibration in the compartments has elapsed. The concentration of the substance in the plasma is computed, taking into account the loss through the urine, the breath, and the skin.

Extracellular water is measured by using substances that do not penetrate cell membranes. Inulin, sucrose, and thiocyanate have been used for this purpose. Plasma water is determined using radiolabeled albumin, red cells, or Evans blue dye. These substances do not allow accurate quantitation, since the albumin and also the Evans blue dye that is bound by albumin will cross the capillary endothelium to a limited degree and enter the interstitial compartment. Methods utilizing red cells also have some inaccuracy because of the uneven distribution of these cells in the plasma of small capillaries. No substances that will become selectively distributed in the interstitial and intracellular compartments have been identified. However, the interstitial space can be calculated as the difference between the extracellular water and the plasma water. The intracellular space can be calculated as the difference between the total body water and the extracellular water.

SOLUTES IN THE FLUID COMPARTMENTS

Sodium is the cation and bicarbonate is the anion of greatest concentration in the extra-

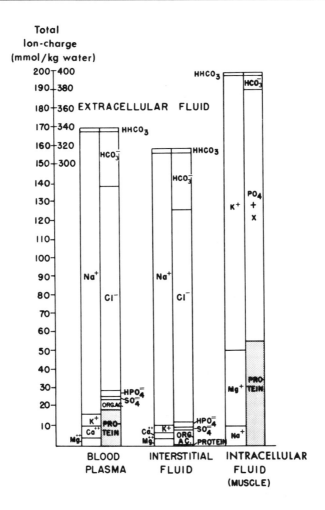

Figure 1.4. Electrolyte composition of blood plasma, interstitial fluid, and intracellular fluid. (From Tietz N, Siggaard-Anderson O: Fundamentals of Clinical Chemistry, 1976, p 948. Courtesy of W.B. Saunders Co.)

cellular fluid. Potassium and magnesium are the cations of greatest concentration in the intracellular fluid, while proteins and organic phosphates are the principal anions. The major difference between the plasma solutes and those of the interstitial fluid is the greater concentration of proteins in the plasma. The barrier of capillary endothelium that prevents protein transport from one compartment to the other establishes a Gibbs-Donnan effect that results in a 5 percent gap between the concentration of diffusible ions in these two compartments (Figs. 1.3, 1.4).

Cells can adjust a difference in osmotic pressure across the membrane by using active transport methods. The distribution of diffusible ions can be practically explained by the effect of the sign and charge of the membrane potential. The explanation is useful when the uneven distribution of the chloride ion in red cells and plasma is considered. Sodium distribution, however, cannot be explained by the membrane potential. Its distribution is explained by an active transport mechanism from the cells to the plasma. Energy for the active transport of sodium undoubtedly is derived from the cellular metabolic processes.

The principal cation of plasma is sodium, whereas the major anions are chloride, bicarbonate, and protein. Some ions are bound to the protein in the plasma (e.g., calcium), and consequently only those that are not bound are diffusible. The binding of ions to proteins is an additional factor contributing to the difference in solute concentrations between compartments. Intracellular fluid has a greater total charge than interstitial fluid because at physiologic pH (7.35 to 7.45) proteins contribute multiple negative charges per molecule.

TRANSUDATES AND EXUDATES

The process of ultrafiltration and formation of interstitial fluid, essentially lymph, is transudation. Transudates may be found in several locations in the body in a healthy person. A list of several ultrafiltrates (transudates) that occur in body cavities is given in Table 1.2. The terms applied to an increased volume of these fluids (effusions) are also listed. When excess transudation occurs into interstitial tissues, it is known as edema. If this excess occurs throughout the body, it is termed anasarca. Edema formation may be a consequence of increased venous pressure, decreased plasma oncotic pressure, increased capillary permeability, lymphatic obstruction, or increased body sodium. Several of the conditions that contribute to these factors are given in Table 1.3.

An exudate is a body fluid resulting when the ultrafiltrate is associated with inflammation. An exudate usually contains leukocytes, a greater concentration of protein, and a higher specific gravity than a transudate.

Fluids are continually being produced in several parts of the body. Many of these are analyzed in the laboratory to gain information that may be useful in diagnosis or treatment of disease. A list of some of these fluids and the sites of their synthesis appears in Table 1.2.

COMPOSITION OF THREE BODY FLUIDS

One of the major chemical constituents of urine is urea. The presence of a high concentration of urea has served to assist in the identification of the source of extraurinary tract fluid suspected of being of renal origin. Table 1.4 gives an indication of the differences in the composition of blood plasma, urine, and cerebrospinal fluid. Although

TABLE 1.2. TRANSCELLULAR ULTRAFILTRATES

Fluid Filtrate	Normal Volume (ml)	Origin	Effusions
Cerebrospinal fluid	150	Choroid plexus (capillaries of brain)	Hydroencephalus
Synovial fluid	0.1–2.0	Synovial membrane and joints	Hydroarthrosis
Pleural fluid	No appreciable amount	Pleural capillaries of lung	Hydrothorax
Pericardial fluid	10–20	Visceral and parietal pericardium	Hydropericardium
Aqueous humor	0.35	Ciliary epithelium of eye	—
Peritoneal fluid	75–100	Peritoneum of the abdominal cavity	Ascites
Lacrimal fluid	0.03	Lacrimal gland	—

TABLE 1.3. FACTORS CONTRIBUTING TO EDEMA

Factor	Condition
Increased venous pressure	Congestive heart failure, venous obstruction from inflammation, thrombosis, neoplasm, cirrhosis
Decreased plasma oncotic pressure	Decreased synthesis of plasma proteins (liver disease, starvation), loss of protein (renal disease, protein-losing gastroenteropathy)
Increased capillary permeability	Anoxia, inflammation, chemical toxins, trauma, burns, irradiation
Lymphatic obstruction	Neoplasms, surgical removal of lymph nodes, filariasis, congenital abnormality
Increased body sodium	Increased aldosterone concentration (decreased perfusion pressure in kidney), congestive heart failure, liver disease, increased concentration of mineralocorticoids (increased secretion from adrenal hyperplasia or exogenous administration)

urine and cerebrospinal fluid represent ultrafiltrates of the plasma, the influence of active transport mechanisms and other non-Starling forces is exhibited by the several striking differences in their composition.

Although the discussion of body fluids in this chapter deals principally with the ion concentrations, it must be stressed that each of the extracellular and transcellular fluids may contain solids or formed elements. The occurrence of cells and other structures in transcellular fluids is associated with inflammation and disease. The cells that occur in these fluids are derived from sloughing of the membranes of the compartment, sites of inflammation and infection (e.g., leukocytes), or bleeding (e.g., red cells). Other structures that may be seen in some fluids are crystals, protein gels or casts, and fibrin clots. The identification of these constituents, particularly the cells, is important in order to determine the cause of the effusion when an increased volume of fluid occurs. Such use has been found in detecting neoplasia, arthritis, meningitis, and glomerulonephritis. A discussion of these structures in body fluids is given in subsequent chapters in this book.

TABLE 1.4. COMPARISON OF SOLUTE CONCENTRATIONS OF CEREBROSPINAL FLUID, BLOOD PLASMA, AND URINE*

	Cerebro-spinal Fluid	Blood Plasma	Urine†
Sodium	227‡	139	183
Chloride	122	105	197
Bicarbonate	7.9	25	2.4
Urea	2.0	4.4	408
Uric acid	0.1	0.3	0.8
Creatinine	0.1	0.1	12.4
Glucose	4.3	5.0	0.6
Protein g/L	0.27	72	0.25
Phosphorus	0.54	1.1	27.1
Potassium	2.4	4.5	64

*Average values based on data in references 3, 4, 5, 6.
†Based on 1,000 ml/day.
‡All values are mmole/L (except for Protein).

Review Questions

One or more responses may be correct.

1. The factor(s) that affect(s) the passage of water, molecules, and ions across a semipermeable membrane is (are):
   A. The product of the diffusible anions and cations on either side
   B. The oncotic pressure on either side
   C. The hydrostatic pressure on either side
   D. The sign and charge of the membrane potential

E. Active transport mechanisms at the membrane

2. What is the net pressure and its direction in terms of ultrafiltration or reabsorption based upon the data below?

	Capillary Pressure (kPa)
Hydrostatic	4.3
Oncotic	3.3
Tissue oncotic (turgor)	2.3
Interstitial	1.3

A. Ultrafiltration occurs at 4.0 kPa
B. Reabsorption occurs at 4.0 kPa
C. Ultrafiltration occurs at 2.0 kPa
D. Reabsorption occurs at 2.0 kPa
E. No exchange occurs at 0 kPa

3. Match the fluids with the following characteristics (Select two fluids if appropriate.):
A. It is a transudate across endothelial capillary walls.
B. Its concentration of sodium is greater than that of potassium
C. It has the highest concentration of potassium
D. It has the lowest concentration of potassium
E. It has the highest concentration of phosphate
F. It has the lowest concentration of protein
   1. Blood plasma
   2. Interstitial fluid
   3. Intracellular fluid

4. Given the initial ion concentrations, what are the expected ion concentrations at equilibrium on both sides of the membrane (//)? (Select only one.)
Initial: 3 Pr^-, 3 Na^+// 3 Cl^-, 3 Na^+
A. 4 Na^+, 1 Cl^-, 3 Pr^-// 2 Na^+, 2 Cl^-
B. 3 Na^+, 2 Cl^-, 3 Pr^-// 2 Na^+, 3 Cl^-
C. 2 Na^+, 2 Cl^-, 3 Pr^-// 4 Na^+, 1 Cl^-
D. 3 Na^+, 3 Pr^-// 3 Na^+, 3 Cl^-
E. 1 Na^+, 3 Pr^-// 5 Na^+, 3 Cl^-

5. Body water is distributed in the following proportions:
A. 30 to 40 percent body weight is intracellular water
B. 30 to 40 percent body weight is extracellular water
C. 20 percent body weight is extracellular water
D. 16 percent body weight is interstitial water
E. 16 percent body weight is intracellular water

6. The osmolality of interstitial fluid normally:
A. Is greater than intracellular fluid
B. Is less than intracellular fluid
C. Is the same as intracellular fluid
D. Is the same as blood plasma
E. Is less than blood plasma

7. Extracellular water may be determined by administering which of the following substances?
A. Antipyrine
B. Tritiated water
C. Radiolabeled albumin
D. Evans blue dye
E. Inulin

8. The cation(s) that differ(s) significantly in concentration between intracellular and extracellular fluids is (are):
A. Sodium
B. Potassium
C. Magnesium
D. Calcium
E. Manganese

9. Match the activity with the effusion:
A. Pleural activity
B. Joint
C. Ventricle of brain
D. Peritoneum
E. Pericardium

   1. Ascites
   2. Hydropericardium
   3. Hydroencephalus
   4. Hydrothorax
   5. Hydroarthroses

10. Which of the following conditions are frequently associated with edema?
A. Increase in interstitial fluid
B. Proteinuria
C. Inflammation
D. Increased venous pressure
E. Increased body sodium

Case Study

An 88-year-old male entered the hospital emergency room in the following condition: cyanosis (bluish discoloration of the skin), increased systemic venous pressure, enlarged liver, decreased urinary output, fatigue, and weakness. The physician noted pitting edema of the feet and ankles and pericardial effusion. The laboratory tests showed a urine of high specific gravity, a 1⁺ protein, one to two casts/low power field in the microscopic examination of the urinary sediment, and a blood serum creatinine of 168 mmole/L (1.9 g/100 ml). He had a blood urea nitrogen (BUN) of 5.8 mmole/L (35 mg/100 ml).

Questions

1. What fluid compartments are affected by fluid retention?
2. What is the most likely primary cause of this condition?
3. What other organs are also contributing to fluid retention?

Answers

1. The fluid compartments affected by fluid retention are the interstitial and pericardium compartments.
2. The most likely primary cause for the condition described is heart failure.
3. Other organs that are contributing to this condition are the liver, stated to be enlarged, which may be unable to produce sufficient albumin to maintain the plasma oncotic pressure, the kidney, which is unable to function properly due to the damage created by insufficient blood supply, and the insufficient blood supply itself.

REFERENCES

1. Starling EH: On the absorption of fluids from the connective tissue spaces. J Physiol 19: 312, 1896.
2. Pitts RF: The Physiology of the Kidney and Body Fluids, 3rd ed. Chicago, Year Book, 1974. p 12.
3. Free AH, Free HM: Urinalysis in Clinical Laboratory Practice. Cleveland, CRC Press, 1975, pp 13–17.
4. Cumings JN, Lascelles PT, Hamilton PB: Physical properties and chemical composition of cerebrospinal fluid. In Altman PL, Dittmer DS (eds): Biology Data Book, 2nd ed. Bethesda, Md, Fed Soc Exp Biol, 1974, pp 1976–1977.
5. Smith C, Wolfe GG, Cartwright GE: Blood and other body electrolytes. I. Man. In Altman PL, Dittmer DS (eds): Biology Data Book, 2nd ed, Bethesda, Md, Fed Am Soc Exp Biol, 1974, pp 1752–1753.
6. Van Pilsun J: Excretion products in urine: Man. In Altman PL, Dittmer DS (eds): Biology Data Book, 2nd ed. Bethesda, Md, Fed Am Soc Exp Biol, 1974, pp 1496–1512.

Doris L. Ross

CHAPTER 2

The Kidneys and Urinary Tract: Anatomy, Physiology, and Disease

Objectives

It is expected that the information presented in this chapter will enable the reader to:

1. Identify the gross anatomic parts of the kidney.
2. List or identify the anatomic parts of the uriniferous tubule.
3. Describe the types of cells that are located in the glomerulus, proximal convoluted tubule, descending and ascending limb of Henle's loop, distal convoluted tubule, and collecting duct.
4. Describe the sequence of urine formation and flow in terms of the anatomic sites.
5. Analyze the relationship of the bladder, urinary tract, and associated structures to the volume and content of urine.
6. Identify the filtration barriers in the glomerulus.
7. Contrast and compare tubular activity for inulin, glucose, and penicillin.
8. Identify the forces present in the glomerulus that contribute to the filtration pressure.
9. Define filtered load.
10. Identify the most common laboratory finding in renal disease.
11. Describe the nephrotic syndrome and identify associated medical laboratory test results.
12. Identify the pathogenesis of most glomerulonephritic disease.
13. Describe one type of glomerulonephritis attributed to circulating antigen-antibody complexes, with particular emphasis on the urinalysis results.
14. Describe one type of glomerulonephritis attributed to antibodies directed to renal tissue.
15. Distinguish between active absorption and passive absorption.
16. List three major functions of the proximal tubule.
17. Identify four events that occur upon hydrogen ion excretion.
18. List two major functions that occur in Henle's loop.

19. Identify the role of urea in the concentration of urine.
20. Identify five major functions that occur in the renal distal tubule or collecting ducts.
21. Identify the fixed acids in the urine.
22. Describe the role that fixed acids play in acid-base balance.
23. Define acidosis and alkalosis.
24. Describe kidney response to metabolic acidosis and metabolic alkalosis.
25. Define renal threshold.
26. Identify the defect in proximal tubular acidosis.
27. Identify the defect in distal tubular acidosis.
28. Compare and contrast the absorption in the proximal and distal tubules.
29. Identify the pathogenesis of pyelonephritis.
30. Identify the abnormal constituents of urine in cases of pyelonephritis.
31. Identify the role of the parathyroid gland in metabolic acidosis.
32. List three important metabolic substances produced in the kidney.
33. Describe the relationship between renal disease and anemia.
34. Describe the relationship of kidney function to calcium metabolism.

It is estimated that over 80 percent of patients entering hospitals in this country have a routine urinalysis test performed. One study has shown that 42 percent of patients with unsuspected membranoproliferative glomerulonephritis were detected by the routine urinalysis.[1] Our understanding of the significance of the volume and contents of urine involves a knowledge of how and where urine is formed in the body. Information about the changes that occur in the characteristics of urine when disease processes occur in the kidney or throughout the body is used in most types of medical practice. It is thus fitting that this chapter on urinalysis begins with the anatomy and physiology of the kidney and urinary tract.

ANATOMY OF KIDNEY AND URINARY TRACT

In the human, there are two kidneys, one on either side of the vertebral column. Embedded in fat, these bean-shaped organs are found against the posterior wall of the abdomen. Major functions of the kidney are:

1. Removal of metabolic wastes and toxic substances from the body.
2. Regulation of volume and composition of body fluids by reabsorption and secretion.
3. Maintenance of acid-base balance.
4. Production of substances important to the metabolism of other body tissues, for example, renin, erythropoietin, vitamin D, and its metabolites.

Although the urine produced leaves each kidney through its separate ureter, these ureters join a common sac, the bladder. Urine is stored in the bladder until it is released from the body through the urethra. In the female, the external end of the urethra is located near the vagina, while that of the male is shared by the seminal canal and has its terminal opening in the glans penis. These anatomic relationships are important to the occasional presence in the urine specimen of substances

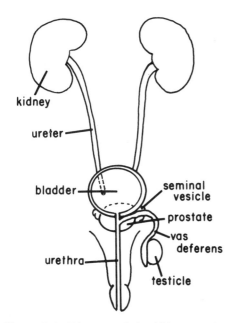

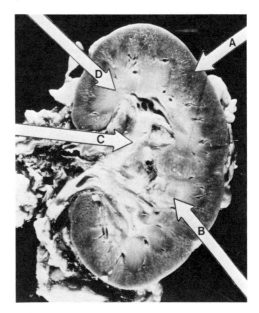

Figure 2.1. Diagram of the kidneys, urinary tract, bladder, and male genital system. (From Kent TH, Hart MN, Shires TK: Introduction to Human Disease, 1979, p 191. Courtesy of Appleton-Century-Crofts.)

Figure 2.2. Cross-section of human kidney. **A.** Cortex. **B.** Pyramid. **C.** Pelvis. **D.** Medulla. (From Bulger R: Diseases of the Kidney, 1979, p 4. Courtesy of Little, Brown, and Co. Copyright 1979.)

arising from these nearby anatomic structures. A diagram of the kidneys, urinary tract, bladder, and male genital system is shown in Figure 2.1.

At the site where the ureter leaves the kidney, the blood supply to the kidney enters through the renal artery. Lymphatics and nerves also enter here. A cross-section of a kidney is shown in Figure 2.2.

The renal cortex (Fig. 2.2) has 6 to 18 pyramids of medullary tissue. The tip of the pyramid is called the "papilla." The papilla is capped by a minor calyx, which is a part of the extrarenal collecting system. The urine is formed by the renal corpuscles located in the renal cortex and is modified by the urinary tubule. Urine is then transported by way of collecting ducts to the ducts of Bellini, which are pinhole openings located at the apex of each papilla. Urine flows from the ducts of Bellini, enters a minor calyx, traverses an inferior or superior major calyx on its way to

the renal pelvis, and goes out through the ureter to the bladder.

The Uriniferous Tubule

The uriniferous tubule is the microscopic, structural, and functional unit of the kidney. There are approximately one million in each kidney (Fig. 2.3). This functional unit includes the nephron and the collecting tubule. A certain degree of heterogeneity exists in the structure and function of nephrons.[2] Current investigation will undoubtedly reveal many differences. However, for the sake of simplicity the nephron will be discussed in general terms of the cortical nephron. A nephron (Fig. 2.3) consists of a capillary network (the glomerulus) and Bowman's capsule, which together are called the renal corpuscle, and a long tubule comprised of segments that have different structures and functions. These segments are the proximal

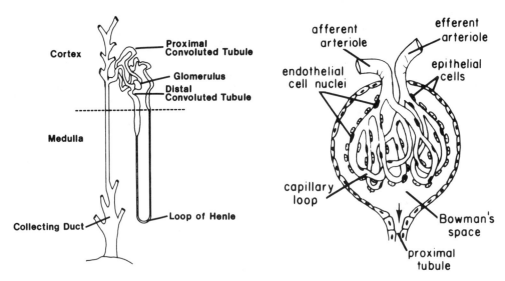

Figure 2.3. Diagram of a urineferous tubule. (From Kent TH, Hart MN, Shires TK: Introduction to Human Disease, 1979, p 192. Courtesy of Appleton-Century-Crofts.)

Figure 2.4. Diagram of a renal corpuscle. (From Kent TH, Hart MN, Shires TK: Introduction to Human Disease, 1979, p 192. Courtesy of Appleton-Century-Crofts.)

convoluted tubule (pars convoluta), the proximal straight tubule (pars recta or descending thin limb of Henle's loop), the narrow hairpin loop of Henle, the distal straight tubule (pars recta or ascending thin limb of the loop of Henle), and the distal convoluted tubule (pars convoluta). The collecting duct plays a complementary role in renal function, although its embryologic origin differs from that of the nephron.

The Renal Corpuscle

The initial event in the formation of urine is the flow of blood to the kidney and into the capillary loops (glomerulus) by way of the afferent arteriole. It is here that the blood is filtered into the space between the layers of Bowman's capsule to form the nascent urine, the glomerular filtrate. The glomerular capillary walls have three layers, an inner endothelial layer, a central basement membrane, and an outer layer of epithelium. Another kind of cell—the mesangial cell—occupies a central position in the renal corpuscle. A diagram of the renal corpuscle is shown in Figure 2.4,

and an electron micrograph is shown in Figure 2.5.

Epithelial Cells. A layer of epithelial cells surrounds the capillary loops like a glove and forms an inner layer of Bowman's capsule. The glomerular epithelial cell has three functions:

1. A role in the synthesis or degradation of the glomerular basement membrane,
2. A barrier to the passage of large molecular weight molecules from the blood into the glomerular filtrate, and
3. Support of the capillary loops.

The epithelial cells, called "podocytes" (Fig. 2.6), have abundant cytoplasm and may extend into long foot processes, trabeculi, which upon further division extend over the capillaries as little feet (pedicels). Neighboring pedicels interdigitate and rest on the glomerular basement membrane. The area between two adjacent podocytes is known as the

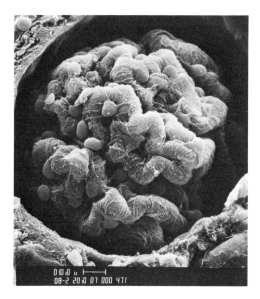

Figure 2.5. Scan electron micrograph of a renal corpuscle. Approximately ×800. (Courtesy of Dr. Dennis Dobyan, Department of Pathology and Laboratory Medicine, The University of Texas Medical School at Houston.)

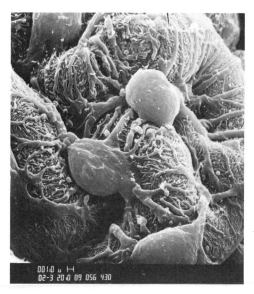

Figure 2.6. Scan electron micrograph of a glomerular capillary loop. Approximately ×2,000. (Courtesy of Dr. Dennis Dobyan, Department of Pathology and Laboratory Medicine, The University of Texas Medical School at Houston.)

"slit pore," which is bridged by a membrane approximately 7 nm thick. Electron microscopic studies have demonstrated these slit pores, which will exclude many proteins in the range of 160,000 to 180,000 daltons and allow those of 40,000 daltons or less to pass freely into the filtrate.[3] Charge effects also play a role in the sieving function of the glomerulus; for example, polyanions are more restricted in their passage than are polycations.[4]

The Basement Membrane. The basement membrane is a continuous structure with an average thickness of about 330 nm.[5] It has been described as a filter composed of a network of fibrils embedded in a gel-like matrix of glycosaminoglycans, principally heparan sulfate.[6] In order to explain the passage of large molecular weight proteins, it has been postulated that when swelling of the basement membrane occurs the fibrils become separated, thus allowing large particles to pass.[7]

The Endothelium. The endothelium is composed of squamous endothelial cells possessing nuclei that protrude into the capillary lumen. The cytoplasm of these cells is spread in a thin sheet to line the capillary walls. Numerous fenestrations or pores are located in the thin cytoplasmic sheet.

The fine structure of the glomerulus indicates that in order for a molecule to enter the filtrate from the blood it must pass through three filtration barriers: (1) The endothelial pores, (2) the basement membrane, and (3) the slit pore. This tripartite structure is referred to as the "glomerular membrane."

Mesangial Cells. Mesangial cells are similar to pericytes seen around endothelial cells in other locations, although the cytoplasm of the mesangial cells differs in its possession of several processes that are enveloped by a material resembling basement membrane. This material is known as the "mesangial matrix." It fills the space between the mesangial cells, capillary endothelial cells, and the capillary basement membrane. The cytoplasm contains rough endoplasmic reticulum, mitochondria, and bundles of fibers. The phagocytic action of these cells is important in maintaining a clean basement membrane. Other functions of these cells are still undetermined, although their importance is indicated by their propensity to divide in certain kidney diseases.[2]

Juxtaglomerular Cells. Endothelial cells and smooth muscle cells compose the afferent arteriolar wall. Just before the afferent arteriole enters the vascular pole of the glomerulus, the smooth muscle cells change. Electron-dense, secretory type granules become noticeable in the cytoplasm. There is also an increase in the rough endoplasmic reticulum. The granules of these secretory cells, known as "juxtaglomerular cells," are considered to contain the hormone renin that is important in the production of angiotensin, a vasopressor substance. The juxtaglomerular cells are sensitive to renal arterial pressure and have been shown to respond to a reduction in pressure by releasing renin.

The Renal Tubules

After the glomerular filtrate is formed, numerous changes occur in the water or the solutes it contains. The changes that occur are created by absorption or secretion by the tubular cells throughout the nephron. Some solutes are neither absorbed nor secreted. An example of this is inulin. Some solutes will be reabsorbed in the tubules to varying degrees so that their concentrations are much less in the urine than they were in the ultrafiltrate. An example for the proximal tubule is glucose. Some ions or molecules will be secreted by the various tubular epithelia into the urine. An example of proximal tubular secretion is penicillin. Secretion may also occur in the distal tubule, for example, hydrogen and potassium ions. Water serves as an example of absorption by the proximal and distal parts of the tubule.

The tubule furnishes the fine tuning of substances that are to be lost to the body and those that are to be conserved after the glomerulus has made the initial coarse adjustment.

The tubules and collecting tubules are enclosed by a continuous basement membrane. The membrane, about 80 nm thick, forms a support upon which the epithelium rests. Associated with the tubules are the peritubular capillaries into which those substances that are reabsorbed return to the circulation and those that are secreted are lost from the circulation.

Proximal Tubules. Immediately following egress through the glomerulus, the glomerular filtrate enters the part of the nephron known as the "proximal tubule." At this point the proximal tubule is serpentine and is referred to as the "proximal convoluted tubule" (pars convoluta). The luminal surfaces of the cells have many fingerlike surface projections, known as the "brush border." The surface area afforded by the brush border contributes greatly to the resorptive area of these cells. Absorption via this covering may require energy to overcome an opposing electrochemical gradient (active) or occur with no expenditure of energy (passive). The basal surface of the cells of the proximal tubules exhibits considerable interdigitation of lateral processes. It is in the proximal tubule that amino acids, glucose, phosphate, sulfate, potassium, urate, and 80 percent of the water are absorbed from the filtrate within the lumen to reenter the circulation via the peritubular capillaries.

Henle's Loop. As the convolutions diminish, the tubule is referred to as the "descending limb of Henle's loop" or pars recta of the proximal tubule. All of the glomeruli in the human are located in the cortex. Cortical nephrons have very short or no thin segments, whereas those nephrons located in the juxtamedullary region of the cortex may have thin loop segments extending as far as the papilla. About 90 percent of the tubules in humans are of the short, looped variety.

The salt concentration in the surrounding interstitium increases as the tubule extends into the medulla. The permeability of the descending limb to water and the increasing salt concentration in the interstitium lead to the passive reabsorption of water as the fluid flows through this part of the nephron. The descending limb or thin segment, if it exists, turns back at a point, forming the loop of Henle. Cells in the thin segment are flattened and thin except at the nucleus, which bulges into the lumen. Microvilli are present in the luminal surface, but they are short and scattered. Past the hairpin loop, the tubule becomes the ascending limb, pars recta (or thin segment if one exists), of the distal tubule. It is impermeable to water. The ascending limb enlarges and becomes a thick segment of the distal tubule. This region actively transports chloride from the filtrate into the interstitium. The distal tubule at this point (pars recta) is straight and courses in a direction toward the parent renal corpuscle where it contacts the afferent arteriole of its glomerulus.

Distal Convoluted Tubule. The tubule is called the "distal convoluted tubule" near the point at which contact is made with the juxtaglomerular cells. At the point of contact with the afferent arteriole of its parent glomerulus, the tubular epithelium adjacent to the arteriole changes. The cells become small and contain deep-staining nuclei, and the cytoplasm has fewer mitochondria than those of the remainder of the distal tubule. These cells are known as the "macula densa" (dense spot) and are a part of the juxtaglomerular complex. The juxtaglomerular cells of the afferent arteriolar wall are the other part of the complex.

The distal tube is shorter than the proximal segment and convolutes in the neighborhood of the afferent arteriole. The cells of the distal tubule, which resemble those of the proximal tubule, are cuboidal and exhibit numerous mitochondria. The luminal surface that does not have a brush border has a few short microvilli that are regularly distributed throughout this part of the tubule. The numerous mitochondria indicate marked enzymatic activity. This is not surprising since the active transport of sodium chloride would utilize enzymatic activity to meet the necessary energy requirements.

Collecting Tubule. The distal tubule empties into a collecting duct which is a connecting tubule for several nephrons. It receives fluid from these distal tubules as it travels through the cortex toward the medulla. In the medulla several collecting ducts join to form one of the papillary ducts that empty at the papillary tip into a minor calyx. The cells of the collecting duct are cuboidal, sparsely granular, and regular with round, uniformly placed nuclei. They increase in height to become columnar cells as the ducts become the papillary ducts. Short microvilli are present on the luminar cell surfaces. No interdigitation occurs, but some basal infolding is present. A light cytoplasm is characteristic of most of the cells of the collecting ducts, although a second cell type called "intercalated" (dark) that contains more mitochondria is noted to appear simultaneously. This cell occurs frequently in the cortical collecting ducts.

The Bladder, Urinary Tract, and Associated Anatomic Structures

A ureter leaves each kidney pelvis and carries the urine to the bladder. No other function has been ascribed to this part of the urinary tract. Peristaltic waves start in the pelvis and ripple along the ureters and into the bladder, furnishing the flow of urine. The frequency of these waves is altered by autonomic impulses and hormones. The muscle tissue of the wall is also important in the flow of urine.

The bladder is a sac lined with transitional epithelium. At the neck of the bladder, a musculature passes around the urethral orifice to function as an internal sphincter. There is an external sphincter that consists of striated muscle. The bladder has two functions: (1) to hold urine and (2) to release its contents via micturition. Micturition depends upon the reflex of the detrussor muscle. This reflex is controlled by the supraspinal part of the nervous system and is reinforced by messages from the urinary tract. The impulse to void generally begins when there is about 150 ml of urine in the bladder.

The urethra of the male passes through the prostate gland and out through the penis (Fig. 2.1). The testis is connected to the urethra via the vas deferens. Sperm produced in the seminiferous tubules are stored in the epididymis and vas deferens and are released during ejaculation by muscular contraction. The neck of the bladder is surrounded by the prostate gland, and inflammation of the gland can interfere with urine excretion, causing oliguria and dysuria. Prostatic ducts empty into the urethra at the point of its encirclement. Prostatic fluid can thus enter the urine. In the female, the urethra leaves the bladder, traverses a urogenital diaphragm, and opens at the urethral meatus, which is located approximately 1 cm proximal to the vagina.

RENAL PHYSIOLOGY AND DISEASE

Although the parts of the kidney function in concert, for purposes of organization, discussion of renal physiology and disease will be in relation to anatomic units where possible.

Glomerular Physiology

Glomerular filtration depends upon the flow of blood entering the kidney by the afferent arterioles. The pressure on the glomerular capillaries supplied by the contraction of the heart is approximately twice that of other capillaries in the body. The permeability of these capillaries is also greater than others. A remarkably constant pressure is maintained by the counterbalance of dilation and restriction of the afferent and efferent arterioles. If pressure falls in the renal artery, the afferent arteriole becomes dilated, and the efferent arteriole constricts in an effort to maintain the usual hydrostatic pressure within the capillaries of 12.0 kilopascals (kPa) (90 mm

Hg).[8] It follows that constriction of the afferent arteriole alone results in a decrease in filtration pressure, whereas a constriction of the efferent arteriole alone results in an increased filtration pressure on the glomerulus.

Most of the autoregulating response of the kidney has been explained by a distal tubule-glomerular feedback mechanism. This response, mediated by the macula densa-juxtaglomerular complex, is to increase the afferent arteriolar resistance whenever the distal tubule is presented with an increase in volume or salt concentration.[9] It has been suggested that the angiotensin effect on filtration is due predominantly to efferent arteriolar action.[8] Micropuncture of rat glomerulus has shown that single nephron glomerular filtration rates and glomerular pressure decrease in response to an increase in the perfusion rate in the distal nephron. In summary, factors that are involved in the control of the glomerular filtration rate are (1) myogenic vascular reflexes, (2) changes in proximal intratubular pressure, (3) local renin-angiotensin activity, and (4) tubule-glomerular feedback.

Other forces exist in opposition to the filtration across the glomerulus. They are the plasma oncotic pressure due to the plasma proteins and the hydrostatic pressure within Bowman's capsule. The oncotic pressure results from the inability of some of the plasma proteins to pass freely through the glomerular filters. This pressure is normally about 3 kPa (25 mm Hg). Whenever there is a significant decrease in blood plasma proteins, the decreased oncotic pressure results in an increasing filtration. The hydrostatic pressure in Bowman's capsule of approximately 2 kPa (15 mm Hg) is due to the pressure of the fluid present in the capsular space.[10]

Approximately 1.2 L of blood flow through the glomerulus each minute. The approximately 600 ml of plasma that is filtered results in 120 ml of fluid entering Bowman's capsule. The rate of this process is called the "glomerular filtration rate" (GFR). The flow rate and composition of the plasma within the af-

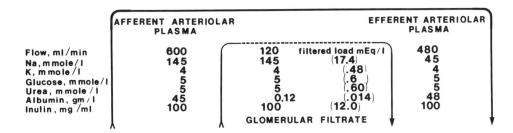

	AFFERENT ARTERIOLAR PLASMA			EFFERENT ARTERIOLAR PLASMA
Flow, ml/min	600	120	filtered load mEq/l	480
Na, mmole/l	145	145	(17.4)	45
K, mmole/l	4	4	(.48)	4
Glucose, mmole/l	5	5	(.6)	5
Urea, mmole/l	5	5	(.60)	5
Albumin, gm/l	45	0.12	(.014)	48
Inulin, mg/ml	100	100	(12.0)	100
		GLOMERULAR FILTRATE		

Figure 2.7. Flow rates and concentrations of certain constituents of the afferent and efferent arteriolar plasma and the glomerular filtrate. (Adapted from Maude DL: Kidney Physiology and Kidney Disease, 1977. Courtesy of J.B. Lippincott Co.)

ferent and efferent arterioles and the flow rate and composition of the glomerular filtrate are shown in Figure 2.7.

The filtered load of a solute is the rate of transfer across the glomerular membranes. It is the product of the plasma concentration of the solute and the glomerular filtration rate. This applies to diffusible solutes of molecular weight of not much greater than 5,000.

Glomerular Disease

Renal disease involving the glomerulus is invariably associated with proteinuria. Normally up to 150 mg of protein is excreted in the urine over a 24-hour period. Proteinuria is the condition resulting from an excretion rate exceeding this value. It is the most common finding in renal disease, including diseases involving the tubules. Proteinuria of glomerular defect is primarily albuminuria because albumin is the protein in greatest concentration in the plasma and has the lowest molecular weight of the major proteins. Whenever the glomerular membranes lose their sieving capacity, a significant amount of albumin enters the tubule and eventually appears in the urine. A concurrent decrease of as much as 25 g/L in the plasma albumin concentration can result from this loss. One of the consequences of this protein shift from the plasma is a decreased plasma oncotic pressure which leads to an increased interstitial fluid and edema. The renin-angiotensin system is triggered by the resulting loss of blood volume and salt and water excretion

decreases. The fluid that is conserved in this manner serves only to increase the tissue fluid.

Edema, hypoalbuminemia of less than 25 g/L, and albuminuria usually greater than 5 g/day are the hallmarks of the nephrotic syndrome.[11] The examination of urinary sediment may show fatty casts. Other manifestations of the nephrotic syndrome are hyperlipidemia and associated increases of plasma concentration of triglycerides and cholesterol. The nephrotic syndrome occurs in several primary glomerular diseases as well as in other diseases with kidney involvement, such as lupus erythematosus, amyloidosis, and diabetes.

Glomerulonephritis

Glomerulonephritis is a term applied to several different diseases of the glomeruli. The pathogenesis of most of the primary glomerulonephritic diseases has a basis in immunologic mechanisms. The immune mechanisms involved in these renal diseases are:

1. The formation of circulating antigen and antibody complexes in response to an infection, foreign protein, or self-antigen and the deposition of these complexes in the glomeruli. This is immune complex glomerulonephritis. This type is seen in primary renal disease and often is secondary to systemic disease accompanied by glomerulonephritis.

2. The formation of antibodies which react with the glomerular or tubular basement membranes. The formation of complexes in the basement membrane in this type of immune mechanism is antibasement membrane disease.

Study at this date shows that these two immune mechanisms may result in similar histopathologic features as described by proliferative glomerulonephritis with crescent formation (Table 2.1).

Serum sickness is an example of renal complication resulting from circulating immune complexes. Persons who have received an injection of foreign protein, for example, antitoxins prepared in an animal species such as the horse, develop soluble antigen-antibody complexes containing the foreign protein. These complexes, when deposited along the epithelial side of the glomerular basement membrane, lead to an acute proliferative glomerulonephritis, causing light proteinuria and microscopic hematuria.

Physicians and scientists have described several types of glomerulonephritis. These types are (1) acute poststreptococcal or postinfectious, (2) membranoproliferative, (3) membranous, (4) minimal change disease, (5) focal or IgA nephropathy, (6) chronic, and (7) rapidly progressive (antibasement membrane disease).

The diagnosis of the specific type of glomerulonephritis is important for the prognosis of the patient. For instance, a child with a diffuse proliferative glomerulonephritis as determined by light microscopy will usually have a good prognosis if it is a postinfectious glomerulonephritis and a much worse prognosis if it is a membranoproliferative glomerulonephritis. Immunofluorescence and electron microscopy studies help to establish the diagnosis because of such features as the humps in postinfectious glomerulonephritis and the subendothelial deposits in the membranoproliferative glomerulonephritis.

Examination of the urine for hematuria by visual inspection or microscopic or chemical analysis and the degree and type of protein-uria assist in the classification of glomerulonephritic types and perhaps is of even greater assistance in the assessment of the degree of renal glomerular impairment.

Poststreptococcal Glomerulonephritis (Postinfectious). This disease generally occurs following an infection by a nephritogenic type of group A beta-hemolytic streptococcus. Most of the infections that lead to this form of glomerulonephritis are located in the pharynx, although skin lesions have also been implicated. The renal involvement is usually seen about one to four weeks after the infection. In all but about 20 percent of the patients with poststreptococcal glomerulonephritis, antibody titers to streptococcal antigen demonstrated by the antistreptolysin O, antistreptokinase, or antihemolysin test increase to a maximum level in one to three weeks after the infection begins.[12] Bacterial cultures may be negative at the time that evidence of renal disease is noticed, and thus negative cultures do not prevent consideration of poststreptococcal glomerulonephritis in the diagnosis. Conversely, the evidence of positive cultures of nephritogenic streptococci does not definitely establish the streptococcal infection as the causative agent in a patient with glomerulonephritis, since such an infection does not necessarily lead to poststreptococcal glomerulonephritis.

The glomerular basement membrane will show deposition of immune complexes of streptococcal antigen and immune globulin. Granular (lumpy) deposits of IgG and C3 can be seen in all glomeruli by immunofluorescent techniques. The inflammation and damage to the membrane in addition to the cellular proliferation lead to the symptoms most commonly seen in these patients: gross hematuria and edema. Erythrocytes and leukocytes pass through the damaged barriers. Some are caught in cast formation in the tubules, and thus when red cell casts are seen in the urine, a glomerular origin can be identified. Nonselective proteinuria also occurs but seldom exceeds 5 g per 24 hours and is generally from 1 to 3 g daily. The reduced glomerular filtration rate leads to retention

TABLE 2.1. CHARACTERISTICS OF GLOMERULONEPHRITIC DISEASES

Type	Histopathologic Change*			Body Fluid Analysis	
	Light Microscopy	Electron Microscopy	Immunofluorescence	Urine	Blood
Postinfectious	Cellular proliferation	Subepithelial, electron-dense deposits (humps)	IgG, C3 in coarsely granular pattern	Nonselective proteinuria (1–3 g/day), leukocytes, gross hematuria, occasional RBC casts, bacteriuria	ASO titer up, azotemia
Membranoproliferative	Mesangial cell proliferation, basement membrane thickening and duplication	Subendothelial electron-dense deposits, basement membrane duplication	IgG, C3 in diffuse pattern in mesangium and basement membrane	Nonselective proteinuria, hematuria, occasional RBC casts	C3 and C5 decreased
Membranous	Diffuse basement membrane thickening	Subepithelial diffuse, small electron-dense deposits (spikes)	IgG, C3 in diffuse granular pattern along basement membrane	Nonselective proteinuria (1 g or less/day), hyaline casts	
Focal proliferative (IgA nephropathy)	Focal mesangial cell proliferation	Electron dense-deposits in mesangium	IgA in mesangium	Nonselective proteinuria (1 g or less/day), gross hematuria	
Minimal change	Normal	Diffuse fusion of the epithelial cell foot processes	Normal (negative)	Selective proteinuria, occasional hematuria; occasional hyaline, granular, fatty casts	Albumin decreased
Rapidly progressive (antibasement membrane)	Cellular proliferation with crescents	No electron-dense deposits	Deposition of IgG, C3 linearly along basement membrane	Nonselective proteinuria, microscopic hematuria, occasional RBC cast	

*Histopathologic change data courtesy of Regina Verani, MD, Department of Pathology and Laboratory Medicine, University of Texas Medical School at Houston.

of the nitrogenous waste substances, urea, uric acid, and creatinine in blood plasma (azotemia). Expansion of the extracellular volume leads to edema formation and, occasionally, to symptoms of congestive heart failure.

In mild cases the morphologic and immunologic studies of the kidney may indicate a disease process even when urinalysis is normal. After recovery, the microscopic hematuria may persist for several years. The urinalysis in these patients thus will often show hematuria, proteinuria, pyuria (leukocytes), and cylinduria (casts). Approximately 5 percent of these patients progress to renal failure.

Membranoproliferative Glomerulonephritis. This type of glomerulonephritis may result in progressive renal disease or renal failure with some periods of remission. Persons diagnosed as having this disease are predominantly children or young adults. In a study,[1] 42 percent of persons diagnosed as having this type of glomerulonephritis were initially detected by routine urinalysis while asymptomatic. The urinalysis in these patients may show marked proteinuria or transient proteinuria of the nonselective type and hematuria. Occasionally, red cell casts will be seen in the chronic course of this disease. The glomerular filtration rate is decreased in about half of the patients, and over half have serum complement levels (C3 and C5) below normal.[13] Complement involvement in this type of glomerulonephritis is by the alternative pathway of complement activation.

The histologic picture shows proliferation of the mesangial cells and thickening of the capillary wall. Complement may be demonstrated on the endothelial lining of the basement membrane.

This form of glomerulonephritis has been subdivided into types I and II, having immune deposits in the mesangium/subendothelial space and glomerular basement membrane, respectively.[13]

Membranous Glomerulonephritis. The course of this disease is variable, and the often spontaneous remission is associated with a reduc-tion in the proteinuria that characterizes this lesion. Otherwise, a slowly deteriorating process continues until death occurs from renal failure. The urinalysis will give evidence of the nonselective proteinuria that is occurring, and occasionally hyaline casts will be seen. Although the etiology of this nephropathy is not known, it has been associated with numerous other diseases, including lymphoma, malaria, syphilis, renal vein thrombosis, and the persistent circulation of hepatitis immune complexes.

Tissue examination reveals a thickening of the glomerular basement membrane associated with inclusion of immune deposits in the epithelial surface layer (Fig. 2.8B). The immune complexes have been demonstrated by immunofluorescence to be granular deposits of IgG and complement.[13]

Minimal Change Disease. There is some speculation about an immunologic mechanism in minimal change disease (nil disease, foot process disease, lipoid nephrosis), but it has not been identified. Investigators are studying the role of abnormal T-cell function in this disease.[14] A variant of this disease is focal glomerulosclerosis in which glomeruli at the corticomedullary junction reveal focal sclerosis. Unlike minimal change disease, this variant does not respond to steroid therapy. This disease is the major cause of nephrotic syndrome of children, especially under 3 years of age. It causes a marked decrease in serum albumin and generalized edema. The prognosis in this disease is good since spontaneous remission frequently occurs and treatment of the patient with antibiotics and steroids has been shown to shorten the duration of the disease.

The urinalysis will indicate the selective proteinuria, predominantly albuminuria, that occurs. Hematuria is seen in up to 30 percent of these patients.[15] Pyuria is not seen, nor does a decrease in glomerular filtration rate often occur. Occasionally, hyaline, granular, or fatty casts may be seen in the urinary sediment. In children the serum albumin may drop to less than 2.0 g/l, and the serum cholesterol often exceeds 12.9

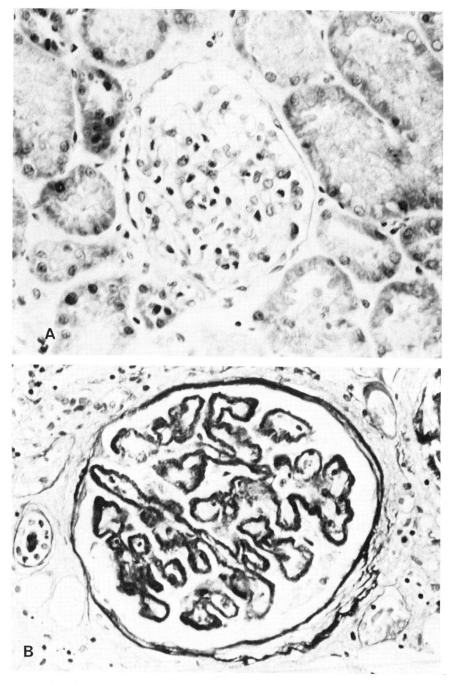

Figure 2.8. The glomerulus as seen in renal biopsy tissue sections by light microscopy. Approximately ×750. **A.** Normal glomerulus. **B.** Membranous glomerulonephritis with thickening of the glomerular basement membrane. (Courtesy of Regina Verani, MD, Department of Pathology and Laboratory Medicine, The University of Texas Medical School at Houston.)

mmole/L (500 mg/dl). The glomeruli are normal upon examination of tissue sections by light microscopy (Fig. 2.8A) and show diffuse fusion of the epithelial cell foot processes by electron microscopy. Immunoglobulins and complement are usually not demonstrable by immunofluorescence.

Focal Proliferative Glomerulonephritis. This form of glomerulonephritis (also called IgA nephropathy) affects some glomeruli and not others (focal), and in those that are affected the changes are seen in only one or two glomerular lobules upon microscopic examination of the tissue. Focal glomerulonephritis can be confused with acute poststreptococcal glomerulonephritis because both show marked hematuria. Focal glomerulonephritis is characterized by its occurrence at the time of a febrile incident. The two diseases differ in that IgA nephropathy or focal glomerulonephritis is not associated with fluid retention nor streptococcal antibodies and is less frequently associated with hypertension. The urinalysis at the time of the attack will show erythrocytes and nonselective type proteinuria of one g or less per day. The glomeruli in this disease are predominantly normal, although a few will show loci of endothelial cell proliferation. Immune complexes and complement deposits can be demonstrated on the otherwise normal-appearing glomerular tissue.

This type of glomerulonephritis can be exhibited in subacute bacterial endocarditis, hereditary nephritis, polyarteritis nodosa, systemic lupus erythematosus, Goodpasture's syndrome, and allergic purpura. The relationship of focal glomerulonephritis, recurrent macroscopic hematuria, and IgA nephropathy as being similar if not identical diseases has been underscored.[16]

Chronic Glomerulonephritis. This condition may become the result of any of the other forms of glomerulonephritis. It is progressive and results in dialysis, renal transplant, or death. Hypertension, nephrotic syndrome, and uremia are common symptoms of patients with chronic glomerulonephritis. Some

patients who have this disease have a history of some form of glomerulonephritis. The urinalysis will show proteinuria and microscopic hematuria. In advanced cases most of the glomeruli have been hyalinized, the tubules are atrophic, and the entire renal mass is markedly reduced.

Proliferative Glomerulonephritis with Crescent Formation. A marked proliferation of epithelial cells of Bowman's capsule with extensive crescent formation characterizes this disease (also called rapidly progressive glomerulonephritis) (Fig. 2.9). Extracapillary proliferation in Bowman's capsular space (crescents) is seen in 50 to 100 percent of the glomeruli. This disease is generally fatal within a few months. The features of this disease are seen in Goodpasture's syndrome (glomerulonephritis accompanying lung hemorrhage) and in immune complex disease (systemic lupus erythematosus, poststreptococcal glomerulonephritis). This type of glomerulonephritis exemplifies that two entirely different immune mechanisms, antiglomerular basement membrane and immune complex disease, can produce identical histologic patterns of glomerular injury. Results of immunofluorescence and electron microscopic analyses of renal glomerular tissue will vary depending upon the etiology of the disease.

Systemic Diseases Affecting the Kidney. Several systemic diseases are complicated by associated glomerulonephritis. Examples of these diseases are diabetes mellitus, amyloidosis, multiple myeloma, gout, hypertension, atherosclerosis, subacute bacterial endocarditis, allergic purpura, and such collagen diseases as systemic lupus erythematosus (SLE), periarteritis nodosa, and scleroderma. SLE, an autoimmune disease involving antibodies to deoxyribonucleic acid and other nuclear material, is an excellent example of the inflammation created in the kidney by circulating immune complexes. Focal, proliferative, and membranous glomerulonephritis are found in patients who have SLE, and it is not uncommon for one

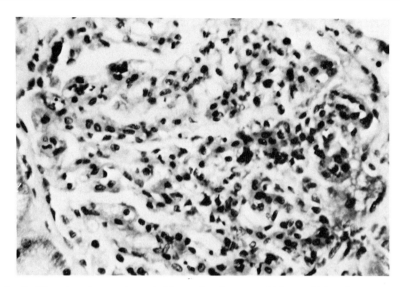

Figure 2.9. Proliferative glomerulonephritis section from renal biopsy, light microscopy, showing proliferation of epithelial cells. ×750. (Courtesy of Regina Verani, MD, Department of Pathology and Laboratory Medicine, The University of Texas Medical School at Houston.)

type of glomerulonephritis to convert to another. The diffuse, proliferative type of disease in persons who have SLE indicates a poorer prognosis.[17] The urinalysis will show proteinuria and microscopic hematuria.

Summary. From the brief descriptions given of the glomerular diseases, it is readily seen that the terminology and classification of these diseases are not well defined. Hopefully the histologic picture, brief description of the symptoms, and the laboratory findings presented here will enable the reader to peruse the literature and learn from sources in pathology and laboratory medicine and nephrology. A summary of the characteristics of several types of glomerulonephritis is given in Table 2.1.

Renal Tubular Physiology

Although filtration and reabsorption occur in all capillaries, there is a difference in the mechanism of reabsorption in the kidney. In addition to the forces described by Starling (Chapter 1, page 3), the renal tubular epithelium provides a mechanism for selective permeability and active transport. These ac-

tivities control the composition of the tubular fluid and, ultimately, that of the urine and the blood. Reabsorption is the term used to indicate the direction of transport from the tubular lumen, through the peritubular interstitium, and into the blood. The reverse transport is secretion.

Passive and Active Reabsorption. A passive mechanism for reabsorption is one that occurs along an electrochemical gradient from the luminal fluid to the peritubular capillary plasma. No energy is required for this mechanism to occur once the initial gradient has been established. An active transport mechanism occurs when a substance is transported against an electrochemical gradient from the luminal fluid to the peritubular plasma or vice versa. Energy is required for this process.

Proximal Tubular Activity. There are two general characteristics of the transport of salt and water by the proximal tubule:

1. Reabsorption of sodium and fluid in the proximal tubule occurs simultaneously with a large passive intercellular

ion movement from the blood into the lumen, and

2. A balance exists between the glomerulus and the proximal tubule in the process of water and salt reabsorption.

These two activities result in the kidney's purge of body wastes and in its equally important role of electrolyte, water, and acid-base balance of the body.

The proximal tubule reabsorbs 80 percent of the volume of fluid filtered by the glomerulus each day. The first event in this process is the reabsorption of sodium chloride, and this is followed by the reabsorption of water. This reabsorption of water does not result in a change in the osmotic pressure of the remaining fluid, and therefore this is known as "isosmotic reabsorption." This term indicates that the osmolality of the proximal tubulal fluid as it moves along the length of the proximal tubule matches that of the plasma of the peritubular capillary. The equality of osmolality is thought to be maintained by a process within the epithelial structure itself.[18] Even though the process results in isosmolar fluid, changes in the concentration of several constituents do occur. For example, glucose is reabsorbed to the extent that its concentration is zero at the end of the proximal tubule. Urea is concentrated twofold although it is partially reabsorbed. Bicarbonate concentration decreases below the plasma value, while there is a corresponding rise in the concentration of chloride of the tubular fluid. Organic acids are introduced into the tubular fluid in the straight segment of the proximal tubule.

Reabsorption of Phosphate, Sulfate, and Organic Compounds. The daily glomerular filtrate (173 L) contains 180 mmole HPO_4, 90 mmole SO_4^-, approximately 864 mmole glucose, and about 400 mmole urea. Urea reabsorption is a direct consequence of water flow and reabsorption. As the urine flow increases, the urea clearance increases. The passive reabsorption of urea is attributed to the permeability of the tubular epithelium primarily in the proximal tubule, although

absorption does occur in distal tubules in antidiuretic states.

Glucose, phosphate, sulfate, lactate, hydroxybutyrate, acetoacetate, vitamin C, and some amino acids are reabsorbed actively by mechanisms that have a capability for processing limited quantities of these solutes in a given time. If more than that amount of solute is present in the tubular lumen, the incapability of its reabsorption results in its appearance in the excreted urine.

Tubular Reabsorptive Maximum and Limited Reabsorptive Mechanisms. These mechanisms are described by two terms, "renal threshold" and "tubular reabsorption maximum" (Tm). Glucose is a good example and will be used to illustrate these terms (Fig. 2.10). Under normal conditions the fasting plasma glucose of approximately 5.5 mmole/L (100 mg/dl) results in 5.5 mmole/L appearing in the glomerular filtrate. The absorption in the proximal tubule results in its complete disappearance from the urine. However, when the plasma concentration exceeds 10 to 11 mmole/L (180 to 200 mg/dl), many of the transport sites in the proximal tubule become occupied, and the renal threshold is exceeded. Glucose, therefore, appears in the excreted urine. The concentration of glucose in the plasma at the time of the appearance of glucose in the urine is the renal plasma threshold for glucose. It is 10 to 11 mmole/L (180 to 200 mg/dl) in human adults, although it can vary from one individual to another. Some persons have lower threshold values, and diabetics of long standing have thresholds higher than 11 mmole/L.

As the number of occupied carrier sites is increased, more glucose is absorbed and more is excreted in the urine. Whenever the transport sites are fully occupied, reabsorption will be occurring at its greatest rate. This is the tubular reabsorptive maximum, which for glucose is about 27.8 to 37.0 μmole/sec (300 to 400 mg/min) in the adult human.[19]

The renal plasma threshold is a result of:

1. Glomerular filtration rate,

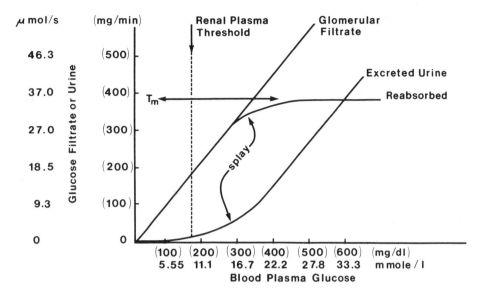

Figure 2.10. The renal threshold and renal tubular absorption maximum (Tm) of glucose.

2. Tubular reabsorptive capacity (reflected by Tm), and
3. Degree of splay in the glucose titration curve. Splay is the result of the affinity of the transport carrier for glucose and/or the difference between nephrons in this activity.

Amino Acids. Plasma amino acid concentrations are consistently about 3 mmole/L. This is near the renal plasma threshold, and amino acids are normally in extremely low concentration in the urine (Table 2.3, page 37). There are at least three transport mechanisms for amino acid reabsorption: one for the reabsorption of the basic amino acids, lysine, arginine, ornithine, cystine, and histidine, another for glutamic and aspartic acids, and a third for the remainder of the amino acids. In several metabolic disorders, for example, phenylketonuria, maple syrup urine disease, Fanconi's syndrome, liver disease, and cystinuria, certain amino acids exceed the renal threshold or the molecular transport mechanisms are missing, and the amino acids appear in the urine.

Phosphate. The plasma concentration of phosphate is maintained at approximately 1 mmole/L (3.1 mg/dl). An increase or decrease in the plasma concentration alters the rate of excretion in the urine. This is regulated by tubular reabsorption. The reabsorption of phosphate is reduced by an increased plasma concentration of cortisone, glucose, calcium, or vitamin D. Parathyroid hormone also increases the urinary excretion of phosphate. A decreased tubular reabsorption of phosphate has been used as an indicator of hyperparathyroidism.

Fixed Acids. About 1 mmole/kg of nonvolatile fixed acid is produced in adult humans daily from the metabolism of carbohydrates, fats, and proteins (Fig. 2.11). The major fixed acid is sulfuric acid. Others are lactic acid, phosphoric acid, citric acid, and α-ketoglutaric acid. The plasma concentration of sulfate is fairly constant at 1 to 1.5 mmole/L. However, when low plasma concentrations occur, reabsorption is complete and active. Glucose, sodium chloride, sodium thiocyanate, and sodium nitrite depress the reabsorption of sulfate. Transportable anions interfere with the reabsorption. The formation of sulfate ions is accompanied by the formation of two hydrogen ions, carbon dioxide, and urea (Fig. 2.11).

Lactic acid is formed in the anaerobic glycolytic metabolism of glucose and appears in the urine. Acetoacetic acid is formed in the oxidation of fatty acids in the liver, and its fate is usually oxidation to carbon dioxide and water. Whenever acetoacetate is released from the liver in a greater amount than can be metabolized in the tissues, aceto-acetate and its metabolites, acetone and β-hydroxybutyric acid, accumulate and appear in the urine. An excess of acetoacetic acid and its metabolites is formed whenever the energy requirements of the body are met primarily by fat metabolism, e.g., in starvation and diabetes.

Citrate is normally excreted in the urine in small amounts. The excretion rate is in-creased in metabolic alkalosis and is reduced in acidosis. The ingestion of fruits and vegetables increases the amounts of salts of these organic acids, e.g., potassium citrate and sodium lactate, and furnishes a mechanism for the removal of free hydrogen ions from the body (Fig. 2.11).

Sodium and Potassium Reabsorption. The active reabsorption of sodium forms the basis for the passive or cooperative transport of other solutes and fluid in the proximal tubule. Sodium transport early in the proximal tubule is via a cotransport system with organic solutes, e.g., glucose, amino acids, and lactic acid.[20] Chloride ions accompany the sodium movement and together create an osmotic influx of water. This activity ultimately results in sufficient hydrostatic pressure to force fluid into interstitial tissue. An Na^+-K^+ ATPase appears to be involved in the active process of sodium ion departure from the cell

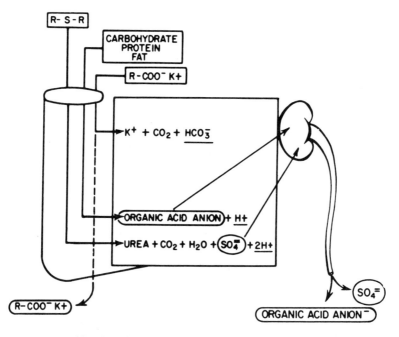

Figure 2.11. Diagram of fixed acid excretion. (From Lennon EJ: In Frohlich ED (ed): Pathophysiology, Altered Regulatory Mechanisms in Disease, 1972, p 256. Courtesy of J.B. Lippincott Co.)

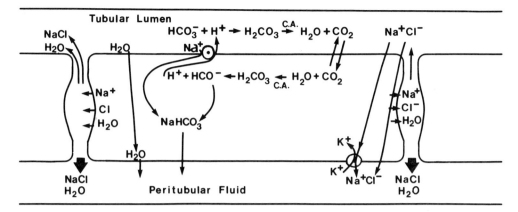

Figure 2.12. The conservation of bicarbonate in the proximal tubule. CA, carbonic anhydrase.

into the peritubular capillaries by way of the lateral intercellular spaces (Fig. 2.12). This is linked to the entrance of potassium ions to the cells. This active transport of sodium is known as the "sodium or cation pump."[21]

Almost all of the potassium in the glomerular filtrate is reabsorbed in the proximal tubule. Thus, urinary potassium results from secretion in the distal nephron. The reabsorption is believed to be an active process since the potassium concentration in tubular fluid is lower than that of the plasma at the time potassium reabsorption is occurring.

Sodium Bicarbonate Reabsorption. The conservation of sodium bicarbonate (HCO_3^-) by reabsorption in the proximal tubule rests upon the hydration of CO_2 by the enzyme, carbonic anhydrase.[22,23] The process is diagrammed in Figure 2.12. Carbonic acid dissociates to give bicarbonate and hydrogen ions. The hydrogen ions are secreted into the proximal tubular fluid, and sodium ions are actively reabsorbed at the same time. The hydrogen ions combine with the bicarbonate ions in the tubular fluid to form carbonic acid, which is transformed to water and carbon dioxide by the carbonic anhydrase of the endothelial brush border. The carbon dioxide enters the cell and once again enters the peritubular plasma along with the sodium ions.

The factors that play a role in the reabsorption of fluid in the proximal tubule are:

1. The Na^+-K^+ ATPase distribution all along the tubular surface,
2. The permeability of the proximal tubular epithelium to salt and water, and
3. The morphologic organization of the proximal tubular epithelium.

Loop of Henle. Salt and water reabsorption in the loop of Henle results in the adjustment of urine osmolality and the maintenance of the glomerulotubular salt balance. The osmolality of fluid in the descending limb increases on its way to the loop and decreases to a hypoosmotic level as it travels the ascending limb. The transport of salt from the fluid has been shown to result in an increasing salt concentration gradient in the surrounding tissue from the cortex to the inner medulla. The highest concentrations are found at the tips of the papillae.[24] This countercurrent multiplier action of the loops is the basis for the concentration of urine.

The countercurrent flow occurs as the tubular fluid flows from the proximal tubule in the cortex to the descending limb of Henle, makes the loop, and travels back toward the cortex in the ascending limb and once again flows toward the papilla and the collecting ducts in the medulla. The parallel arrangement of the looped tubules (Fig. 2.3) and the collecting tubule allows a concentration differential to be established and multiplied as the urine flows toward the collecting ducts.

The active transfer of salt from the lumen of the *ascending* thick limb is responsible for the hypotonicity of the fluid that enters the distal tubule, the hypertonicity of the interstitium, and the diffusion of salt into the fluid in the *descending* thin limb. Water moves passively down a concentration gradient from the distal tubule and cortical collecting duct into the surrounding capillaries in the cortex. Urea concentration is increased in the cortical collecting duct for two reasons: this part of the tubule *is not* permeable to urea and, in the presence of ADH, *is* permeable to water. The water diffuses out of the lumen.

In the medullary collecting duct, the urea diffuses out into the interstitium. This concentration of urea and salt causes water to be lost from the lumen of the descending thin limb and transferred to the surrounding blood vessels. Thus the concentration of the salt and urea in the descending thin limb increases. Urea diffuses into the descending thin limb. This cycling of urea back to the thin limbs from the medullary collecting ducts results in the concentration of urea in the fluid of the medullary collecting duct.

The fluid moving into the ascending limb at the papilla is more concentrated than is the interstitial fluid. As the fluid moves up the ascending limb, salt diffuses out to the more dilute interstitium. All of this results in a high salt and urea concentration in the medullary interstitium, which promotes water reabsorption from the collecting duct.

This countercurrent or recycling system results in the formation of a small volume of concentrated urine.

Micropuncture studies of superficial loops show that 25 percent of the sodium in the glomerular filtrate is reabsorbed in the loop.[25] Less than 15 percent of the water is reabsorbed. This results in a dilute tubular urine as it leaves the loop of Henle. The rate of salt reabsorption in the loop is proportional to the salt load entering the loop. This is true also for the proximal tubule. The prin-

cipal event in the concentrating mechanism of the human kidney is attributed to the active transport of chloride across the almost water-impermeable epithelial layer of the tubule segment known as the "ascending thick limb" of the loop or the pars recta of the distal tubule.

The volume of urine necessary for the excretion of a given amount of solute is lower when urea is the principal solute.[26] This is reflected by the increase in the concentration of urine when the diet contains large amounts of protein. Urea promotes the concentration of nonurea solutes by increasing the salt concentration in the descending loops and by increasing the salt departure from the ascending limbs into the interstitium. The resulting increase in medullary interstitial salt concentration leads to water reabsorption by the medullary collecting ducts, thereby concentrating the nonurea solutes of the urine.

Reabsorption of urea has been demonstrated by the difference in the urea clearance and the glomerular filtration rate and also by the change in urea clearance values with urine flow during a constant glomerular filtration rate. Urea is recycled from medullary collecting ducts into the loop of Henle concomitantly with the reabsorption of water in the collecting ducts. Whenever the urea/creatinine ratio exceeds the usual 15:1, lower nephron disability should be considered.[27]

Distal Tubules and Collecting Ducts. The distal tubule transports small quantities of solute and water. Sodium reabsorption is by active transport, and the rate is about one-third the rate in the proximal tubule. The sodium pump in the distal tubule can maintain a greater electrochemical gradient due to the tight junctions between cells and a small shunt path compared with the proximal convoluted tubule. Unlike the proximal tubules, the distal convoluted tubule maintains its load-dependent reabsorption of salt even when there is an increase in the extracellular fluid volume. The rate of sodium reabsorption and potassium secretion in the distal convoluted tubule is affected by hormones from the adrenal glands called "mineralocorticoids." Adrenalectomized rats cannot lower the intraluminal sodium concentration, but the administration of aldosterone reverses this in about 60 minutes. The Na^+-K^+ ATPase of the distal tubular epithelium has been shown to be stimulated at that time, thus suggesting a mechanism for the influence of aldosterone.[28]

Water Reabsorption. Approximately 8 percent (2.4 nl/min) of the filtered load of water is reabsorbed. The permeability of the distal convoluted tubule to water is only half that of the proximal tubulal epithelium.[29] In antidiuresis, where levels of antidiuretic hormone (ADH) are high, the collecting tubules in the cortical and medullary regions and the collecting ducts become highly permeable to water, and water is absorbed from the tubular lumen as the tubule traverses the concentrated medullary interstitium. In diuresis, the epithelium of the collecting duct becomes much less permeable to water.

Chloride. The net reabsorption of chloride by the distal convoluted tubule is 6 to 7 percent of the filtered chloride.[30] After administration of sodium bicarbonate or sodium sulfate, chloride concentration in the distal tubular fluid drops significantly. This serves to illustrate that the presence of poorly permeable anions in the distal tubule reduces the chloride concentration within the lumen. The transport of chloride differs in the early and late distal tubule. The mechanism for chloride transport in the early part of the distal tubule is thought to require energy because the electrochemical gradient is not great enough to be a factor. Thus, sodium and chloride appear to be actively transported in the early segment. In the late portion, chloride transport is passive.

Tubular Secretion. All potassium appearing in the excreted urine originates from secretion by the distal convoluted tubules and collecting ducts. Exceptions are the excretion of potassium in osmotic diuresis, large extracellular volume expansion, or after the administration of furosemide. Net reabsorption

of potassium is seen after dietary potassium restriction, and net secretion can be increased above normal by a diet containing large amounts of potassium.

Increased flow rates are accompanied by high rates of potassium ion secretion. Whenever the proximal tubular reabsorption of sodium is reduced, the secretion of potassium in the distal tubule is enhanced. This relationship can be explained by the combined effects of the load dependency of sodium ions and the flow dependency of potassium ions. Metabolic or respiratory acidosis is associated with a decreased potassium excretion, and alkalosis results in increased loss of potassium into the urine.

pH. The distal nephron contributes to the acid-base balance through its reabsorption of sodium bicarbonate and by secretion of ammonium and titratable acid to the tubular fluid (Fig. 2.13). Secretion of some 10 to 15 percent of the hydrogen ions that are secreted takes place in the distal tubule. This reduces the pH of the urine from about 6.8 to approximately 6.0.[31]

Carbonic anhydrase is absent from the luminal cells of the distal tubule. Bicarbonate reabsorption is a consequence of hydrogen ion secretion. Principal factors that control hydrogen ion secretion by the distal convoluted tubule are (1) the load of bicarbonate delivered to the distal tubule, (2) CO_2 tension of the peritubular blood, and (3) intracellular pH. Bicarbonate reabsorption and hydrogen ion secretion are increased when additional bicarbonate is delivered to the distal convoluted tubule. When intratubular buffer loads are high, the tubular fluid remains relatively alkaline, and hydrogen ion secretion can proceed against small pH gradients by active transport. The *net* rate of hydrogen ion secretion is determined by (1) the pH of the cell, (2) the back diffusion of hydrogen ions from the blood, and (3) the strength of the hydrogen pump located in the luminal cell membranes.

Kidney Response to Acidosis and Alkalosis. Acidosis and alkalosis are terms applied to variations of the blood pH value below and

Tubular Fluid   **Peritubular Fluid**

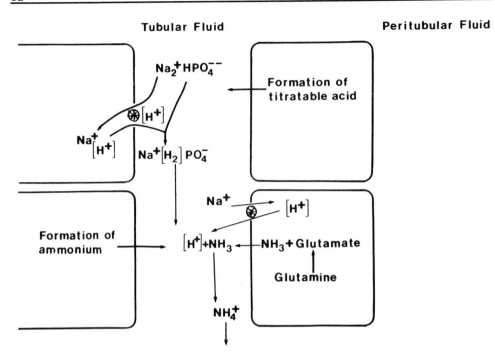

Figure 2.13. Secretion of ammonium and titratable acid in the distal tubule. (From Maude DL: Kidney Physiology and Kidney Disease, 1977, p 61. Courtesy of J.B. Lippincott Co.)

above 7.36 to 7.44 (normal range), respectively. In metabolic acidosis an abnormal anion gap occurs in the blood serum. The anion gap is the difference between the sum of the measured serum cations (Na, K, Ca) in milliequivalents per liter and the sum of the measured serum anions (HCO_3 and Cl) in milliequivalents per liter. Normally the gap is from 8 to 12 mEq/L (unmeasured anions, e.g., lactic acid). However, in acidosis the gap is usually more than 22 mEq/L. Metabolic acidosis in the presence of a normal anion gap is indicative of:

1. An increase in the unmeasured anions of the serum, i.e., the fixed acids,
2. An abnormal serum chloride ion concentration, or
3. An abnormal water loss.

The method selected for treatment of the acidotic condition will depend upon which of the above conditions has caused the anion gap.

With an increase in unmeasured ions, the production of fixed acid in the body leads to the excretion of urine with a pH of 5 to 6 that contains titratable acid and ammonium ions. When the acid load is increased, as in acidosis, there is a concomitant increase in hydrogen ion secretion, and a urine of pH near 4.5 results. Maximal values of titratable acid excretion are near 1.5 mmole/kg body weight per day. Sustained acidosis leads to a fivefold increase in excretion of ammonium ions (as ammonium chloride) or about 300 nmoles/day.[31]

In alkalosis the normal renal mechanisms for the reabsorption of bicarbonate, acidification of phosphate buffer salts, and secretion of ammonium chloride are modified to accomplish an increase in the excretion of base with a resulting increase in the urine pH. In some cases this may be as high as pH 7.8. The hydrogen ion secretion drops to a point where the titratable acidity is near zero, and the reabsorption of sodium bicarbonate is reduced.

In summary, the distal nephron accomplishes the following:

1. It creates a high concentration gradient between blood plasma or the peritubular capillaries and the urine. An example is the conservation of salt in salt deprivation by the excretion of limited sodium ions. Conversely, the sodium concentration of urine can be twice that of the blood when salt intake is high and the intake of water is low. A second example is the steep hydrogen ion gradient that is formed as a result of a large acid load (acidosis). This can result in a collecting duct urine with a pH as low as 4.5.
2. It creates a high osmolar concentration gradient between urine and blood plasma. In diuresis the osmolality of urine may be 40 times less than that found in water deprivation and one-tenth that of blood plasma.
3. It responds to the level of circulating antidiuretic hormone (ADH) by altering its permeability to water. In hydropenia, ADH concentration is high, and the permeability of the distal tubule and collecting ducts is increased.
4. It reabsorbs water passively in a manner dependent upon the osmotic forces between tubular fluid, interstitial fluid, and the peritubular blood plasma.
5. It secretes potassium by a mechanism that is influenced by dietary intake, the load of fixed acid, flow rate, and sodium reabsorption in the proximal tubule.

Table 2.2 shows the transport of water and some solutes in the various parts of the renal tubule and the collecting ducts. It serves as a summary of the results of the reabsorption and secretion that occur.

Renal Tubular Disease

Renal Tubular Acidosis. Renal tubular acidosis is a disease of the kidney that results in the increased excretion of bicarbonate. It may be recalled that the normal kidney responds to metabolic alkalosis by an increase of bicarbonate in urine, an increase in urinary pH, a low ammonium ion excretion, and a low titratable acid excretion. This occurs because the tubular secretory capacity is overcome by the increased filtered load of plasma bicarbonate. In renal tubular acidosis, the bicarbonate excretion may also occur when the maximum tubular capacity for the secretion of hydrogen ions is blocked or abnormally low. In distal tubular acidosis, the ability to create a normal hydrogen gradient is lost. However, the amount of bicarbonate lost is small, usually less than 15 percent of the fluid load. Urine pH is fixed high.

TABLE 2.2. WATER AND SOLUTE TRANSPORT IN THE RENAL TUBULE AND COLLECTING DUCT

Flow and Content	Glomerular Filtrate	Midproximal	End Proximal	Early Distal	Late Distal	Collecting Duct
Flow (ml/sec)	2	1	0.4			
Total solute (mOsm/L)	285	285	285	140	140–285	100–1,000
Na^+ (mmole/L)	145	145	145	50	30–70	1–300
K^+ (mmole/L)	4	2		0.4	0.8	
Cl^- (mmole/L)	105	120	120			
HCO_3^- (mmole)	25	10	10			
Glucose (mmole/L)	5	2	0			
Urea (mmole/L)	5	8	10	15	15–30	15–200
H_2O filtered load remaining (%)			20	20	2–15	0.5–15

After Maude DL: Kidney Physiology and Kidney Disease, 1977. Courtesy of J.B. Lippincott Co.

In proximal tubular acidosis, the rate of hydrogen ion secretion is limited, resulting in a large excretion of bicarbonate. In this case, if the filtered load is reduced, some reabsorption occurs in the proximal tubule, and the distal secretory capacity may be able to process most of the remaining bicarbonate.

Uremic acidosis may be partly due to bicarbonate wastage rather than a retention of acid. A defect in bicarbonate absorption is a constant finding in glomerular or uremic acidosis. The tubular defects resulting in renal tubular acidosis (RTA) have been classified as type I (distal), type II (proximal), and types III and IV, which are variants. A fifth classification has been proposed and a suggestion made that since so many variants exist, the system should be abandoned in favor of describing RTA in a functional way. For example, type I would be described as a no-threshold RTA with minimal wasting, and type II would be described as RTA with gross bicarbonate wasting.[32] The steady state plasma bicarbonate concentration is controlled by the load at which the tubular threshold for bicarbonate reabsorption is set in renal disease.

Acute Tubular Cell Injury. Tubular necrosis, i.e., the destruction of the tubular epithelial cells, occurs fairly rapidly in the following conditions:

1. Whenever the blood supply to the renal tubules is halted (ischemia),
2. In allergic or hypersensitivity reactions (interstitial nephritis), and
3. On exposure to chemicals (nephrotoxic tubular necrosis).

The glomerular filtration rate is reduced, and oliguria or anuria occurs. The tubular functions, e.g., the reabsorption of sodium, glucose, and the secretion of potassium and hydrogen ions, are impaired. In addition to the changes in the urine volume and composition, a retention of nitrogenous waste products creates azotemia.

The loss of blood supply has its greatest impact upon the pars recta of the proximal tubule. The tubular epithelium dies, but if the cell death is not too extensive, regeneration can occur. Interstitial swelling occurs. Tubular injury can result from trauma accompanied by muscle damage (crush syndrome), hemorrhage, reduction in plasma volume, intravascular hemolysis, sepsis, and other causes of shock. Cortical necrosis can occur when prolonged loss of renal blood supply occurs.

Nephrotoxic tubular injury is also caused by the ingestion of certain chemicals, e.g., cadmium, mercuric chloride, and ethylene glycol, or from the administration of certain drugs. Medications known for their nephrotoxicity include some antibiotics, e.g., gentamicin and kanamycin.

Papillary necrosis can occur whenever urinary tract obstruction occurs or there is a loss of blood supply to the kidney. The pathogenesis may involve acute pyelonephritis, abuse with alcohol or analgesic medications, such as aspirin or phenacetin, diabetes, sickle cell disease, or renal calculi.

Medications that induce an allergic response in some persons are one of the causes of an inflammatory reaction in the renal interstitium. The drugs that are common offenders are sulfonamides and methicillin. Other causes of interstitial nephritis excluding primary renal disease are staphylococcal and streptococcal septicemia, sarcoidosis, and Sjögren's syndrome.

Urinary Tract Infection. Growth of bacteria in the tissues of the urinary tract or in the urine constitutes urinary tract infection (bacteriuria). The urine in the bladder is normally sterile. This may seem surprising since the urine can serve as an appropriate culture medium and the microorganisms for colonization lie at the anterior urethra. This is particularly amazing in the female where there is such a short distance from the bladder to the urethra and also where the vaginal orifice affords an additional source of microbes. Colonization of the urinary tract is considered to be demonstrated by the presence of greater than 10^5 organisms per ml in the urine. Contamination is considered to be the source of organisms in urine when the concentration is less than 10^3 per ml.[33] Occasionally, urinary tract infection occurs without the symptoms of frequency of micturition and burning (dysuria).

Asymptomatic bacteriuria can set the stage for subsequent tissue infection and the development of cystitis (bladder infection) and pyelonephritis. For example, in one study, one third of the pregnant women who had bacteriuria subsequently developed acute pyelonephritis which could be prevented by antibiotic treatment.[34] Although bacteriuria is the most common expression of urinary tract infection, it may be absent when the infection is barricaded from the urine, for example, in hematogenous pyelonephritis, obstruction of the infected part of the tract, or whenever antibiotic therapy has been less than totally effective.

Pyelonephritis. Pyelonephritis can occur as an active infection, in which case it is called "acute pyelonephritis," or it can be the disease of a kidney damaged by a preceding but no longer active infection.

In acute pyelonephritis, the bacterial infection causes inflammation of the renal pelvis and calyces and progresses via the collecting ducts to the tubular cells of the corticomedullary junction. Leukocytes are found in the lumen. Small abscesses form which obliterate the infected nephrons. Generally, the involvement is patchy, and there is little or no effect on the glomerular filtration rate. Chills, fever, and bacteriuria often accompany this disease.

The urine will exhibit white cells in clumps, white cell casts, and large numbers of bacteria. Proteinuria is not a common event. Hematuria may occur in severe inflammation of the bladder. Bacteriuria, in addition to being detected in the urine by microscopic examination, may be detected by using one or more chemical spot tests for nitrite or a dip-slide culture method. However, bacteriologic culture methods are the recommended procedure for the detection of bacteriuria. Asymptomatic bacteriuria in adults has been a comparatively benign condition in the ab-

sence of preexisting renal abnormalities.[35] One of the correlatives of bacterial infection in renal tissue is the formation of kidney stones composed principally of calcium phosphate and magnesium salts.

HORMONES AND THE KIDNEY

Hormones Produced by the Kidney

The kidneys are known to be the major participants in the production of erythropoietin, a hormone that stimulates erythrocyte production. It is not known how this occurs. It is thought that renal tissue synthesizes erythrogenin that catalyzes the formation of active erythropoietin from a circulating substrate. The stimulation of erythropoietin production occurs when there is a decreased oxygen supply to the kidney. When there is an occlusion of the flow of blood to the kidney, e.g., in neoplasm, cysts, or renal arterial stenosis, erythropoietin may be synthesized in excess. An excess of erythropoietin has resulted in an abnormally high production of erythrocytes (polycythemia). Conversely, chronic renal disease is often accompanied by anemia, and the decrease in erythropoietin is a participant in this associated condition.[36,37]

Prostaglandins E_1 and F_2 and perhaps A are synthesized in the collecting ducts and cells of the medullary interstitium. These compounds are considered to be attenuators, modulators, or enhancers of hormone activity. Entrance into the urine is through Henle's loop. The administration of prostaglandin E and A results in increased renal plasma flow and an increased salt and water excretion in some animals but not in others.[38] Although the possibility exists for the involvement of prostaglandins in the control of hypertension, no role has been established.

The active form of vitamin D (1,25-dihydroxy vitamin D_3) is produced exclusively in the kidney by a reaction catalyzed by 25-hydroxy vitamin D_3 hydroxylase. This vitamin is now considered by many to be a hormone with target tissues of bone, kidney, and intestine. This then would place the kidney among the endocrine organs. Vitamin D production is intimately associated with the mobilization of calcium and phosphate. Synthesis of this hormone-vitamin is regulated inversely by the circulating calcium concentration.[39] Parathyroid hormone is also involved in the stimulation of vitamin D synthesis in the kidney.[40] Patients who have hypercalcemia, hyperparathyroidism, hypervitamin D, and chronic renal failure lose the ability to control calcium homeostasis through vitamin D synthesis.

In response to changes in blood volume and low sodium concentration, the juxtaglomerular cells of the kidney produce and secrete renin.[41] Renin acts upon angiotensinogen to produce angiotensin I, which in turn is converted by enzymatic action to angiotensin II, an active vasoconstrictor agent. Angiotensin II stimulates the secretion of aldosterone by the adrenal gland. Thus renin is a hormone that is produced in the kidney that also indirectly acts upon the kidney through aldosterone.

Hormones that Act upon the Kidney

Hyperparathyroidism and the resulting increase in the concentration of circulating parathyroid hormone are accompanied by a loss of bicarbonate via poor absorption by the renal tubules. This loss is sufficient to trigger metabolic acidosis. Parathyroid hormone deficiency is accompanied by a marginal metabolic alkalosis. The maximal renal threshold for bicarbonate is clearly increased, and an increase in plasma bicarbonate results. Parathyroid hormone must, therefore, be considered one of the regulators of metabolic acid-base balance. A feedback mechanism for the control of this process rests upon the alteration of plasma ionized calcium by a change in blood pH. Calcium ions determined by an ion-selective electrode decreased by 0.08 mmole (0.32 percent) upon a change from pH 7.2 to 7.4.[42] This level of diminishing Ca ions is sufficient to double the circulating plasma concentration of parathyroid hormone.[43]

The mineralocorticoid aldosterone produced in the adrenal gland causes sodium retention and loss of potassium in the urine.

It acts upon the distal tubule, causing sodium reabsorption in exchange for hydrogen and potassium indirectly through the production of new protein.[44]

Antidiuretic hormone (arginine vasopressin) is synthesized in the hypothalamus and stored in the posterior lobe of the pituitary gland. It causes an increased permeability of the distal convoluted tubules and the collecting ducts to water. Several pharmacologic agents, as well as pain and emotional stress, affect the release of ADH. The agents that stimulate release are anesthetics, barbiturates, and nicotine. Ethanol is known to suppress the release of antidiuretic hormone.

COMPOSITION OF URINE

The activities of the human kidney, some of which have been discussed, normally result in the production of urine that contains pigments, electrolytes, vitamins, lipids, carbohydrates, amino acids, mucopolysaccharides, peptides, proteins, purine and pyrimidine metabolites, nonprotein nitrogenous compounds, various organic compounds, nonsteroid and steroid hormones, and water. Abnormal values for any of these substances under circumstances of normal diet, usual climate, and personal habits are generally associated with some disease process.

Over 403 nonsteroid and 122 steroid compounds have been determined in human urine.[45] Some of the compounds excreted in larger amounts and of medical importance are given in Table 2.3.

In addition to the solutes in urine there are structural constituents present. These are the cells, bacteria, crystals, and casts. Normally there are few cells present in the urine. These are the red cells and white cells that are introduced into the urine during the normal activity of cell death and regeneration in the kidney and urinary tract. Other cells seen are cells originating in the urinary tract or kidney. The most common cell occurring in the sediment is the squamous epithelial cell that is sloughed from the terminal urethra as a con-

TABLE 2.3. TYPICAL URINARY EXCRETION OF CERTAIN SOLUTES

Solute	Amount Excreted/Kg Body Weight/Day
ELECTROLYTES	
Chloride	1.1–5.1 mmole
Sodium	1.1–4.1 mmole
Potassium	0.4–1.4 mmole
Sulfur, inorganic	0.1–0.6 mmole
Bicarbonate	0.01–0.2 mmole
Phosphorus, inorganic	0.3–0.48 mmole
Calcium	0.001–0.28 mmole
VITAMINS AND RELATED COMPOUNDS	
Inositol	1.1 μmole
Niacinamide	0.16 μmole
Ascorbic acid	0.56–2.3 μmole
Pantothenic acid	0.21 μmole
Choline	0.65 μmole
CARBOHYDRATES	
Glucose	0–7.8 μmole
Oligosaccharides as fructose	3–14 μmole
Mannitol	0–4 μmole
Arabitol	0–4 μmole
AMINOSUGARS/MUCOPOLYSACCHARIDES	
Oligosaccharides (as hexosamine)	1,030–2,570 μg
Amino sugars, bound	200–700 μg
Sialic acid, bound	367–795 μg
Acid mucopoly-saccharides	30–140 μg
AMINO ACIDS/PEPTIDES/PROTEINS	
Proteins, total	0.5–2.0 mg
Amino acids, total	20–40 mg
IgA	10–70 μg
IgG	20–90 μg
Glycoprotein (Tamm-Horsfall)	250–500 μg
MISCELLANEOUS	
Coproporphyrin	0.4–0.9 nmole
Porphobilinogen	40–130 nmole
Urobilin and Urobilino-gen	2–70 nmole
Urea	3.3×10^6 nmole
Ketone bodies as acetone	10.3×10^4 nmole
Purine bases as adenine	1–7.4×10^3 nmole

sequence of cellular aging. Other cells of renal origin may be helpful diagnostically, for example, bits of tissue may be seen in renal papillary necrosis. In malignancy of the urinary tract or kidney, cells with abnormal cytologic features will be seen. The numbers of cells and their significance will be discussed in subsequent chapters.

Bacteria are not normally present but may be introduced during the collection of the specimen from external contamination. The presence of crystals depends upon the pH of the urine as well as the concentration of the components of the crystal. Generally very few, if any, crystals are present in healthy persons. The presence of certain crystals in large numbers may be helpful diagnostically. Casts are present but rarely seen in random urine specimens.

The examination of urine and the measures to be taken in assuring valid results that can be of diagnostic or therapeutic importance in the assessment of disease and pursuit of health are discussed in several subsequent chapters.

Review Questions

1. Match the name of the part of the kidney with the part of the diagram.

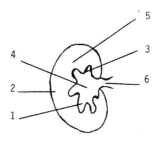

A. Medulla
B. Cortex
C. Major calyx
D. Minor calyx
E. Pyramid
F. Ureter

2. Match the name of the part of the uriniferous tubule with the part in the diagram.

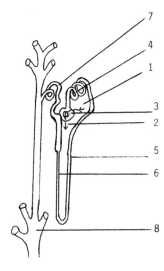

A. Distal tubule (pars convoluta)
B. Afferent arteriole
C. Proximal tubule (pars convoluta)
D. Proximal tubule (pars recta)
E. Ascending limb loop of Henle
F. Bowman's space
G. Collecting duct

3. The following cell type(s) is (are) normally found in the glomerulus:
A. Podocytes
B. Mesangial
C. Epithelial
D. Endothelial
E. Histiocyte

4. The formation of urine occurs in the following sequence:
A. Proximal convoluted tubule, hairpin loop, distal tubule, collecting tubule
B. Glomerulus, Bowman's space, proximal convoluted tubule, proximal tubule, loop, distal tubule, distal convoluted tubule, collecting duct
C. Bowman's space, glomerulus, proximal convoluted tubule, proximal tubule, loop, distal tubule, distal convoluted tubule, collecting duct

D. Glomerulus, Bowman's space, proximal tubule, proximal convoluted tubule, loop, distal tubule, distal convoluted tubule, collecting duct
E. Bowman's space, glomerulus, proximal tubule, proximal convoluted tubule, loop, distal tubule, distal convoluted tubule, collecting duct

5. Prostatitis usually has the following effect on urine excretion:
A. No effect
B. Polyuria
C. Oliguria
D. Anuria
E. Dysuria

6. The filtration barrier(s) in the glomerulus is (are):
A. Basement membrane
B. Endothelial pores
C. Mesangial matrix
D. Juxtaglomerular complex
E. Slit pore

7. The glomerular epithelial cell performs the following function(s):
A. Secretes potassium
B. Synthesizes glomerular basement membrane
C. Supports capillary loops
D. Forms barriers to passage of high molecular weight substances
E. Forms mesangial matrix

8. The substance(s) that is (are) useful in determining glomerular filtration rate because it (they) is (are) neither absorbed nor secreted:
A. Penicillin
B. Urea
C. Glucose
D. Inulin
E. Potassium

9. Selective passage of molecules through the glomerulus depends on:
A. The charge of the molecules
B. The size (molecular weight)
C. The flow of urine
D. The concentration in the blood
E. The arteriolar pressure

10. The most common laboratory finding in renal disease is:

A. Glucosuria
B. Creatinuria
C. Increased volume of urine
D. Proteinuria
E. Increased numbers of red cells in urine

11. The filtered load of a substance is the:
    A. Rate of transport of a substance across glomerular membrane
    B. Amount of substance in the efferent arteriole to be filtered
    C. Amount of substance in the efferent arteriole after filtration
    D. Rate of excretion of a substance in the urine
    E. Amount of substance above which filtration does not occur

12. The following results for laboratory tests are found frequently in the nephrotic syndrome:
    A. Proteinuria
    B. Oliguira
    C. Hypercholesterolemia
    D. Polyuria
    E. Red cell casts

13. The pathogenesis of the majority of the different types of glomerulonephritic diseases is:
    A. Infection
    B. Circulating immune complexes
    C. Inherited renal defect
    D. Improper diet
    E. Heart failure

14. Urine from individuals who have membranous glomerulonephritis will often exhibit:
    A. Gross hematuria
    B. Proteinuria
    C. Cylinduria
    D. Bacteriuria
    E. Increased white cells

15. Which of the following renal diseases is (are) ascribed to antibodies directed to renal tissue?
    A. Goodpasture's syndrome
    B. Nephrotic syndrome
    C. Acute glomerulonephritis
    D. Tubular necrosis
    E. Renal tubular acidosis

16. Active absorption is defined as transport:
    A. Against an electrochemical gradient
    B. Not requiring energy
    C. In the direction of the electrochemical gradient
    D. That requires energy
    E. Based on simple diffusion

17. Three major functions of the proximal tubule are:
    A. Isosmotic reabsorption
    B. Reabsorption of sodium
    C. Reabsorption of potassium
    D. Secretion of potassium
    E. Secretion of ammonia

18. Hydrogen ion excretion in the distal nephron is accompanied by:
    A. A decrease in urine pH to near 4.5
    B. An increase in bicarbonate reabsorption
    C. Increased excretion of ammonium ions
    D. Decrease in titratable acidity
    E. An increased anionic gap

19. Two major functions that occur in Henle's loop are:
    A. Active transport of chloride
    B. Absorption of about 80 percent of water in fluid
    C. Bicarbonate excretion
    D. Excretion of ammonium ions
    E. Reabsorption of about 25 percent of the sodium in the glomerular filtrate

20. The role of urea in the concentration of the urine is to:
    A. Increase the secretion of potassium
    B. Increase the reabsorption of water
    C. Decrease the reabsorption of bicarbonate
    D. Decrease the reabsorption of glucose
    E. Increase the reabsorption of amino acids

21. The major fixed acids of the urine are:
    A. Lactic acid
    B. Phosphoric acid
    C. Citric acid
    D. α-Ketoglutaric acid
    E. Nitric acid

22. Which of the following are major functions of the distal tubule or collecting duct?
    A. Secretion of potassium
    B. Secretion of ammonium ion
    C. Active reabsorption of sodium
    D. Respond to ADH by increased reabsorption of water
    E. Secretion of approximately 10 to 15 percent of hydrogen ions

23. Fixed acids in the case of acidosis:
    A. Are increased in the urine
    B. May explain a normal anion gap
    C. Are in the same concentration as in alkalosis
    D. Lead to urine with a pH of 3 to 4
    E. Are converted to hydrogen ions and salts

24. Alkalosis is a condition in which the:
    A. Blood pH is greater than 7.44
    B. Anion gap is greater than 22 mEq/L
    C. Hydrogen ion secretion is increased
    D. Urine pH is approximately 4.5
    E. Ammonium ion secretion is increased

25. Renal threshold is defined as:
    A. The molecular size that can pass the filtration barrier
    B. The concentration of a substance in the urine
    C. The ratio of urine concentration to plasma concentration
    D. The maximal concentration that can be excreted
    E. The concentration of a substance in the blood at the time of its appearance in the excreted urine

26. Proximal tubular acidosis may occur from the following defect:
    A. A block in the maximal tubular capacity for secretion of hydrogen ions
    B. Inability to create a normal hydrogen ion gradient
    C. An abnormal mechanism for hydrogen ion secretion
    D. Decreased carbonic anhydrase
    E. Decreased ammonia excretion

27. Distal tubular acidosis is attributed to:
    A. A block in the maximal tubular capacity for the secretion of hydrogen ions
    B. Decreased carbonic anhydrase
    C. Increased ammonia excretion
    D. The loss of ability to create a normal hydrogen ion gradient
    E. An abnormal mechanism for hydrogen ion secretion

28. In the blanks below place an "X" if the activity is greater in the proximal than in the distal tubule and a "Y" if the activity is greater in the distal tubule.
    ___ Isosmotic reabsorption
    ___ Glucose reabsorption
    ___ Secretion of potassium
    ___ Secretion of organic acids
    ___ Sodium reabsorption
    ___ Response to ADH
    ___ Maintenance of high osmolar gradient between blood and urine

29. The pathogenesis of pyelonephritis is principally:
    A. Proteinuria
    B. Hematuria
    C. Bacteriuria
    D. Leukocytosis
    E. Cylinduria

30. The following are often observed in the examination of urine in pyelonephritis:
    A. White cells in clumps
    B. Large numbers of bacteria
    C. Large numbers of red cells
    D. Proteinuria
    E. Red cell casts

31. The role of the parathyroid gland in acidosis is:
    A. Hyperparathyroidism is caused by consistent acidosis
    B. Hyperparathyroidism is accompanied by a loss of bicarbonate
    C. Hypoparathyroidism is accompanied by a loss of bicarbonate
    D. Hypoparathyroidism is caused by consistent acidosis
    E. Hyperparathyroidism prevents acidosis from occurring

32. Four hormones that are produced in

the kidney are:
A. Prostaglandins
B. Parathyroid hormone
C. Erythropoietin
D. Renin
E. Vitamin D

33. The relationship between renal disease and anemia is:
A. Persistent anemia results in renal disease
B. Azotemia causes the red cells to disintegrate
C. Leukocytosis depresses red cell production
D. Azotemia depresses the formation of red cells
E. Erythropoietin is decreased in renal disease

34. The relationship of the kidney to calcium metabolism is explained by which of the following?
A. Feedback control of vitamin D synthesis in the kidney by the circulating calcium concentration
B. Parathyroid hormone stimulates vitamin D synthesis in the kidney
C. Vitamin D production determines calcification of bone
D. Vitamin D depresses erythropoietin synthesis
E. The excretion of calcium is by active transport

(See Appendix for answers.)

Case Study

A 25-year-old man with a history of seasonal allergies was admitted for renal biopsy. He had been treated for a urinary tract infection six years before. One year prior to admission, he had developed a flu-like illness with nausea and malaise, then fever and a cough productive of yellow-green sputum, then high fever, shaking chills, low back pain, and chest pain. On the third day of illness, he developed dark urine, which progressed to gross hematuria. Oral cephalexin was be-

gun, and the patient was admitted to the hospital. The physical examination was unremarkable, but urinalysis revealed 2^+ proteinuria, the microscopic examination showed 30 to 40 red blood cells (RBC)/high-power field, 30 white blood cells (WBC)/high-power field, no RBC casts, and a urine culture was negative. Urines had 2.9 g protein, then 1.2 g protein per day. Serum creatinine was 1.0 mg/dl (88.4 μmole/L). Repeat urinalysis revealed RBC casts. The patient improved in a week, refused renal biopsy, and was discharged.

At six month follow-up, the patient was well, but proteinuria persisted at 0.5 g/day. An antinuclear antibody test was negative. At 10 months, he had 0.4 g protein/day and serum creatinine was 1.1 mg/dl (97.2 μmole/L).

At 11 months, the patient developed an abscessed tooth, for which he was given penicillin and a combination analgesic containing oxycodone. Again he developed fever, malaise, yellow-green sputum, headache, and dark urine. Outpatient urinalysis showed greater than 100 RBC/high-power field, 25 WBC/high-power field, and RBC casts. Serum creatinine was 1.1 mg/dl (97.2 μmole/L). He had 4.7 g protein/day in his urine. His condition improved in several days, but admission was scheduled a month later for renal biopsy.

Admission history was similar to the above, including a history of seasonal rhinitis, conjunctivitis, sinusitis, and occasional asthmatic attacks. The physical examination was normal except for prominent tonsils. Blood pressure was 120/60, and there was no edema. Urinalysis showed many RBC/high-power field, 2 to 6 WBC/high-power field, and rare RBC casts. BUN/creatinine was 21/1.2. A 12-hour urine implied a creatinine clearance of 156 ml/min, and 0.3 g protein/day. C3 was normal at 80 mg/dl (normal 55 to 120), and C4 was normal at 30 mg/dl (normal 20 to 50). Coagulation studies and platelet count were normal. A renal biopsy was done. The light microscopic examination of the biopsy showed fibrosis of the cortex, two sclerosed glomeruli, and an increased diffuse mesangium. The electron microscopic analysis showed electron-dense deposits in the mesangium with slight thickening in some glomeruli.

Immunofluorescent studies showed IgA and C3 deposits mainly in the mesangium.

Questions

1. What does the blood urea nitrogen (BUN)/creatinine ratio indicate?
2. Why was an antinuclear antibody test done?
3. What information appears to be the most helpful in determining the type of glomerulonephritis?

Answers

1. The blood urea nitrogen/creatinine ratio is greater than 15/1, and thus lower nephron disability should also be considered.
2. The antinuclear antibody test was done to rule out systemic lupus erythematosus as the cause of the renal disease.
3. The information most useful in this case is that obtained from the light, electron, and the fluorescent microscopic analysis in particular. Although the degree of proteinuria was atypical, the diagnosis was IgA nephropathy.

REFERENCES

1. Habib R, Kleinknecht C, Gubler MC, Levy M: Idiopathic membranoproliferative glomerulonephritis in children. Report of 105 cases. Clin Nephrol 1:194, 1973.
2. Bulger RE: Functional architecture of the kidney. In Kidney Disease—Present Status. IAP Monograph No 20. Baltimore, Williams & Wilkins, 1979, pp 162–201.
3. Venkatachalam MA, Karnovsky MJ, Fahimi HD, Cotran RS: An ultrastructural study of glomerular permeability using catalase and peroxidase as tracer proteins. J Exp Med 132:1153, 1970.
4. Chang RLS, Deen WM, Robertson CE, Brenner BM: Permselectivity of the glomerular capillary wall. III. Restricted transport of polyanions. Kidney Int 8:212, 1975.
5. Jorgensen F, Bentzon MW: The ultrastructure of the normal human glomerulus: Thickness of glomerular basement membrane. Lab Invest 18:42, 1968.
6. Kanwar YS, Farquhar MG: Presence of heparan sulfate in the glomerular basement membrane. Proc Natl Acad Sci USA 76:1303, 1979.
7. Rhodin JAG: Structure of the kidney. In Strauss MB, Welt LG (eds): Diseases of the Kidney, 2nd ed. Boston, Little, Brown, 1971, pp 1–30.
8. Hollenberg K: The physiology of the renal circulation. In Black D, Jones NF (eds): Renal Disease, 4th ed. Oxford, Blackwell, 1979, pp 30–63.
9. Schnermann J, Levine DZ: Tubular control of glomerular filtration rate in single nephrons. Can J Physiol Pharmacol 53:325, 1975.
10. Pitts RF: Physiology of the Kidney and Body Fluids, 3rd ed. Chicago, Yearbook, 1974, p 42.
11. Maude DL: Kidney Physiology and Kidney Disease. Philadelphia, Lippincott, 1977, p 108.
12. Maude DL: Kidney Physiology and Kidney Disease. Philadelphia, Lippincott, 1977, p 142.
13. Fish AJ, Michael AF: Immunopathogenesis of renal disease. In Earley LE, Gottschalk CW (eds): Strauss and Welt's Diseases of the Kidney, 3rd ed. Boston, Little, Brown, 1979, p 561.
14. Mallick NP: The pathogenesis of minimal change nephropathy. Clin Nephrol 7:87, 1977.
15. Cameron JS, Turner DR, Ogg CS, Sharpstone P, Brown CB: The nephrotic syndrome in adults with "minimal change" glomerular lesions. Q J Med 43:461, 1974.
16. Berger J: IgA glomerular deposits in renal disease. Transplant Proc 1:939, 1969.
17. Walker WG, Solez K: Renal involvement in disorders of connective tissue. In Earley LE, Gottschalk EW (eds): Strauss and Welt's Diseases of the Kidney, 3rd ed. Boston, Little, Brown, 1979, p 1263.
18. Valtin H: Renal Function: Mechanisms Preserving Fluid and Solute Balance in Health. Boston, Little, Brown, 1973, p 107.
19. Maude DL: Kidney Physiology and Kidney Disease. Philadelphia, Lippincott, 1977, p 74.
20. Kokko JP: Proximal tubular potential difference. Dependence on glucose, bicarbonate and amino acids. J Clin Invest 52:1362, 1970.
21. Skou JC: Enzymatic basis for active transport of Na^+ and K^+ across cell membranes. Physiol Rev 45:596, 1965.
22. Pitts RF, Lotspeich WD, Schiess WA, Ayer JL: The renal regulation of acid-base balance in man. I. The nature of the mechanism for acidifying the urine. J Clin Invest 27:48, 1948.

23. Rector FC Jr, Carter NW, Seldin DW: The mechanism of bicarbonate reabsorption in the proximal and distal tubules of the kidney. J Clin Invest 44:278, 1965.

24. Maack T, Windhager EH: Electrolyte transport in the nephron. In Black D, Jones NF (eds): Renal Disease, 4th ed. Oxford, Blackwell, 1979, p 133.

25. Maack T, Windhager EH: Electrolyte transport in the nephron. In Black D, Jones NF (eds): Renal Disease, 4th ed. Oxford, Blackwell, 1979, p 117.

26. Gamble JL, McKhann CF, Bulter AM, Tuthill E: An economy of water in renal function referrable to urea. Am J Physiol 109:139, 1934.

27. Maude DL: Kidney Physiology and Kidney Disease. Philadelphia, Lippincott, 1977, p 119.

28. Hierholzer K, Wiederholt M: Some aspects of distal tubular solute and water transport. Kidney Int 9:198, 1976.

29. Khuri RW, Wiederholt M, Strieder N, Giebisch G: Effects of graded solute diureses on renal tubular sodium transport in the rat. Am J Physiol 228:1262, 1975.

30. Gottschalk CW: Renal tubular function: lessons from micropuncture. Harvey Lect 58:99, 1962.

31. Maude DL: Kidney Physiology and Kidney Disease. Philadelphia, Lippincott, 1977, pp 60–62.

32. Muldowney FP: Renal acidosis. In Black D, Jones NF (eds): Renal Disease, 4th ed. Oxford, Blackwell, 1979, p 596.

33. Kass EH: Asymptomatic infections of the urinary tract. Trans Assoc Am Physician's 69:56, 1956.

34. Kass EH: Bacteriuria and pyelonephritis of pregnancy. Arch Intern Med 105:194, 1960.

35. Asscher AW, Chick S, Radford N, et al.: Natural history of asymptomatic bacteriuria (ASB) in non-pregnant women. In Brumfitt, W, Asscher AW (eds): Urinary Tract Infection. London, Oxford University Press, 1973, pp 51–61.

36. Fisher JW, Busuttil R, Rodgers GM et al.: The kidney and erythropoietin production: A review. In Nakao K, Fischer JW, Takaku F (eds): Erythropoiesis. Tokyo, University of Tokyo Press, 1975, p 315.

37. Naets JP: Hematologic disorders in renal failure. Nephron 14:181, 1975.

38. Hollenberg NK: The physiology of the renal circulation. In Black D, Jones NF (eds): Renal Disease, 4th ed. Oxford, Blackwell, 1979, p 52.

39. Boyle IT, Gray RW, De Luca HF: Regulation by calcium of in vivo synthesis of 1,25-dihydroxycalciferol and 24,25-dihydroxycholecalciferol. Proc Natl Acad Sci USA 68:2131, 1971.

40. Fraser DR, Kodicek E: Regulation of 25-hydroxycholecalciferol-1, α-hydroxylase activity in kidney by parathyroid hormone. Nature New Biol 241:163, 1973.

41. Granger P, Dahlheim H, Thurau K: Enzyme activities of the single juxtaglomerular apparatus in the rat kidney. Kidney Int 1:78, 1972.

42. Moore EW: Ionized calcium in normal serum, ultrafiltrates, and whole blood determined by ion-exchange electrodes. J Clin Invest 49:318, 1970.

43. Reiss E, Canterbury JM, Bercovit MA, Kaplan EL: The role of phosphate in the secretion of parathyroid hormone in man. J Clin Invest 49:2146, 1970.

44. Edelman IS, Fimongari GM: On the biochemical mechanism of action of aldosterone. Recent Prog Horm Res 24:1, 1968.

45. Van Pilsun J: Excretion products in urine and man. In Altman PL, Dittmer DS (eds): Biology Data Book, 2nd ed. Bethesda, Md, Federation of American Society for Experimental Biology, 1974, pp 1496–1511.

Kathleen Becan-McBride

CHAPTER 3

Tests to Evaluate Renal Function

Objectives

It is expected that the information presented in this chapter will enable the reader to:

1. Define clearance as it is used in renal glomerular filtration rate.
2. Identify criteria for substances to be used to quantify renal glomerular filtration rate.
3. Calculate a creatinine clearance.
4. Relate glomerular clearance to the plasma concentration of metabolic waste products and other urinary solutes.
5. Identify variables that affect the glomerular filtration rate and relate these variables to disease states.
6. List the functions of the renal tubules.
7. Describe and compare the tests employed in the laboratory investigation of the renal tubule.

Maintenance and distribution of water, electrolytes, calcium, phosphate, and acid-base equilibrium are essential for the survival and well-being of man. The homeostatic function is performed primarily by the kidneys. In adapting to the task of maintaining a near constant internal environment, the kidney has evolved a series of physiologic mechanisms to excrete or conserve water and solutes, as discussed in Chapter 2.

This chapter considers various renal function tests and their importance in determining if the kidneys are diseased and if the disease is progressive.

GLOMERULAR FILTRATION RATE

Glomerular filtration rate (GFR) is a valuable clinical parameter for the assessment of renal function. In most renal diseases, the GFR can provide a rather accurate measurement of the degree of renal damage. In addition, most of the methods utilized to evaluate glomerular filtration are fairly simple, safe, and reliable. In order to understand clearly the meaning of GFR, the nature of normal glomerular filtration will be reviewed.

The initial event in the process of urine formation is the separation of a protein-free filtrate of plasma by the glomerular capillary walls. As shown in Figure 3.1, the glomerulus is a network of blood capillaries covered by epithelial cells and encased in Bowman's capsule. Pressure of the plasma in the glomerulus causes fluid to filter into Bowman's

capsule, from which it flows first into the proximal tubule. From the proximal tubule, the fluid passes into the renal tubule and finally flows into the collecting tubule, which collects fluid from several nephrons.

The basic function of the nephron is to clear the blood plasma of unwanted substances as it passes through the kidney. The substances that must be cleared include end-product metabolites, such as creatinine, urea, uric acid, and urates, and sodium ions, potassium ions, chloride ions, and hydrogen ions that have accumulated in the body in excessive amounts.

The nephron clears the plasma of unwanted substances by filtering the plasma through the glomerular membrane into the tubules of the nephron, and as this filtrate passes through the tubules, the unwanted end-product metabolites are not reabsorbed, but the wanted substances (i.e., sodium ions, water) are reabsorbed back into the plasma. Thus, the wanted substances are returned to the blood while the waste products are passed into the urine. A second mechanism by which the nephron clears the plasma of unwanted substances is by secretion. Substances are secreted from the plasma into the tubular fluid. Thus, the urine that is formed is composed of filtered substances and secreted substances.

The ability of the glomeruli to filter soluble constituents from the blood can be measured by clearance tests. These tests are based upon the rate at which kidneys remove a substance from the plasma. The rate of fluid filtration is determined by the following factors:

1. The balance of hydrostatic and oncotic pressures acting across the capillary wall—Bowman's space oncotic and glomerular capillary hydrostatic pressures favor filtration, whereas Bowman's space hydrostatic and glomerular capillary oncotic pressures retard filtration,[1]
2. The total surface area and permeability characteristics unique to the walls of the glomerular capillaries, and
3. The plasma flow rate entering the glomerulus.

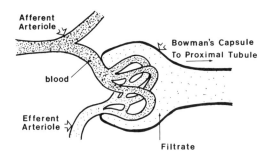

Figure 3.1. Glomerular filtration.

Examples of causes for a decreased GFR include:

1. Hypotensive shock in which the glomerular hydrostatic pressure is reduced.
2. Multiple myeloma in which the plasma oncotic pressure rises to abnormally elevated levels.
3. Obstruction of the ureters by calculi, inflammation, or neoplasm causing increased Bowman's space hydrostatic pressure,
4. Progressive renal disease, which reduces the glomerular capillary permeability and/or total surface area for filtration as glomeruli are damaged, and
5. Cardiac failure, which decreases the plasma flow rate entering the glomerulus.

The rate at which the glomerular filtrate is formed can be quantified by determining clearance of any substance that has the following ideal characteristics:

1. It is freely filtrable (molecular weight is less than 10,000),
2. It is not bound to protein,
3. It is not secreted by the tubule, and
4. It is not reabsorbed in passage through the tubule.

The concept of clearance is based on the premise that the rate of removal (filtration) from the plasma of a substance having the above four properties will be equal to the simultaneous rate of excretion of that substance into the urine. Wherever this is the case, the clearance of a substance remains relatively constant even though its blood plasma concentration and rate of excretion may vary considerably. The units of clearance are volume/time, usually expressed as volume (ml) of blood plasma from which a certain mass of substances (mg) is removed in a unit of time (min) and excreted in the urine, for:

$$C = \frac{UV}{P}$$

where

C = clearance of the substance being studied in ml cleared/min,

U = urine concentration of the substance in mg/dl,

V = urine excreted in ml/min, and

P = plasma concentration of the substance in mg/dl.

INULIN CLEARANCE

Inulin, a fructose polysaccharide (average molecular weight 3,000 to 4,000), is one of several substances used in the measurement of GFR.[2] This inert and nonmetabolizable substance can be recovered quantitatively in the urine following parenteral administration. The measurement of inulin clearance is an accurate and reproducible method of estimating GFR. However, in order to perform inulin clearance measurements, crystalline inulin must be dissolved, and about two hours of infusion is required before a stable plasma level is achieved. Accurate measurement of the urinary excretion rate usually requires bladder catheterization or several blood samples and timed urine collections. Because of the difficulties in clinical laboratory analysis, inulin clearance is mainly a research tool and has been replaced in clinical practice by other substances that are nearly as good indicators of glomerular filtration and are easier to measure.

CREATININE CLEARANCE

The measurement of creatinine clearance is the most popular test for estimating GFR. Several features of creatinine metabolism make it a useful indicator for monitoring GFR. Creatinine is eliminated from the plasma predominantly by glomerular filtration, and this measurement of its rate is relatively accurate and useful. The blood level of creatinine, formed from muscle creatine and phosphocreatine, depends on skeletal muscle mass and is relatively constant in any individual from day to day. For these reasons, measurement of creatinine clearance requires only a timed urine collection and blood sample. No parenteral administration is required in this procedure.

A drawback of the creatinine clearance procedure is that the renal tubules secrete a small amount of creatinine, and the creatinine clearance measurement, therefore, is slightly higher than the true GFR. However, this drawback is partially compensated by the error of the Jaffé alkaline picrate reaction that is used to measure the creatinine present in the blood and urine. Chromogens other than creatinine that are measured in the Jaffé reaction occur in the plasma but not in the urine, and this results in an offsetting underestimation of the creatinine clearance.

Procedure for Creatinine Clearance Test

In order for a creatinine clearance test to be run, the nursing staff must prepare the patient in the following manner:

1. Hydrate the patient by administering at least 600 ml of water. Withhold tea, coffee, and medications the rest of the day;
2. Have the patient void and discard the specimen;
3. Collect a 4-, 12-, or 24-hour specimen and record the exact times of starting and completing the collection;
4. Record the height and weight of the patient for the body surface area collection.

The laboratory procedure for the creatinine clearance test involves the following steps:

1. Collect a specimen of oxalated or clotted blood during the urine collection period. Since creatinine values are relatively constant, the blood specimens can be collected at any time during the urine collection;
2. Measure the volume of the 4-, 12-, or 24-hour urine specimen;

3. Determine the creatinine concentration in the serum or plasma and an aliquot of the well-mixed urine specimen; and
4. Calculate the rate of urine flow in milliliters/min as follows: total volume of urine in milliliters by the number of minutes in the collecting time.

As shown in Figure 3.2, the clearance in milliliters of plasma cleared of creatinine per minute can be calculated by:

$$C = \frac{UV}{P} \times \frac{1.73}{A}$$

where
    C = endogenous creatinine clearance corrected to average body surface area,
    U = mmole creatinine/L urine,
    V = ml urine excreted/min,
    P = mmole creatinine/L serum,
    A = body surface area in sq m, and
    1.73 = average body surface area in sq m.

Normalization of Clearance Data

As expected, creatinine clearance is not the same in a child as in an adult, and clearance data must be normalized to body surface area in order to derive a relatively constant range for the measured population. The standard 70-kg man has a body surface area of 1.73 sq m, and it has become customary to normalize creatinine clearance in this area (Fig. 3.3). In order to correct for size, the volume in milliliters excreted per minute must be

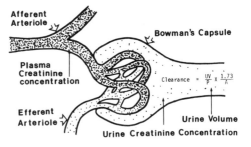

Figure 3.2. Calculation of creatinine clearance.

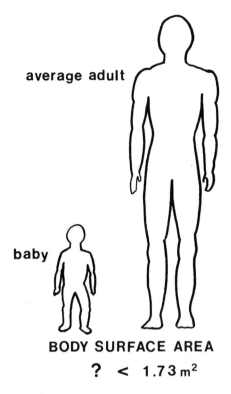

average adult

baby

BODY SURFACE AREA

? < 1.73 m²

Figure 3.3. Size correction factor.

multiplied by a size correction factor. The factor may be derived by calculating the patient's surface area according to the following formula:

$$\log A = (0.425 \log W) + (0.725 \log H) - 2.144$$

where
    A = body surface area in sq m
    W = weight of patient in kg
    H = height of patient in cm

Another approach to obtaining the patient's surface area is to use a nomogram, as illustrated in Figure 3.4. After obtaining the patient's height and weight, place a ruler on the surface area nomogram of Dubois at the height and weight of the patient and read the surface area from the middle column. For example:

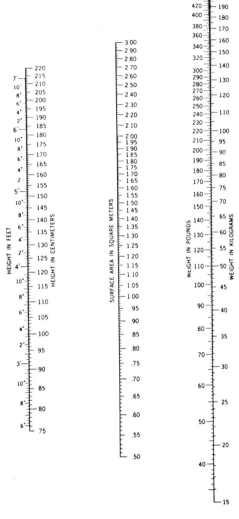

Figure 3.4. Surface area nomogram (Dubois). (From Boothby W, Sandiford RB: N Engl J Med 185:337, 1921. Reprinted by permission.)

1. The patient is 4 feet 4 inches tall and weighs 69 pounds. By placing a ruler at these points, a surface area of 1.06 sq m is noted.
2. To obtain the size correction factor, divide 1.73 sq m, the standard surface area, by the derived surface area, 1.06 sq m.

$$\text{Size correction factor} = \frac{1.73}{1.06} = 1.63$$

3. Multiply the size correction factor by the milliliters of urine excreted per minute. Normal values are as follows:

Adult male: 105 ± 20 ml/min (milliliters of blood cleared of creatinine per minute)

Adult female: 95 ± 20 ml/min (ml of blood cleared of creatinine per minute)

Children have about the same normally expected creatinine clearance value. For example, in one study, children of ages 3 to 13 years had mean creatinine clearances of 113 to 118 ml/min.[3] Creatinine clearance values decrease with age after adulthood. Patients over 60 years of age had mean creatinine clearances of 72 and 63 ml/min for males and females, respectively.[4]

Sources of Error in Creatinine Clearance Tests

To avoid erroneous results in the creatinine clearance test, the patient should not exercise vigorously before or during the test, since this increased exertion may cause changes in the clearance rate. If the patient does not drink enough water to ensure a urine flow of 2 ml/min or more, the creatinine clearance results will not reflect the correct filtration rate for the patient.

The most common sources of error in clearance tests are incorrect timing and improper collection of the urine specimen.

UREA CLEARANCE

Urea, the most abundant end product of protein metabolism, is distributed throughout the intracellular and extracellular body fluids in equal concentrations. The process of urea synthesis occurs almost exclusively in the liver. Most of it is excreted from the body by the kidneys.

Although urea is cleared by the glomeruli, it is partially absorbed by the tubules (Fig. 3.5)

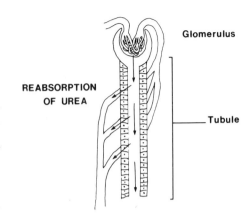

Figure 3.5. Urea excretion.

at an average rate of 40 to 50 percent of that filtered. The rate of reabsorption, which is a process of passive diffusion, varies with the amount of water reabsorbed. Thus, the urea clearance test is not a measure of the glomerular filtration rate (although it has been used for this purpose) but is an index of overall renal function. For the measurement of glomerular filtration, it has been replaced by the more accurate creatinine clearance test.

OTHER METHODS TO ASSESS GLOMERULAR FILTRATION RATE

In recent years, there has been extensive research in developing methods for measuring GFR that are as accurate as the inulin clearance test but simpler to carry out. Substances with clearance rates approximately that of inulin that can be labeled with radioisotopes have been used in estimating GFR. Chromium-51 EDTA has been widely studied, but research has shown that it significantly underestimates GFR.[5,6] Other substances, such as sodium diatrizoate, sodium iothalamate, stannous DPTA, and vitamin B_{12}, have been labeled with radioisotopes and utilized in clearance measurements. Even though most of these recently developed methods provide reasonably accurate measurements of GFR, their utility has not been expanded to most clinical laboratories. The drawbacks of using these radioisotope-labeled substances for clearance tests include:

1. They must be administered intravenously or subcutaneously, and
2. They are expensive.

Thus, the most popular test has been the endogenous creatinine clearance test.

TUBULAR FUNCTION

Without the reabsorptive activity of the tubules, the high rate of filtration by the glomeruli would rapidly eliminate all water and water-soluble constituents from the body. By reabsorption and secretion, the tubules maintain the volume, osmolality, and electrolytes of body fluids within normal limits. While they act to conserve water and essential solutes in a manner dependent on the dietary intake and storage requirements, they excrete waste products and other substances not needed by the body.

MEASUREMENT OF PLASMA FLOW AND BLOOD FLOW THROUGH THE KIDNEYS

The total renal blood flow is that volume which enters the renal arteries each minute (approximately 1,200 ml). The effective renal flow, or renal plasma flow, is that amount which perfuses the functional renal tissue each minute. Decrease in effective renal blood flow can result from:

1. Decrease in cardiac output or arterial blood pressure (e.g., coronary occlusion, congestive heart failure, shock),
2. Organic disease of the renal vascular system (e.g., renal arteriosclerosis, glomerulosclerosis, glomerulonephritis, periarteritis nodosa),
3. Increased local resistance to blood flow (e.g., vasoconstriction, early hypertension), and
4. Decrease in mass of functioning kidney

tissue (e.g., polycystic disease, malignancy, tuberculosis).

Measurement of the effective renal plasma flow can be obtained through the utilization of para-aminohippurate (PAH) if tubular function is normal.

PAH

Para-aminohippurate (PAH), like inulin, is filtered through the glomerulus. However, it is different from inulin in that in addition to being filtered through the glomerular membrane, it is also removed by the kidney via tubular secretion (Fig. 3.6). Approximately 10 percent of the original PAH remains in the plasma after a single passage through the kidney. Thus, the rate of PAH excretion is equal to the plasma concentration multiplied by the renal plasma flow. PAH clearance can be a good indicator of renal plasma flow as long as the plasma concentration does not exceed the capacity of tubular secretion.

In order to obtain PAH clearance and renal plasma flow values, PAH must be infused into the blood in the same manner as inulin. At the present time, PAH is used mainly in investigative procedures and not in routine clinical ones.

TUBULAR SECRETORY FUNCTION TEST

Phenolsulfonphthalein (PSP) shares a common secretory mechanism with PAH. To measure renal tubular secretion, PSP (also called "phenol red") is injected intravenously in a single dose. Provided tubular saturation is not exceeded, 60 to 70 percent of this dye is extracted from the plasma during one passage of blood through the kidneys. Of the total quantity removed by the kidneys, 94 percent is removed by tubular excretion and 6 percent by glomerular filtration.

Under optimal conditions, 25 to 50 percent of the injected dye is secreted in the first 15 minutes, and an additional 15 to 25 percent is secreted in the next 15 minutes. The critical measurement is the 15-minute dye excretion.

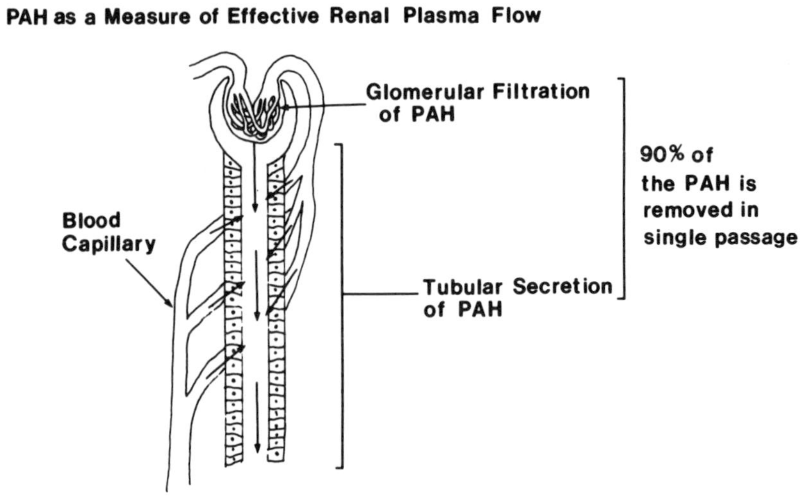

PAH as a Measure of Effective Renal Plasma Flow

Figure 3.6. PAH as a measure of effective renal plasma flow.

After alkalizing the urine, the dye is measured spectrophotometrically at 540 nm. If the dye excretion during the first 15 minutes is 25 percent or less, kidney function is most likely impaired. The PSP excretion is usually decreased in chronic glomerulonephritis, chronic pyelonephritis, congenital polycystic kidney disease, nephrosis, and advanced essential hypertension.

The PSP test can be used to test separately the function of each kidney if the 15-minute specimens are collected by means of ureteral catheters. However, in terms of total renal function, the PSP test results give about the same clinical information as the creatinine clearance test, since glomerular and tubular dysfunction usually occur together in acute and chronic kidney damage. The creatinine clearance seems to be replacing the PSP test in renal function testing.

CONCENTRATING ABILITY OF THE KIDNEYS

Regulation of the concentration of urine is one of the principal functions of the renal tubules and is often diminished in renal disease. The formation of hypertonic urine by the distal tubule and collecting tubule is fun-

damental to the concentrating mechanism. In such diseases as pyelonephritis and glomerulonephritis, the concentrating mechanism decreases prior to the retention of nitrogenous waste products. Measurements of the kidneys' concentrating ability are carried out by determining the osmolality, the specific gravity, or the refractive index of the urine.

Specific Gravity

As discussed in Chapter 5 on the Routine Examination of Urine, the specific gravity is the ratio of the weight of a solution compared with the weight of an equal volume of water. Urine specific gravity has a wide range of 1.003 to 1.035, reflecting either a dilution or concentration ability of the kidneys.

Osmolality Measurements

A more sensitive indication of the dilution and concentration ability of the kidneys can be obtained through osmolality measurements. As discussed in Chapter 5, osmolality is a measure of the number of dissolved solute particles in a solution and is generally determined by means of freezing point depression of dewpoint analysis. Urinary specific gravity and urine osmolality measurements usually correlate with one another in patients having normally functioning kidneys. However, in patients with diabetes mellitus or other diseases that lead to the excretion of increased numbers of high molecular weight substances in the urine (e.g., proteins), the urine specific gravity usually has no correlation with urinary osmolality. The major cause for the noncorrelation is that osmolality depends only on the number of dissolved particles in solution and not on their size or shape as do specific gravity determinations. The reference values for urine osmolality normally range between 300 and 900 mOsm/kg water in conditions of dehydration and between 40 and 80 mOsm/kg water during water diuresis. Usually, the first morning urine specimen will have an osmolality greater than 800 mOsm/kg water.

Pitressin Test

Another measurement of the kidneys' concentrating ability can be obtained through the Pitressin test. This test involves 12 to 14 hours of dehydration and the subcutaneous administration of Pitressin (vasopressin), followed by four 1-hour urine collections. The highest value obtained from these urine specimens is the maximal osmolality.[7] The results should be corrected for age since urinary concentrating ability decreases with age. Thus, a young adult will usually have a normal value of over 800 mOsm/kg water, whereas an adult older than 50 will have a normal value of approximately 600 mOsm/kg water.

The values obtained in the Pitressin test should be compared to other renal function test results in order to evaluate the renal dysfunction process. In diseases affecting the glomerulus more so than the tubules (e.g., glomerulonephritis), the GFR is decreased more than is the concentrating ability. In diseases primarily affecting the tubules (e.g., pyelonephritis), the concentrating ability is decreased to a greater extent than is the GFR.

Ratio of Urine Osmolality to Serum Osmolality

Serum osmolality has a much narrower range than does urine osmolality, 285 to 290 mOsm/kg water. Normally, the ratio of urine osmolality to serum osmolality:

$$\frac{U_{osm}}{S_{osm}}$$

is between 1.0 and 3.0. In diabetes insipidus, severe pyelonephritis, and water intoxication, the ratio is usually equal to or less than 1.0. In acute glomerulonephritis and congestive heart failure, the ratio is generally greater than 1.2.[3] After fluid restriction, the ratio may rise above 3.0.

Free Water Clearance

Free water clearance may be defined as the amount of distilled water that must be increased or decreased in urine formation so that the urine is isosthenuric (i.e., urine osmolality is equal to plasma osmolality). This clearance (C_{H_2O}) value can be expressed in the following equation:

$$C_{H_2O} = V - C_{osm},$$

where

V = total urine volume and
C_{osm} = the osmolal clearance, or:

$$\frac{U_{osm} \times V}{P_{osm}}$$

When urine is formed that is more dilute than plasma (i.e., hyposthenuria), the free water clearance value is positive. Alternatively, when urine is formed that is more concentrated than plasma (i.e., hyperosthenuria), the clearance has a negative value. For example, a hyperosmotic urine of 940 mOsm/kg water is formed, the urine flow is 0.4 ml/min, and the plasma osmolality is 300 mOsm/kg water. Therefore:

$$C_{H_2O} = \frac{0.4 \text{ ml}}{\text{min}}$$

$$- \left(\frac{940 \text{mOsm}}{\text{kg}} \times \frac{0.4 \text{ ml}}{\text{min}} \times \frac{\text{kg}}{300 \text{ mOsm}} \right)$$

$$C_{H_2O} = -0.85 \text{ ml/min}$$

PROTEINURIA

Urine protein is usually an important indicator of renal dysfunction. Minute amounts of protein are present in normal urine, and the term proteinuria is reserved for values in excess of normal. Protein excretion is abnormal when the value exceeds 150 mg per 24 hours. The methods for detecting urine protein concentration are discussed in Chapter 5.

Normal urine contains approximately 30 proteins, the most prominent among these being the high molecular weight mucoprotein, the Tamm-Horsfall protein. It is formed in the cells of the loop of Henle's distal convoluted and collecting tubules and is the major protein constituent of renal casts. In addition to this large protein, other proteins are produced in the lower urinary tract and from seminal and prostatic secretions.

The filtrate from the glomeruli contains no plasma proteins above the molecular weight of albumin. Proteins that filter through the glomerular membrane, such as β_2-microglobulin and light chains, have low molecular weights and are largely reabsorbed in the tubules. Normally, they are found in only trace amounts in the urine.

Four possible mechanisms that cause abnormal quantities of protein to enter the urine are:

1. A defect in the membrane of the glomerular capillary increases filtration of high molecular weight proteins (e.g., diabetes, glomerulonephritis, pregnancy, and nephrosis);
2. Protein is secreted into the tubules (i.e., pyelonephritis, ureteral obstruction);
3. Abnormally elevated plasma levels of low molecular weight proteins surpass the threshold level and thus filter across the glomerular capillary membrane (e.g., multiple myeloma), and
4. Tubular reabsorption of the low molecular weight proteins that are normally filtered by the glomerulus (e.g., renal tubular acidosis, acute renal insufficiency) is decreased.

It can be seen that the quantitation of urine protein can aid in the diagnosis of renal diseases. The extent of proteinuria can best be quantified by measuring the protein from a 24-hour specimen. Overall, urine protein measurements can be used with other renal function tests to assess renal disease processes. A discussion of the tests used for defining the types of proteinuria and their use in the diagnosis and treatment of renal disease is given in Chapter 8.

Review Questions

One or more responses may be correct.

1. Given the following what is the creatinine clearance for this patient?

   Characteristic and results
   Blood creatinine: 371.3 μmole/L (4.2 mg/dl)
   24-hour urine volume: 840 ml
   Urine creatinine: 2828.8 μmole/L (32 mg/dl)
   Height: 132 cm
   Weight: 31.4 kg

   A. 2.7 ml/min
   B. 7.2 ml/min
   C. 27 ml/min
   D. 72 ml/min
   E. 111 ml/min

2. The glomerular filtration rate can be quantified by determining the clearance of any substance that is:
   A. Freely filtrable (MW <10,000)
   B. Not bound to protein
   C. Not secreted by the tubules
   D. Not reabsorbed in passage through the tubules

3. Which of the following statements is (are) correct concerning urea? It is:
   A. Partially reabsorbed by the tubules
   B. The most abundant end product of purine metabolism
   C. Formed in skeletal muscle mass
   D. An accurate measure of tubular function

4. The hormone that controls the volume and concentration of urine is:
   A. ACTH
   B. ADH
   C. TSH
   D. GH

5. The renal plasma flow may be estimated by using which of the following procedures?
   A. Pitressin test
   B. Para-aminohippurate excretion
   C. Free water clearance
   D. ^{51}Cr-EDTA clearance
6. The phenosulfonphthalein (PSP) test is utilized as a measure of:
   A. Liver blood flow
   B. Urine flow
   C. GFR
   D. Free water clearance
   E. Renal tubular secretion
7. The ratio of urine osmolality to serum osmolality $U_{osm}:S_{osm}$ is normally from:
   A. 0.5 to 4.0
   B. 1.0 to 3.0
   C. 2.5 to 5.5
   D. 4.0 to 8.0
8. When urine is formed that is more dilute than plasma, this can be referred to as:
   A. Hyperosthenuria
   B. Isosthenuria
   C. Hyposthenuria
(See Appendix for answers.)

Case Study

A 58-year-old woman was admitted to the hospital with complaints of polyuria and nocturia. Her past medical history revealed numerous urinary tract infections. Over the past year, she had consistently had specific gravity readings below 1.010 for all of her urine specimens collected after water restriction. The following laboratory studies were performed: plasma urea nitrogen 27 mmole/L (78 mg/dl), plasma creatinine 265 μmole/L (3 mg/dl), urine specific gravity 1.007, one to two white blood cell casts per low power field in the microscopic examination of the urinary sediment, inulin clearance 28 ml/min (average normal value is 115 ml/min in women), and urine volume 2860 ml/dl.

Questions
1. What might be a possible cause of this condition?
2. Why is the urine volume so high with such a low inulin clearance?

Answers
1. The most probable cause for this condition is chronic pyelonephritis. This disease process begins by invading the renal medulla and eventually destroys tubular function. This involves a decrease in the effectiveness of the medullary countercurrent concentrating mechanism, resulting in decreased concentration of solute.
2. The low inulin clearance is a result of the inadequate number of functional nephrons in this woman. The urine volume is elevated, since the tubular damage prevents the efficient reabsorptive characteristics of the kidneys.

BIBLIOGRAPHY

Beeson P, McDermott W, Wyngaarden J: Cecil Textbook of Medicine. Philadelphia, Saunders, 1979, pp 1336–1340.
Black D, Jones N: Renal Diseases. London, Blackwell, 1979.
Brenner B, Rector F (eds): The Kidney. Philadelphia, Saunders, 1976.
Greenhill A, Gruskin A: Laboratory evaluation of renal function. Pediatr Clin North Am 23:661, 1976.
Guyton A: Textbook of Medical Physiology. Philadelphia, Saunders, 1976, pp 438–455.
Henry J (ed): Clinical Diagnosis and Management by Laboratory Methods. Philadelphia, Saunders, 1979, pp 138–143.
Pitts R: Physiology of the Kidney and Body Fluids. Chicago, Year Book, 1974.
Tietz N (ed): Fundamentals of Clinical Chemistry. Philadelphia, Saunders, 1976, pp. 975–1013.
Wilson D: Urinalysis and other tests of renal function. Minn Med 58:9, 1975.

REFERENCES

1. Deen W, Troy J, Robertson C, Brenner B: Dynamics of glomerular ultrafiltration in the rat. IV. Determination of the ultrafiltration coefficient. J Clin Invest 52:1500, 1973.

2. Maude D: Kidney Physiology and Kidney Diseases. Philadelphia, Lippincott, 1977.
3. Barratt TM, Chantler C: Clinical assessment of renal function. In Rubin MI, Barratt TM (eds): Pediatric Nephrology. Baltimore, Williams & Wilkins, 1975, pp 55–83.
4. Kampmann J, Siersback-Nielsen K, Kristensen M, Hansen JM: Rapid evaluation of creatinine clearance. Acta Med Scand 196:517, 1974.
5. Heath D, Knapp M, Walker W: Comparison between inulin and Cr-labelled edetic acid for the measurement of glomerular filtration rate. Lancet 2:1110, 1968.
6. Stamp T, Stacey T, Rose G: Comparison of glomerular filtration rate measurements using inulin, ^{51}Cr-EDTA, and a phosphate infusion technique. Clin Chim Acta 30:351, 1970.
7. Maxwell M, Kleeman C: Clinical Disorders of Fluid and Electrolyte Metabolism. New York, McGraw-Hill, 1962, p 148.

Diana Garza

	CHAPTER 4

Urine Collection and Preservation

Objectives

It is expected that the information presented in this chapter will enable the reader to:

1. Identify factors affecting the quality of a specimen.
2. Determine the importance of a properly collected urine specimen.
3. Describe the method of urine collection most suitable for most types of laboratory analysis.
4. Describe the proper procedure for collecting random, midstream, clean-catch, and 24-hour urine specimens.
5. Identify commonly used preservatives and know advantages and disadvantages of their use.
6. List the basic rules for urine collection.

Urine has been used for centuries in various ways. It has been used in some countries for fertilizer because of its nitrogen and mineral content. At one period in history, urine was used to diagnose diabetes. It was collected, poured over sand, and observed. Insects were attracted to sand that had been exposed to urine from diabetic patients. Aside from this simplistic but effective analysis, urine has been collected and analyzed by a variety of methods. Uroscopists often used clear round-bottom flasks for visual examination. It is known that collection cups came in numerous sizes and shapes and occasionally were made of silver or gold.[1] The fact remains that urine collection and evaluation have been and will remain essential to health care.

Urine collection is relatively easy and convenient. Normal adults void approximately a liter of urine per day, theoretically allowing for a convenient and ample specimen for almost any type of constituent analysis. It must be remembered, however, that different types of specimens are suitable for certain tests. Some analyses involve timed periods for specimen collection, some specimens are collected at particular hours of the day, and some tests are based on specific methods of collection.[1]

A laboratory analysis is only as good as the specimen used, and, in turn, a specimen is only as good as the container used for collection. It is necessary at all times to monitor the quality of specimens in order to assure excellence in any laboratory system. Unlike most specimens for laboratory analysis, urine collection is not directly supervised by laboratory personnel. Several people may be involved in the collection procedure, i.e., a nurse or aide, possibly a ward clerk, and often a human or mechanical transportation system. The quality of the specimen may be affected by these people as well as by time factors, the type and integrity of the container, and the manner in which it was collected. When it is properly collected, however, a urine sample can provide a wealth of useful information.

CONTAINERS

The ideal container for any urine specimen is a sterile or chemically clean wide-mouthed bottle of appropriate size. The container must be sterile if the specimen is to be submitted for culture. Many commercial containers are available on the market today. Most hospitals prefer the clear disposable plastic type of 6- to 10-ounce capacity, with a tight-fitting lid and an attached label.

Collection containers should be chemically clean without residues of previous contents, sanitizing agents, and benzylkonium or other quaternary ammonium compounds used for cleaning, since these may cause misleading reactions. Specifically, cleaning compounds can cause false positive reactions with colorimetric procedures for proteins, or they may inhibit the growth of microorganisms to be cultured.[1]

It is generally preferred that a container be clear so as to make visual determination of urine color easier. This also allows for easy detection of yellow foam after shaking, which is indicative of bilirubin in the urine. Bilirubin, urobilinogen, and porphyrins are light sensitive, and when being quantitatively analyzed, specimens should be protected from light. Use of an amber bottle or covered container will minimize the breakdown of these substances.

The ideal container may not be what the patient likes or uses, however. Specimens have been known to arrive at the hospital or clinic in such containers as perfume bottles, soda bottles, paint buckets, liquor or wine bottles, mayonnaise or jelly jars, bleach containers, and hand cream jars, just to name a few.

TYPES OF SPECIMENS

Generally, the most frequently used urine specimen is the spot or random test. Specimens of this nature vary considerably in concentration of constituents even though they provide a vast amount of information. Some methods of collection avoid this variability in concentration simply by collection during a specified time. This may be a 24-hour specimen or a known period of time when the particular substance to be measured is in high concentration. Normal variations, which are often rythmic, may be due to such factors as water consumption, diet, or circadian, diurnal, or 24-hour excretion periods.[1] Table 4.1 gives examples of several urine components with defined periods of maximum excretion. Table 4.2 lists types of specimens and their uses.

Random or Spot Specimens

Random specimens are the most common and convenient type used because they are voided at any time. The method simply involves collecting a portion of the urine in a clean container. No prior preparation of the patient is necessary. These specimens are satisfactory for routine urinalysis. However, due to the variations in water intake, diet, and the time of collection, results must be interpreted with these factors in mind.

First Morning Voiding

Urine that is voided in the early morning is best for routine examinations. Assuming that the patient did not void during the night and that this is the first morning voiding, as the name states, it is the most concentrated type of specimen. First morning specimens are more apt to contain pus and mucus in the presence of infection. In addition, they are most likely to have an acid pH, show dysfunction of the kidneys' concentrating ability, and are generally more uniform. First morning urine should be examined within one hour after voiding. If circumstances do not allow this, specimens with a specific gravity below 1.010 should be recollected if possible, especially if the urine is alkaline. Alkalinity and hypoosmolality promote deterioration of casts and red blood cells.[2] First morning specimens are less likely to indicate threshold sub-

TABLE 4.1. VARIATIONS IN URINARY EXCRETION

Urine Constituent	Low Excretion Period	High Excretion Period
Potassium	4-6 AM 23 mmole/min	10 AM-noon 99 mmole/min
Sodium	4-6 AM 85 mmole/min	10 AM-noon 237 mmole/min
Chloride	4-6 AM 91 mmole/min	Noon-2 PM 299 mmole/min
17-Hydroxycortico- steroids	2-6 AM 6.5 mmole/min	10 AM-noon 12.3 mmole/min
Water	8-10 PM 0.45 ml/min	10 AM-noon and 4-6 PM 1.32 ml/min
Catecholamine	Morning 8.6 mg/100 ml	Afternoon 11.9 mg/100 ml
Urobilinogen	Unspecified	2-4 PM Maximum

Adapted from Free AH, Free HM: Urinalysis in Clinical Laboratory Practice, 1975, p 23. Copyright The Chemical Rubber Co, CRC Press, Inc.

TABLE 4.2. SPECIMENS AND THEIR USES

Specimen	Analysis	Reason for Use
First morning	Protein	Most concentrated
	Microscopic	Good recovery of cellular constituents and casts
	Bacteria nitrite	Increase time needed for bacteria to metabolize nitrate
Random or spot	Routine urine analysis	Ease and convenience
2-4 PM	Urobilinogen	Better differentiation of normal and abnormal results
12-hour	Addis count	Pattern of formed elements is seen better with long collections
24-hour	Quantitative metabolic determinations	Overcomes fluctuations in concentration
Clean-catch catherization, suprapubic	Culture	Avoids contamination
Fasting	Glucose	Suggests severe disturbances in carbohydrate metabolism
Postprandial	Glucose	Suggest moderate disturbances in carbohydrate metabolism

Adapted from Free AH, Free HM: Urinalysis in Clinical Laboratory Practice, 1975, p 22. Copyright The Chemical Rubber Co, CRC Press, Inc.

stances related to diet and metabolism, such as glucose and proteins.[3] Morning specimens collected in clinics or private offices are often from patients who have recently eaten, so that they are likely to contain proteins and reducing substances. The morning specimen is used for a variety of routine tests as well as for cultures. This specimen is especially useful for culturing acid-fast bacilli. With the exception of a catheterized specimen, a first morning urine specimen is superior to a 24-hour specimen for the culture of acid-fast bacilli because of the toxicity of urine to the organisms during a 24-hour period.

Two-hour Specimens
Because of concentration fluctuations, some specimens may be collected during known hours of maximum concentration. Watson and co-workers proposed a two-hour afternoon collection because it is known that urobilinogen excretion is at its maximum level in the midafternoon or evening.[4] This collection procedure involves instructing the patient to empty his/her bladder and discard the urine at approximately 2 PM. All urine from 2 to 4 PM is saved, with a final voiding at 4 PM. Hence, one has a two-hour specimen. It is mandatory that these specimens be collected and labeled properly. The time of collection should be among the items on the label.

Postprandial Specimens
Postprandial specimens are not commonly used. Occasionally they are requested for diabetic screening.[3] The procedure involves collection of a spot specimen at a given time after a meal.

Twenty-four-hour Specimens

The use of a 24-hour urine specimen reduces the variability caused by a fluctuation in the concentration of constituents to be tested (e.g., diurnal variations in hormones). In general, the results of an analysis are first expressed in units/time. The concentration of a substance can easily be tabulated by multiplying the units/time (mmole/24 hours) by the total volume collected in liters to give mmole/liter. Taking the analysis a step further, one can estimate the clearance of a particular substance by comparing the amount in urine per 24 hours with the concentration of that substance in the blood. It must be kept in mind that the accuracy of these results depends largely on proper specimen collection.[5]

The container for a 24-hour specimen should be of adequate size. A 1-gallon bottle is sufficient. Easy, concise instructions should be given to the patient by someone who fully understands the procedure. Written instructions are frequently given to the patient as a reminder of the verbal instruction. The collection process usually begins between 6 and 8 AM. The bladder must be emptied at this time and the urine discarded. It is most important to note the time and date on the container. In a hospital setting the ward clerk or nurse must be sure not to predate or pretime the container, since it is improbable that the patient will urinate at a specified time. All urine should be collected during the next 24-hour period. The patient should be reminded to void at the end of the collection period and include that specimen with the collected urine. Again, the time and date should be noted on the container. If the time exceeds 24 hours by a few minutes it is acceptable only if the exact time is indicated on the container. Indication of the exact timing period is of utmost importance to the validity of the results.

In addition to proper labeling, there are other precautions. The urine container should be refrigerated, and each specimen should be added to it throughout the 24-hour period. When using bed pans, patients should be instructed to urinate before having bowel movements. Fecal contamination will make the specimen unacceptable. Patients should also be warned of any preservatives in the container. Substances such as hydrochloric acid are very corrosive if accidentally spilled or if contact is made during collection. Hydrochloric acid is frequently used for 24-hour vanillylmandelic acid determinations.[2] Simple directions should be used for the patients, since, for example, many do not understand the term "void." They should be reminded to include all specimens during the 24-hour period. The most common errors in this procedure are loss of voided specimens, addition of the first voided specimen which should have been discarded, and insufficient amounts of preservative.[6]

Fasting Specimens

Fasting specimens are occasionally used in glucose studies. The patient is instructed to void four hours after eating and discard the urine. The next voided specimen should be collected and labeled as a "fasting specimen."[7] In most cases, fasting is considered to be a condition of no food or beverage except water for a period of 14 to 16 hours.

Midstream Specimens

Midstream specimens are commonly used for routine urinalysis. The patient is instructed as follows: after voiding approximately one half of the urine into the toilet, a portion is collected in a readily available container, and the rest is allowed to pass into the toilet.

Clean-catch Specimens

Clean-catch specimens may be used for microbial cultures as well as routine urinalysis. This procedure minimizes contamination by bacteria normally present in the genital and rectal areas. Women should clean the vulvar area with a mild antiseptic soap and water. Holding the labia apart and after allowing some urine to pass, the patient should void into a sterile bottle. A sterile, tight-fitting lid should be placed on the container, and it should be taken directly to the laboratory. Men should clean the meatus and surrounding part with soap and water and collect a midstream specimen.[7]

Catheterized Specimens

Catheterized specimens are obtained by inserting a flexible tubular instrument into the bladder through the urethra and withdrawing urine. These specimens are used for microbial culturing purposes. Because this procedure involves the risk of infecting the bladder, it is avoided when possible.

Infant Specimens

Catheterized specimens are common for urine from infants. However, if a child is too small for catheterization, a specimen may still be collected by first washing the area with an antiseptic or sterile saline and attaching with adhesive tape a sterile test tube or polyethylene urine collector over the penis or the urethral meatus. This type of specimen will not be sterile.[8] Suprapubic needle aspirations are used for sterile urine collections from infants and children.

Suprapubic Needle Aspiration

Suprapubic needle aspiration involves withdrawing bladder urine by needle aspiration. Using sterile technique, the needle is inserted just above the suprapubic arch. The procedure adds the risk of bladder infection. However, this method of collection, when used for bacterial culture, may be of value in determining more exactly the site of a urinary tract infection, especially in females where vaginal contamination presents a problem.

Three-glass Test

This type of specimen is used to localize pathologic sites in males. The patient voids sequentially into three bottles. The first specimen will detect abnormalities in the urethra, the second will reflect the bladder and upper urinary tract, and the third will have larger amounts of prostatic secretion.

Specimen for Cytologic Evaluation

Cytologic evaluation of urine for the identification of tumor cells requires a freshly collected specimen. Fresh specimens allow for easiest differentiation of normal and abnormal cells.[1] Various fixatives, such as alcohol

(50 to 70 percent), Esposti fixative, Mucolex, and Saccomanno's fixative (isopropyl or ethyl alcohol with 2 percent polyethylene glycol) preserve and/or minimize cellular degeneration.[9]

PRESERVATIVES

Ideally, urine should be analyzed immediately after voiding. This is highly unlikely and not very feasible in most facilities. Preservatives should only be used whenever it is not possible to obtain fresh specimens. If an analysis must be delayed more than one hour, some form of preservation is necessary. There is no single preserving compound acceptable for all tests. The selection of preservatives depends on the procedure to be performed on the specimen. Microbiologic or pregnancy tests do not require preservatives.[3] When they are necessary, preservatives are valuable to chemical analysis, and, occasionally, to the microscopic analysis of urine.

Refrigeration

Refrigeration at about 4C is the most acceptable method of preservation, particularly when used along with chemical preservatives. Suprapubic aspirates may be refrigerated for six hours, whereas random specimens, especially those for bacteriologic and microscopic examinations, should be analyzed within three hours.[10]

Specimens may also be frozen, especially if they are to be transported, as is often the case when specimens are to be sent to a reference laboratory.

Toluene

Toluene works as a preservative by forming a layer over the surface of the specimen, thereby excluding exposure to air. It also inhibits bacterial growth. Toluene is not widely used because of its flammable nature and the difficulty one has pipetting through the layer to the specimen. When used, however, it preserves acetone, diacetic acid, reducing substances, and proteins.[2]

Thymol

Thymol is an adequate preservative, although not widely used. It may cause false positive results for protein with heat and acetic acid. However, it does not affect reagent strip chemical tests that are based on protein error of indicators.[2]

Chloroform

Chloroform is not recommended as a preservative, although it is used for determination of aldosterone levels.[11] It settles to the bottom of containers, interferes with microscopic examinations, and, if ingested, will cause liver damage.[2]

Formaldehyde

Formaldehyde is a 37 percent solution of formalin. It is excellent for preserving formed elements for microscopic analysis, although it cannot be used for preserving specimens to be used for evaluating glucose excretion.[2]

Acidification

Acids are excellent preservatives if they do not interfere with testing. The acid is added to the container prior to urine collection. Both hospitalized and ambulatory patients should be warned verbally and by container labels of the danger of acids and their fumes. The less concentrated forms of acid are recommended because of the consequence of adding aqueous urine to acid.

Acids are particularly useful in the determination of steroids, catecholamines, and vanillylmandelic acid, since these substances are only stable in acidic solutions. Approximately 10 ml of concentrated hydrochloric acid (HCl) or 25 ml of 6N HCl is added per 24-hour volume.[2] Before analysis in the laboratory, the urine should be tested for acidity (pH 3), and, hence, for proper preservation.

It should be mentioned that formed elements in the urine are readily destroyed in urine acidified by HCl. In addition, if there is an excess of acid, uric acid may precipitate out.[2]

Boric acid preserves chemical as well as formed elements, inhibits the growth of bacteria but not yeast, and may also precipitate uric acid. Approximately 5 mg should be added per 30 ml of urine.[2]

Sodium Carbonate

Sodium carbonate is useful for preserving porphyrins which require an alkaline solution for stability. About 4 to 5 g of sodium carbonate should be sufficient for 2 L of urine. It is preferable to use a brown bottle as a specimen container because of the destruction of porphyrins by light. Often it is recommended that about 100 ml of petroleum ether be added to the specimen. This forms a layer over the top, thereby preventing oxidation. These preserved specimens may also be used for urobilinogen determinations.[6]

Urinary Preservative Tablets

Urinary tablets are used by insurance companies for preserving specimens that must be transported. These tablets, originated by Francis Kingsbury, are excellent for routine analyses and for formed elements. They may not be used in determinations for sodium, potassium specific gravity, and hormone studies. The tablets are acidic and will buffer all but strongly alkaline urines. Each tablet will preserve about 56.7 ml (2 ounces) of urine. The primary constituents are potassium acid phosphate, sodium benzoate, benzoic acid methenamine, and sodium bicarbonate.[2]

Chlorhexidine

Recent evidence indicates that chlorhexidine gluconate (200 g/L solution) can be used to prevent bacterial growth and preserve urine for glucose determinations by the hexokinase method for six-week periods. The urine may be stored at 4C or 24C with no significant change in glucose values. Use of 50 ml per 10 ml of urine has been suggested.[12]

Table 4.3 shows the advantages and disadvantages of different methods of preservation.

TABLE 4.3. URINE PRESERVATIVES

Method	Advantage	Disadvantage
Refrigeration	For periods of time from 3-6 hours	For prolonged periods, additional preservatives must be used
Freezing	For specimen transport	May destroy formed elements
Toluene	Preserves acetone, diacetic acid, reducing substances, proteins	Flammable, difficult to separate from specimen
Thymol	Adequately preserves most constituents	Not widely used because it causes false positives for proteins with heat and acetic acid test
Chloroform	Preserves urine for aldosterone levels	Settles to bottom of containers
Formaldehyde	Preserves formed elements	Interferes with glucose evaluation
Acids HCl	Stabilizes steroids, catecholamines, and vanillylmandelic acid	Fumes and liquid are hazardous, formed elements are destroyed by HCl
Boric acid	Preserves chemical and formed elements	Uric acid may precipitate out with HCl or boric acid
Preservation tablet	Preserves urine for routine examinations and formed elements when transportation is necessary	Not method of choice, unsuitable for sodium, potassium, and hormone analysis
Chlorhexidine	Preserves urine for glucose determination by hexokinase method for up to 6 weeks	Useful only for glucose preservation
Sodium carbonate	Preserves porphyrins and urobilinogen	Interferes with other urine constituents

SUMMARY

Many interfering factors influence the quality of any urine specimen, among which a few have been mentioned. If one remembers the following basic rules of urine collection, these factors will have a minimal effect[1]:

1. Urine should be collected at the best time for constituent analysis. (*Not* necessarily the most convenient time for patient, physician, or technologist.)

2. A clean disposable container is preferable.
3. The proper preservative should be used when necessary.
4. The specimen container should be properly labeled with vital information (i.e., name, date, patient identification number, time of collection, and specific information about the collection procedure and/or the preservative used, if any).

Review Questions

Match the best container with each situation listed:
A. Clean, clear plastic container
B. Sterile, clear container
C. Brown bottle
D. Sterile test tube
E. Clean glass jar

1. ___ Routine urinalysis on a premature newborn
2. ___ Diabetic urine screening for a community organization
3. ___ Bacterial culture on a hospitalized patient
4. ___ Quantitative analysis of bilirubin in urine
5. ___ First morning specimen on an outpatient

6. List problems associated with the following preservatives:
   A. HCl
   B. Formaldehyde
   C. Thymol
   D. Toluene
7. Briefly describe the method of collection of a 24-hour urine specimen.
8. What type of specimen would one collect for the following conditions:
   A. Routine urinalysis and bacterial culture
   B. Routine urinalysis only
   C. Urine urobilinogen analysis
   D. Porphyrin screen
   E. Detection of urine abnormalities in the prostatic area
   F. Cytologic examination of urine

(See Appendix for answers.)

Case Study

A physician is setting up a small clinic in a rural area. He needs a basic urinalysis laboratory and supplies for sending urine specimens to various reference laboratories. All of the patients will be seen on an outpatient basis and will frequently be asked to collect urine specimens at home. Included in the laboratory will be facilities for routine bacteriologic studies.

Questions

1. What type(s) of specimen would be most useful for this environment?
2. What type of specimen would be appropriate for both routine urinalysis and bacteriologic culture?
3. What essential supplies for collection purposes should be recommended?
4. What preservative(s) would be most useful and why?

Answers

1. Random or spot specimens are useful for routine urinalysis.
2. Clean-catch specimens are useful for both routine urinalysis and bacteriologic studies.
3. Supplies should include clean containers for random specimens, sterile containers for bacteriologic culture, and larger brown bottles for 24-hour specimens. All containers should have labels and, if necessary, warning labels. Written instructions for collection should be available.
4. Refrigeration and/or freezing are useful because they interfere with the least number of tests. Freezing is good for transportation purposes. Formaldehyde is useful for preserving formed elements. Hydrochloric acid is useful for preserving many chemical constituents.

REFERENCES

1. Free AH, Free HM: Urinalysis in Clinical Laboratory Practice. Cleveland, CRC Press, 1975, pp 21–25.
2. Freeman JA, Beeler MF: Laboratory Medicine—Clinical Microscopy. Philadelphia, Lea & Febiger, 1974, p 169.
3. French R: Guide to Diagnostic Procedures. New York, McGraw-Hill, 1975, p 19.
4. Watson CJ, Schwartz S, Sborov V, Bertie E: A simple method for quantitative recording of Ehrlich's reaction as carried out with urine and feces. Am J Clin Pathol 14:605, 1944.
5. Zilva J, Pannal PR: Clinical Chemistry in Diagnostic Treatment, 2nd ed. Chicago, Year Book, 1975, p 465.
6. Tietz N (ed): Fundamentals of Clinical Chemistry. Philadelphia, Saunders, 1976, p 52.
7. Free AH, Free H: Urodynamics and Concepts Relating to Urine Chemistry. Elkhart, Ind, Ames Division, Miles Laboratories, 1978, p 19.
8. MacFate R: Introduction to the Clinical Laboratory, 3rd ed. Chicago, Year Book, 1972, p 41.
9. Schumann GB: Urine Sediment Examination. Baltimore, Williams & Wilkins, 1980, p 17.
10. Bailey RR, Little PJ: Suprapubic bladder aspiration in diagnosis of urinary tract infection. Br Med J 1:293, 1969.
11. Race GJ, White MG: Basic Urinalysis. New York, Harper and Row, 1979, p 10.
12. Worth RD, Harrison J, Skillen AW: Stability of glucose in urine. Clin Chem 26:789, 1980.

Barbara Smith Michael

CHAPTER 5

The Routine Examination of Urine

Objectives

It is expected that the reader, using the information presented in this chapter, will be able to:

1. Recognize normal and abnormal colors of urine and relate them to possible causes/conditions.
2. Identify the principal causes of turbid urine.
3. List and compare methods used to measure urine concentration.
4. Define terms used to describe urine volume output, such as anuria, oliguria, and polyuria.
5. Relate and correlate the origin and significance of the chemical constituents usually determined in urine by multitest reagent strip methodology, i.e., pH, protein, glucose, ketone, bilirubin, blood, nitrite, and urobilinogen.
6. Describe the test principle and reactants for each urinary reagent strip test.
7. Relate sensitivity and specificity for each chemical test, particularly as they apply to the occurrence of false positive or false negative reactions.
8. Describe procedures used as confirmatory methods for protein, reducing substances, and bilirubin.
9. List and discuss at least three variables inherent in the current methods used to prepare urine for sediment examination.
10. Outline a standardized procedure for the preparation of urinary sediment, including a grading system for reporting formed elements.
11. List the three microscopic techniques most frequently used in urine sediment examination and explain the underlying principle and the advantage provided by each type.
12. Discuss why the identification of the normal as well as the abnormal constituents found during the microscopic examination of urinary sediment is important.

13. Name the two broad categories into which urine sediment constituents may be classified and give examples.
14. Describe how the morphology of cells found in the urine is influenced by the tonicity of the urine.
15. Distinguish among erythrocytes, leukocytes, and renal tubular cells and explain the significance of their presence in elevated numbers.
16. Distinguish among squamous epithelial cells, transitional epithelial cells, and renal tubular epithelial cells.
17. Suggest two techniques to aid in the identification of fat droplets and oval fat bodies.
18. Explain the significance of bacteria found in urine and suggest two other techniques to help identify (classify) and quantitate the microorganisms.
19. Describe the morphologic characteristics of yeast and distinguish them from red blood cells and oil droplets.
20. Define cylinduria and discuss its significance.
21. List three factors that determine the appearance of a particular urine cast.
22. Identify and describe the different types of casts found in the urine.
23. Discuss two explanations for the genesis of granular casts.
24. List at least four crystals found in normal urine and describe their morphology and solubility characteristics.
25. List and describe at least three abnormal crystals found in urine.
26. Associate crystal type with urinary pH where found.
27. List at least three artifacts or contaminants found in urine and their significance.
28. Explain why a properly collected and promptly processed specimen is particularly important in urine sediment examination.
29. Correlate physicochemical/microscopic sediment findings in selected clinical conditions.

Urinalysis is the term used to describe a group of qualitative or semiquantitative tests performed most frequently on a random, nontimed urine specimen. While the examination of urine dates back many centuries (Hippocrates even mentions urinalysis in his writings), it continues to be very important because of the relative simplicity of the test, the ease of collection and availability of the specimen, and because of the wealth of clinical information that can be derived from one routine examination.

Hayashi[2] and others[3-9] have discussed three important reasons for performing urinalysis: (1) its use as a screening test for the detection of various endocrine or metabolic abnormalities in which the kidneys are functioning properly but excreting abnormal amounts of a specific metabolic end product; (2) urinalysis provides useful information concerning the presence or absence of renal and other diseases, i.e., it assists in diagnosis; and (3) urinalysis on a routine basis is a very simple method for monitoring the course of a disease as well as the efficacy of treatment.

Modern urinalysis consists of several physicochemical measurements in addition to the microscopic examination of the urinary sediment. Like other laboratory procedures, urinalysis should and can be standardized, i.e., all specimens can be handled in an identical manner so that any data obtained will be reproducible and consistent with prior test results and from laboratory to laboratory. Unfortunately, in many laboratories, the examination of urine is frequently assigned to the most inexperienced personnel who commonly have inadequate supervision and training.

As Brody and associates state[10]:

> The future of laboratory medicine is concerned with two goals . . . to provide accurate and significant information for the use of computer methods. . . . Secondly, since modern medicine will be more involved . . . with early detection and prevention of chronic disease, the laboratory must respond with appropriate rapid, simple, and accurate detection techniques for screening large populations. Workers in urinalysis now must be concerned with the development of new and more accurate quantitative techniques.*

PHYSICAL CHARACTERISTICS OF URINE

Color, appearance or turbidity, indices of urine solute concentration (specific gravity, refractive index, and osmolality), and volume are important physical properties of urine. While the significance of the macroscopic examination of urine (color and turbidity) is frequently overlooked, it can provide the clinician with useful diagnostic information if it is done accurately and objectively. Schumann and Greenberg[11] have reported that a macroscopic analysis of urine which also includes reagent strip chemical tests is a sufficient screening procedure and that microscopic analysis, i.e., urinary sediment examination, is only necessary in specimens with abnormal macroscopic or chemical findings and/or in patients with known renal or urinary tract disease.

*Brody LH, et al: Urinalysis and the urinary sediment. Med Clin North Am 55:243, 1971.

Color

In a healthy individual, urine is usually a clear fluid ranging in color from pale to dark yellow, with the intensity of color depending on the urine concentration and hence on the hydration of the person. Its color is due to a mixture of normal metabolic end products. One of the major sources of color is urochrome, a derivative of the degradation of the pigment heme. Urobilin and uroerythrin are pigments also present in small amounts in normal urine.

Various dietary or food pigments also may contribute to the color of urine, such as the red pigment of beets. In addition, certain drugs and their metabolites and dyes may give specific coloration.

Certain pathologic disease states (renal and metabolic disorders) are associated with abnormal urine coloration, and a change in normal urine color may be the first indication. One interesting condition in which both the color and turbidity of the urine are altered is chyluria.[1] The urine, especially after a fat-containing meal, has a characteristic milky appearance. Chyluria, the appearance of chyle (a mixture of lymph and emulsified fat) in the urine, is due to the obstruction of proper lymphatic drainage by parasites or other conditions. A few of the possible conditions that can alter urine color and appearance are summarized in Table 5.1.

Appearance or Turbidity

While abnormal numbers of erythrocytes (red blood cells, RBC), leukocytes (white blood cells, WBC), and bacteria or the presence of fat can impart turbidity, the appearance of urine by itself is usually of limited diagnostic significance. For instance, turbidity might be due to mucus from vaginal contamination or precipitation of phosphates in alkaline urine, both of which are normal occurrences.

Urine may be turbid upon excretion or become turbid upon standing. The formation of turbidity occurs when the normally present soluble constituents are rendered insoluble due to changes in urinary pH, temperature, or because of their precipitation from a

TABLE 5.1. APPEARANCE AND COLOR OF URINE

Appearance	Cause	Remarks
Colorless	Very dilute urine	Polyuria, diabetes insipidus
Cloudy	Phosphates, carbonates	Soluble in dilute acetic acid
	Urates, uric acid	Dissolve at 60C
	Leukocytes	Insoluble in dilute acetic acid
	Red cells (smoky)	Lyse in dilute acetic acid
	Bacteria, yeasts	Insoluble in dilute acetic acid
	Spermatozoa	Insoluble in dilute acetic acid
	Prostatic fluid	
	Mucin, mucous threads	May be flocculent
	Calculi gravel	Phosphates, oxalates
	Clumps, pus, tissue	
	Fecal contamination	Rectovesical fistula
	X-ray media	In acid urine
Milky	Many PMN (pyuria)	Insoluble in dilute acetic acid
	Fat	
	Lipuria, opalescent	Nephrosis, crush injury—soluble in ether
	Chyluria, milky	Lymphatic obstruction—soluble in ether
Yellow	Acriflavine	Green fluorescence
	Mepacrine	
	Nitrofurantoin	Antibiotic
	Riboflavin	Large doses
Yellow-orange	Concentrated urine	Dehydration, fever
	Urobilin in excess	No yellow foam
	Bilirubin	Yellow foam
	Pyridium	Color increases with HCl
Yellow-green	Bilirubin-biliverdin	Yellow foam
Yellow-brown	Bilirubin-biliverdin	Beer brown, yellow foam
	Senna, rhubarb, cascara	In acid urine

(Continued)

supersaturated solution. Free and Free[3] have demonstrated that the incidence of turbidity of urine is over 50 percent following refrigeration and that about 10 percent of voided specimens are turbid.

Usually turbidity is evaluated using subjective criteria, such as clear, slightly turbid, moderately turbid, or very turbid. However, Schumann and Greenberg[11] state in their report that an accurate assessment of turbidity should be made on a clean-catch specimen, and they used nephelometry to determine turbidity objectively.

Indices of Urinary Solute Concentration

The life-sustaining functions of the kidney include (1) the excretion of excess body water and the elimination of waste or nonessential products of metabolism and exogenous foreign substances, (2) the retention of essential substances required for proper bodily activities, and (3) the control or regulation of electrolyte homeostasis and osmotic pressure of body fluids.[12] These important tasks are carried out by the functional/structural units of the kidney, the nephrons.

The ultimate excreted product of the kidneys is the fluid commonly referred to as urine. About 95 percent of urine is the solvent water, and the remainder is comprised of various solids. The major solutes in urine include calcium, chloride, creatinine, phosphates, potassium, sodium, sulfates, urea, and uric acid.[12] The ability of the kidneys to produce a concentrated urine is frequently the first function to fail in renal disease. Hence, the measurements of urine solute

TABLE 5.1. APPEARANCE AND COLOR OF URINE (Cont.)

Appearance	Cause	Remarks
Red	Hemoglobin	o-Tolidine positive
	Red blood cells	o-Tolidine positive
	Myoglobin	o-Tolidine positive
	Porphyrin	o-Tolidine negative, may be colorless
	Phenindione	Anticoagulant
	Amidopyrine	
	Fuscin, aniline dye	Foods, candy
	Beets	Yellow alkaline, genetic
	Menstrual contamination	Clots, mucus
Red-pink	Phenolsulfonphthalein	In alkaline urine
	Penolphthalein	In alkaline urine
	Sulfobromophthalein	In alkaline urine
	Santonin	In alkaline urine
	Rhubarb, senna, cascara	In alkaline urine
Red-purple	Porphyrin	May be colorless
Red-brown	Red blood cells	
	Hemoglobin on standing	
	Methemoglobin	
	Myoglobin	
Brown-black	Methemoglobin	
	Homogentisic acid	On standing, alkaline
		Alkaptonuria
	Melanin, methyldopa	On standing
	Phenols	Reduce Benedict's reagent
Blue-green	Methylene blue	In drugs
	Indigo-carmine	Decolorize with alkali
	Indicans	Intestinal putrefaction
	Pseudomonas infection	
Dark brown	Levodopa	Large dose

From Bradley M, et al.: Examination of urine. In Henry JB (ed): Todd-Sanford-Davidson Clinical Diagnosis and Management by Laboratory Methods, 16th ed, 1979, p 574. (Courtesy of W.B. Saunders Co.)

concentration and urine volume itself are important indicators of kidney function.

Three measured properties of urine that are dependent on its solute concentration include specific gravity, refractive index, and osmolality. While these properties are closely related and an increase in solute concentration will result in an increased value of each of the properties, they also vary independently, and the observed increases are not necessarily proportional. This is because some of the dissolved solids (solute molecules and ions) influence each of these properties differently.[13-15]

Specific Gravity. Specific gravity has been the most widely used index of urine concentration.[3,12,13,16] It is the ratio of the density (mass per unit volume) of a liquid (the urine) compared to the density of an equal volume of pure (solute-free) water at a specific temperature. Pure water, the point of reference, has a specific gravity of 1.000. While specific gravity depends upon the number, density, and weight of dissolved particles (solute molecules and ions) in the urine, it is primarily a comparison of weights. Therefore, it is not an exact quantitation of the number of solute particles present because different atoms and molecules do not have the same weight.

Although the specific gravity of plasma is very constant in health (1.010 to 1.012), the normal specific gravity of urine is quite variable over a 24-hour period. It ranges from 1.003 to 1.035 due to such factors as fluid intake, environmental temperature, and activity and is usually highest in the first morning specimen.

Under standardized conditions of dehydration or hydration, specific gravity measurements can be used to assess the concentrating ability of the kidneys. In a typical concentration test, the patient is requested to avoid all fluids after the evening meal. Any urine voided during the night is discarded, and the first morning specimen is then tested for specific gravity. A value of 1.025 or higher indicates normal concentrating ability. In patients with diabetes insipidus, for example, there is a loss of effective concentrating ability, and urine specific gravity remains low. This is caused by the impairment of the normal water reabsorption in the kidney, which is dependent on the action of antidiuretic hormone (ADH) secreted by cells in the hypothalamus gland. Patients with various renal diseases in which there has been actual renal tubular damage (water reabsorption occurs in the distal segment of the tubules of the nephron) also will not be able to concentrate urine.

Specific gravity can be measured with a urinometer, a special type of hydrometer that has been modified to measure specific gravity in urine. It is a glass float weighted with mercury at the bottom with an air bulb above the weight with a graduated stem (usually 1.000 to 1.050) on the top. The test consists of inserting the urinometer into a cylinder filled with urine (usual volume is around 15 ml), twirling it slightly, and then noting the scale reading at the meniscus when it equilibrates.

Urinometers are calibrated to read 1.000 in pure distilled water at a given temperature. Therefore, if the temperature of the urine is either higher or lower than this calibration temperature, positive or negative errors are introduced. The reading must then be corrected or adjusted by adding 0.001 for each 3C that the specimen is above the given temperature or subtracting 0.001 for each 3C below this temperature. In addition to the correction for temperature effects, it is also

necessary to correct for the presence of abnormal amounts of dissolved substances in urine, e.g., by subtracting 0.003 for each g/dl of protein and 0.004 for each g/dl of glucose. The presence of exogenous materials, such as x-ray contrast media injected for radiologic examination of the urinary system and later excreted by the kidneys, can cause abnormally elevated specific gravity values. In these cases, values higher than 1.050 have been observed, and unusual crystals frequently are seen in the urine sediment.

Refractive Index. Refractive index[12,13,15,17] refers to the velocity or speed of light passing through air compared to the velocity of light passing through a solution. The degree to which a beam of transmitted light is refracted and its velocity is impeded as it passes through a solution is determined by the total solute content. The refractive index of urine is similarly influenced by the content of the dissolved particles present and is easily measured by a simple hand instrument, a refractometer, which is calibrated to read urine density or specific gravity.

The specific gravity of urine and the refractive index are not identical. A specific gravity reading on the same specimen using a refractometer would be around 0.002 lower. However, for clinical purposes, this difference is not significant, and refractometry has become the preferred method. A refractometer is easier to calibrate, use, and clean, and it requires only one or two drops of urine (especially helpful in pediatric or oliguric patients) and is temperature compensated over the temperature range of 60 to 100F. Correction for proteinuria and glucosuria is still required, however.

Osmolality. Osmolality is a measurement of the effective number of dissolved particles (ions and molecules) in a solution.[12,13,15,18,19] It does not depend on the weight of the particles and is a more accurate physiologic indicator of the renal concentrating ability of the kidneys. Techniques for measuring osmolality require a special instrument, an osmometer, and therefore determination of osmolality is not a routine procedure in many laboratories.

The principle of the method frequently used to determine osmolality is the reduction in the freezing point of a solution below that of pure water, i.e., freezing point depression. Recall that solutes change the physical properties of a solution, the so-called colligative properties that include osmotic pressure, vapor pressure, boiling point, and freezing point. One osmole of a solute will lower the freezing point of 1 kg of water 1.858C. One mole of a substance dissolved in 1 kg of water that does not dissociate (glucose for example) has an effective osmolality of 1 osmole. However, such a substance as sodium chloride which dissociates into two ions has an osmolality of 2 osmoles.

Whereas osmolality and specific gravity values are similar in nondisease states, they do not correlate very well in pathologic conditions. This is particularly true in diseases associated with proteinuria and glucosuria. This is because osmolality is not as disproportionately affected by the presence of these high molecular weight substances, and the values, therefore, do not have to be corrected.

Adults on a normal diet and fluid intake will produce a urine with an osmolality in the range of 500 to 800 mOsm/kg of water. The normal kidney is able to produce osmolalities ranging from 40 to 80 mOsm/kg (hydration conditions) to 800 to 1,400 mOsm/kg (dehydration conditions).

Volume

Urine volume measurements[13,16] are usually not a part of a routine urinalysis. However, volume determinations on timed specimens collected under specified conditions and used in conjunction with other measurements may provide valuable diagnostic information. Normal daily urine volumes depend on several variables, such as fluid intake, environmental temperature, activity, and age. The average urine volume of an adult is 600 to 1,600 ml/24 hours. Children excrete smaller daily urine volumes, but based on kilogram of body weight, they actually excrete three to four times that of an adult. Terms frequently used to describe urine volume output are given in Table 5.2.

CHEMICAL CHARACTERISTICS OF URINE IN HEALTH AND DISEASE

In many clinical laboratories the basic qualitative or semiquantitative screening of urine is done using the rapid and convenient colorimetric, multitest solid-state reagent, dipstick system.[20–23] Dipsticks are plastic strips to which are attached various reagent-

TABLE 5.2. URINE VOLUME OUTPUT

Term	Definition	Possible Cause/Condition
Anuria	Cessation of excretion of urine—essentially no urine output	Renal disease or failure, obstruction
Diuresis	Increased excretion of urine—volume increase is usually temporary	Pharmacologic agents—diuretics
Nocturia	Excessive urination at night (volume greater than 500 ml), normal day to night ratio is 4:1	Renal disease
Oliguria	Excretion of diminished amount of urine in relation to fluid intake	Renal disease or ischemia, dehydration
Polyuria	Excretion of a large volume of urine in a given period (more than 2,000 ml/24 hours)	Metabolic or renal disease

impregnated areas that test for specific constituents. Depending on the system used, as many as eight chemical determinations can be made in less than two minutes, including pH, protein, glucose, ketone, bilirubin, blood, nitrite, and urobilinogen. In addition to the reagent strip systems, various tablet test systems are available to test for reducing substances (Clinitest*), protein (Bumintest*), and bilirubin (Ictotest*).

Dip-and-read systems are easy to use. However, it is important that the user be familiar with the proper use of a particular system and with the problems that can occur. Free and Free[24] have published an excellent article on the use and misuse of these rapid and convenient tests. They emphasize the importance of avoiding errors in urine testing, beginning with proper urine collection. Users should closely follow the product insert sheets provided by the manufacturer in order to achieve reliable test results and to be aware of any improvements or changes.

A typical procedure is[23]:

1. Briefly (less than 1 second) dip the reagent test strip into a well-mixed, uncentrifuged, fresh urine specimen. A refrigerated specimen must be allowed to equilibrate to room temperature before analysis. All reagent areas must be completely immersed.
2. As the strip is removed from the urine, draw the edge of the strip along the rim of the specimen container to remove excess urine. Hold the strip in a horizontal position to prevent reagent runover.
3. Compare the color changes of the test areas to the color blocks on the color chart at the times indicated for obtaining the results.

Brereton et al[25] have evaluated the results obtained on patient and contrived urines at different time intervals to assess whether the timing of reactions is actually a critical factor

*Ames Division, Miles Laboratories, Inc., Elkhart, Indiana.

in the quantitation of compounds present in urine. They found that a quantitatively positive dipstick reading will not become negative at any time up to 120 seconds. They also found that a few urine specimens negative on initial reading became trace-positive at 60 seconds. However, they did not feel that this was of great clinical significance since they felt any positive findings would be substantiated by additional testing. Their conclusion was that where strict timing schedules are not possible, the reagent dipstick system test results would be best used as qualitative tests only.

Some laboratories are now using a semi-automated system (based on the principle of reflectance) to replace visual reading of urinalysis dipsticks. Peele et al[26,27] have evaluated the instrument readings versus visual readings. It is their contention that while the chemistry or color reactions are subject to the same errors, the semi-automated method does minimize interpersonnel variation, and subjective interpretation of the colorimetric reactions and improved reproducibility is achieved. Refer to Chapter 8 for a further detailed discussion of the quality control process and monitoring in urinalysis.

pH

Origin and Clinical Significance. Whereas the normal blood pH range is confined to narrow limits (7.34 to 7.42), the pH of freshly voided normal urine may vary widely from 4.5 to around 8.5.[3,13,21,23] Urinary pH, a reflection of the homeostatic acid-base regulating role of the kidneys, varies considerably with individual metabolic status, type of diet, and with disease and drug therapy. The pH of urine for a healthy individual reflects largely the acid or alkaline composition of the diet. For instance, individuals on high protein diets excrete a more acidic urine specimen than do those on a predominantly vegetarian diet.

The pH range of normal urine is the same as that seen in disease states. However, urinary pH can still provide important information on the acid-base status of a patient if used as part of the total clinical picture and in conjunction with other laboratory measurements. Acidity (decreased pH) is noted in patients with severe diarrhea, dehydration, or fever. Patients with renal tubular acidosis, for example, are not able to excrete a very acid urine because of the decreased ability of the renal tubules to secrete an acid load, i.e., hydrogen ions. While the urine pH remains around neutral, an excess of acid builds up in the body and acidosis results.

High (alkaline) pH values may be caused by acute and chronic renal disease, severe vomiting, or respiratory alkalosis. However, a very alkaline, ammoniacal urine specimen usually means the growth of urea-splitting bacteria in an improperly collected specimen or delayed processing. The presence of a true urinary tract infection will also cause an alkaline pH urine and must be confirmed. Hence, the importance of testing only freshly voided specimens if the pH determination is to be relevant.

An estimation of urinary pH using reagent strip systems is usually satisfactory. However, when an accurate pH measurement is needed, as in special renal function tests, the urine specimen should be collected under oil or in a closed container on ice, and the pH determination should be made with a pH electrode without delay.

Test Principle. The pH test is based on a double indicator principle with the reagent area impregnated with the pH indicators, bromthymol blue and methyl red.[28,29] Timing is not critical and the test may be read immediately with N-Multistix* and Chemstrip†.

Specificity. There are no known interferences.[28,29] However, a phenomenon called "runover" may occur if excess urine is left on the strip after it is removed from the specimen (N-Multistix). A false drop in pH may result when the acid buffer from the protein reagent runs over onto the adjacent pH area.

*Ames Division, Miles Laboratories, Inc., Elkhart, Indiana.
†Bio-Dynamics/bmc, Division of Boehringer Mannheim, Indianapolis, Indiana.

It is most noticeable in specimens with a pH of 7 or greater.

Protein

Origin and Clinical Significance. The kidneys normally excrete a minimal amount of protein daily (up to 150 mg/24 hours). However, an increased amount of protein in the urine is most often one of the first indications of renal disease.[3,13,21,23,31] Proteinuria may vary from minimal to marked and be continuous or intermittent depending on the nature of the disorder. It may also be due to physiologic or functional conditions. The so-called orthostatic or postural proteinuria is an example.

About one third of urinary protein is albumin that is identical to serum albumin. The majority of urinary proteins, however, are globulins that are closely related to the serum globulins. Tamm-Horsfall protein, a high molecular weight mucoprotein, is unique to urine only. Bence-Jones protein is a low molecular weight protein with the unusual property of coagulating upon heating at temperatures between 45C and 60C and then redissolving upon heating to the boiling point. It may be found in the urine of patients with multiple myeloma or macroglobulinemia.

Test Principle. The detection of urinary proteins is based on Sorenson's principle of the "protein error of indicators."[28,29] The reagent area is impregnated with tetrabromphenol blue (N-Multistix) or tetrachlorophenol-tetrabromosulfophthalein (Chemstrip) buffered at a constant acidic pH. A sequential color change from yellow-green through green to blue occurs in the presence of protein. The test area remains yellow in the absence of protein. Timing is not critical, and the reaction may be read immediately.

Sensitivity. The reagent solid-state systems are primarily reactive toward albumin with 0.05 to 0.2 g/L (5 to 20 mg/dl) detected as a trace amount.[28,29,32–34] The lack of sensitivity of these strips to other urinary proteins, such as globulin, Bence-Jones protein, and mucoprotein, is well known. The difference in the sensitivity of the dipstick indicators for protein other than albumin is based on the binding characteristics of the indicators with these other proteins. Therefore, negative to trace reactions do not necessarily rule out proteinuria. Consequently, alternate methods, such as the sulfosalicylic acid semiquantitative procedure which accurately detects albumin as well as other kinds of protein, are recommended as confirmatory tests. (page 81).

Specificity. False positive results may be obtained in highly alkaline urine specimens (pH greater than 9), during certain drug therapy, or due to contamination with quaternary ammonium compounds from residues of disinfectants or detergents in specimen collection containers. However, the colorimetric dipstick method is not subject to some of the other interferences that can cause positive reactions with the sulfosalicylic acid method of protein precipitation, such as turbidity, presence of radiographic contrast media, or the urine preservative thymol.[24,28,29,33]

Glucose

Origin and Clinical Significance. Like protein, a minute amount of glucose is excreted daily, although its concentration in normal urine is below the detection limits of the methods routinely employed.[3,13,21,23,35] The appearance of glucose in the urine occurs in such disease states as diabetes mellitus, or it may occur in a benign condition called renal glucosuria. Glucosuria occurs whenever the blood sugar level exceeds what is known as the renal threshold. At this point the renal tubules are unable to handle the load, i.e., they reabsorb the glucose, and it then spills over into the urine. Glycosuria is occasionally accompanied by bacterial or fungal organisms in the urine, high specific gravity, positive test for ketones, and proteinuria in cases of long-standing diabetes.

Test Principle. Glucose is determined by a double sequential reaction, the specific glucose/peroxidase enzymatic method[28,29]:

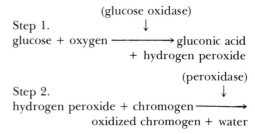

N-Multistix uses potassium iodide chromogen with a resultant color change from green to brown. Chemstrip employs the chromogen C1-APAC (amino-chloro-dimethyl-tetra-bromo-sulfophthalein). A positive reaction is demonstrated by a color change from yellow to orange-brown/brown.

Sensitivity. The N-Multistix can detect glucose concentrations as low as 6 mmole/L (0.1 g/dl). Qualitative results may be obtained at 10 seconds or semiquantitative results at 30 seconds. Concentrations of 2.22 mmole/L (40 mg/dl) or greater produce a positive result with the Chemstrip system (reaction read at 60 seconds). Both systems are affected if large amounts of ascorbic acid are present in the urine, e.g., concentration of 0.425 mmole/L (75 mg/dl) or greater, and the concentration of glucose is low, e.g., less than 5.6 mmole/L (100 mg/dl).[19,28,29,36–38] Inhibition of the enzyme reaction occurs which leads to a false negative result. A high urinary specific gravity in combination with an alkaline pH may also reduce the test's level of detection and could in the presence of low glucose concentration result in a false negative reaction.

Specificity. The enzymatic reaction is specific only for glucose and does not react with other sugars, such as lactose, galactose, or fructose.[19,28,29,37,38] Because glucose oxidase reacts only with glucose, it is recommended that specimens from pediatric patients be routinely screened with another system, such as Clinitest, a tablet test system that reacts with various reducing substances (page 82). Screening tests on children for certain sugars and other reducing substances are used to detect inborn errors of metabolism, such as galactosemia, fructosuria, and alkaptonuria. Tests for these conditions, some of which are associated with mental or neurologic disorders, are discussed in greater detail in Chapter 6.

The glucose oxidase-specific test does not react with the reducing metabolites of such drugs as salicylates. However, residues of strong oxidizing agents (hydrogen peroxide or hypochlorite) used to clean urine specimen containers can cause false positive reactions.

Ketone

Origin and Clinical Significance. The term "ketone bodies" includes acetone, acetoacetic acid, and β-hydroxybutyric acid, although the latter is not a ketone.[3,13,21,23,39] Ketone bodies, the products of incomplete fat metabolism, are normally not detectable in urine. However, ketonuria can even occur in normal individuals on fasting or starvation diets. It frequently occurs in children in a variety of conditions, such as in a febrile state in which the child is not eating and/or is vomiting. The presence of ketone bodies is also indicative of acidosis which may occur with carbohydrate metabolism abnormalities, such as diabetes mellitus. Before serum ketone levels are elevated, ketones may be excreted in the urine in large amounts.

Test Principle. The test is based on Legal's method in which sodium nitroferricyanide (nitroprusside), glycine, and buffer react with acetone and acetoacetic acid in an alkaline medium to form a violet dye complex.[28,29] A positive reaction results in a color change from beige to violet. The reaction is read at 15 seconds with N-Multistix and at 60 seconds with Chemstrip.

Sensitivity. The test detects as little as 0.49 mmole/L (5 mg/dl) of acetoacetic acid (N-Multistix) and a concentration of 8.8 mmole/L (9 mg/dl) or greater with Chemstrip.[24,28,29] The test is less sensitive to acetone, but a concentration of 68.6 mmole/L (70 mg/dl) or greater produces a positive result with Chemstrip. Beta-hydroxybutyric

acid is not detected. Ketone test results can be reported in specific mg/dl using N-Multistix with the new ketone test instead of in relative amounts. The improved ketone test is also reported to be more stable.

Another critical factor is the extreme sensitivity of the ketone reagent to moisture—it becomes nonreactive if left exposed to room humidity for any length of time. The reagent area may even become discolored and difficult to read. Hence, it is very important to protect the reagent strips from moisture and to discard any strips with a discolored reaction area. The necessity of testing a fresh specimen cannot be overstressed. While it is not true that acetoacetic acid rapidly converts to acetone which then volatilizes and disappears, it is true that the growth of bacteria which metabolize acetoacetic acid in a urine specimen can cause a false negative reaction.

Specificity. The Chemstrip test reacts with the ketone bodies acetoacetic acid and acetone in urine. N-Multistix with the new ketone test reacts only with acetoacetic acid. It is reported that some low pH, high specific gravity urines may give trace reactions (0.49 mmole/L or 5 mg/dl), and therefore clinical judgment is needed to determine the significance.[24,28,29] False-positive color reactions can be produced by compounds used in renal and liver function tests, such as bromsulphalein (BSP) or phenolsulfonphthalein (PSP). It can also occur in urines containing metabolites of the drug L-dopa, used to treat patients with Parkinson's disease, or in the presence of large amounts of phenylketones. In general, however, other drug interference is minimal.

Bilirubin

Origin and Clinical Significance. Bilirubin, the principal bile pigment, is derived primarily from the degradation of hemoglobin in senescent erythrocytes. In the liver, free, unconjugated bilirubin, bound to the plasma protein albumin, is converted to water-soluble bilirubin diglucuronide. This conjugated form of bilirubin is normally excreted by the liver with the rest of the bile into the intestinal tract where it is reduced by the action of intestinal microorganisms.[3,13,21,23,40,41]

The detection of bilirubinuria, which may occur before yellow pigmentation of the skin (jaundice), is an important early indicator of hepatitis. Bilirubin is usually not detectable in urine, but when there is an increased amount of water-soluble conjugated bilirubin in the blood, increased excretion in the urine will occur. This can be due to liver cell damage or to obstructive biliary tract diseases. Increased formation of unconjugated bilirubin with elevated blood levels is also associated with diseases, such as hemolytic anemias, but an increase of bilirubin in the urine is not noted in these cases. This is because the unconjugated form of bilirubin is not water soluble and, hence, cannot be excreted by the kidneys.

Test results for bilirubin alone and used in conjunction with urobilinogen levels can be very helpful to the clinician in differential diagnosis. For example, in hepatic diseases, urine bilirubin may be positive or negative, and urine urobilinogen is increased. In patients with biliary obstruction, urine bilirubin is positive, but the urine urobilinogen level is decreased. Bilirubinuria is often accomplished by a yellow-brown color in the urine and stained (deep yellow) structures in the urinary sediment.

Test Principle. The detection of bilirubin is based on a diazo reaction where bilirubin couples with a diazonium salt in a strongly acidic medium.[28,29] N-Multistix uses diazotized 2,4-dichloroaniline. Color reactions, read at 20 seconds, range from buff through various shades of tan. The stable diazonium salt used in Chemstrip is 2.6-dichloro-benzene-diazoniumfluoroborate. A color change from buff to tannish purple, proportional to the bilirubin concentration, occurs. The reaction is read at 30 to 60 seconds.

Sensitivity. The level of detection with N-Multistix is 3.4μmole/L to 6.8μmole/L (0.2 to 0.4 mg/dl). Bilirubin levels as low as 8.5 μmole/L (0.5 mg/dl) will produce a positive result with Chemstrip. Test sensitivity may be lowered by the presence of elevated levels of ascorbic acid from dietary or medicinal sources or nitrite due to urinary tract infection. False negative reactions can also occur if testing is performed on urine that has been allowed to stand for any length of time after voiding or is exposed to light, since bilirubin will be oxidized to form nonreactive biliverdin. A fresh specimen protected from light is, therefore, highly recommended. When the detection of very low levels of bilirubin is important, as in the early stages of viral hepatitis, another more sensitive method should be used (page 83).

Specificity. False positive reactions may occur in patients receiving certain drugs, such as chlorpromazine. On the other hand, pyridiumlike drug metabolites may produce a reddish coloration of the strip and mask any reaction.[24,28,29,40]

Blood

Origin and Clinical Significance. Hematuria, the presence of intact erythrocytes in the urine, occurs in patients with urinary tract bleeding and is frequently found in urine from females because of gynecologic bleeding or menstruation. Hematuria is also found in patients with renal disease, and in these patients it is usually accompanied by significant proteinuria and casts in the urine. Bleeding can be extensive and noted macroscopically (gross hematuria). However, in many cases the blood can be detected only by some physical procedure, such as microscopic examination of the urinary sediment or a chemical test, in which instance the bleeding is called occult or hidden. Both the chemical and microscopic tests for blood are usually positive in cases of hematuria.[3,13,21,23,42-44]

Hemoglobinuria, the presence of free hemoglobin in urine, reflects intravascular hemolysis such as occurs in transfusion reactions or paroxysmal nocturnal hemoglobinuria (PNH). However, the lysis of intact red blood cells in urine of low specific gravity (less than 1.010) or due to mechanical trauma also releases hemoglobin. Therefore, a misdiagnosis of hemoglobinuria could be made.

Myoglobinuria, the presence of myoglobin in urine, is uncommon. Myoglobin, a small protein present in muscle, can be released into the circulating blood and subsequently excreted in the urine by the kidneys. Crushing injuries or trauma to muscle, including myocardial infarction, will release myoglobin, and it is found in the urine of patients with various familial diseases. Since myoglobin has chemical properties similar to hemoglobin, it can be detected by methods identical to those used to confirm the presence of hemoglobin. To differentiate between myoglobinuria and hemoglobinuria is difficult based on the examination of the urine alone. The chemical tests will be positive, and the microscopic findings negative in both conditions. Blondheim's method[45] of salt precipitation using an 80 percent saturated ammonium sulfate solution to precipitate hemoglobin is a useful method to confirm the presence of myoglobin. Other methods are separation of the smaller protein, myoglobin, by ultrafiltration or electrophoresis and identification and quantitation by immunoprecipitation.

Test Principle. The detection of blood in urine is based on the peroxidase-like action of hemoglobin, which catalyzes the oxidation reaction of the color indicator by the organic peroxide present in the test area.[28,29] In N-Multistix the chromogen is o-Tolidine, and it produces colors ranging from orange through green to dark blue. Chemstrip, which uses another indicator, is yellow in the absence of blood and green in its presence. Both systems now have separate color blocks to allow the differentiation of intact red blood cells (nonhemolyzed blood) and free hemoglobin. Intact erythrocytes that are hemolyzed by the lysing agent in the strip show up as small dots or spots on the reaction area.

$$\begin{array}{c} \text{hemoglobin} \\ \text{Hydrogen peroxide} \;\downarrow\; \text{oxidized chromogen} \\ + \text{ chromogen} \;\longrightarrow\; + \text{ water} \\ \text{(color indicator)} \;\uparrow\; \text{(highly colored)} \\ \text{peroxidase activity} \end{array}$$

The reaction is read at 45 seconds and 60 seconds for N-Multistix and Chemstrip, respectively.

Sensitivity. The test is most sensitive to free hemoglobin and myoglobin but can still detect intact erythrocytes.[24,28,29,44] N-Multistix is capable of detecting levels of 0.15 by 10^{-3} g/L to 0.45 by 10^{-3} g/L (0.015 to 0.045 mg/dl) of free hemoglobin or 5 to 15 intact red blood cells per microliter. (A normal red blood cell contains approximately 30 pg of hemoglobin.) The chemical test should be used, however, in conjunction with a microscopic examination of the urinary sediment to detect the presence of intact red blood cells that might have resisted hemolysis.

The level of detection is reduced in urines with elevated specific gravities or high protein levels. False negative results may also occur in urines containing levels of ascorbic acid of 0.567 mmole/L (10 mg/dl) or greater or due to the presence of formalin as a urine preservative. Recall that ascorbic acid is a reducing agent. Bradley et al[13] recommend that if the microscopic examination of the urine sediment reveals 4 to 8 RBC/high power field or greater and if the chemical screening test for blood is negative, it is useful to further test for the presence of ascorbic acid. C-Stix* reagent strips impregnated with phosphomolybdates which are reduced to a blue color by ascorbic acid are available. As mentioned previously, the presence of ascorbic acid decreases the sensitivity of the glucose-oxidase-peroxidase reactions as well as the diazo reaction for bilirubin.

Specificity. Intact erythrocytes, hemoglobin, and myoglobin all give positive reactions.[23,24,28,29] However, false positive reactions can occur if residue from a strong oxidizing agent is present, such as bleach used to clean urine specimen containers. Peroxidase produced by some pathogenic microorganisms could also cause a false positive result.

---

*Ames Division, Miles Laboratories, Inc., Elkhart, Indiana.

Nitrite

Origin and Clinical Significance   The presence of a critical number of bacteria in the urine (organisms in excess of 10^5/ml) in a fresh, clean-catch, midstream urine specimen is usually indicative of a significant urinary tract infection.[3,13,21,23,46–48] Nitrite is normally not detectable in the urine of healthy individuals and does not appear even after ingestions of high levels of nitrite from processed foods. However, most of the organisms associated with urinary tract infections are capable by enzymatic action of reducing nitrate in the urine derived from dietary sources to nitrite. The nitrite test based on the detection of nitrite in the urine can, therefore, be used to screen for significant bacteria.

Test Principle.   The nitrite method is based on the well-known Griess nitrite test.[28,29] Nitrite, if present in the urine in significant quantities, reacts at an acidic pH with paraarsanilic acid to form a diazonium compound which couples with 1,2,3,4-tetrahydrobenzo(h)quinolin-3-ol to produce a pink azo dye (N-Multistix).

Sensitivity.   The detection level of nitrite in urine of normal specific gravity with N-Multistix is 6.52 μmole/L to 13.04 μmole/L (0.03 to 0.06 mg/dl). Chemstrip detects a concentration of 10.87 μmole/L (0.05 mg/dl). Both tests are read at 30 seconds.[21,23,28,29]

There are several factors that can reduce test sensitivity, and therefore, a negative result by itself does not rule out the presence of a clinically significant number of bacteria. For instance, urine must be incubated in the bladder for a minimum period of time (four to six hours) to allow the conversion of nitrate to nitrite to occur. Therefore, examination of the first morning specimen is recommended.

If nitrate, which is entirely derived from dietary sources, is absent from the urine, nitrite formation is not possible. In addition, such organisms as *Enterococcus* which do not form nitrite might be the pathogen present. A false negative result can occur in patients receiving antimicrobial drugs as well as in the presence of ascorbic acid levels of 25 mg/dl (1.42 mmole/L) or greater.

Specificity.   This test is specific for nitrite, but the presence of a red dye in the urine from drugs containing phenazopyridine can cause a false positive color reaction.[24,28,29] Growth of contaminating organisms in stale urine can also result in a positive reaction.

Urobilinogen

Origin and Clinical Significance.   Urobilinogen is the name given to the colorless compounds (mesobilirubinogen, stercobilinogen, and urobilinogen) that are derived from the reduction of conjugated water-soluble bilirubin, the principal pigment of bile.[3,13,21,23,49] These end products of bilirubin metabolism secreted by the liver into the intestine are oxidized by bacterial action in the intestinal tract to produce brown compounds. A portion of the products formed is automatically eliminated in the feces in a normal individual. The rest of the reduction products are then reabsorbed into the bloodstream via the portal vein and re-excreted by the liver cells. However, a small portion of the urobilinogen escapes re-excretion, reaches the peripheral blood circulation, and then is excreted in the urine. Concentrations from about 1 to 5 μmole/day (0.5 to 2.5 mg/24 hour) are found in the urine of a healthy adult. There is a diurnal variation with levels usually higher in the afternoon.

Elevated levels of urinary urobilinogen can occur in liver disease where the hepatocytes are unable to reabsorb or re-excrete the urobilinogen, i.e., decreased removal. Increased amounts are also noted in hemolytic disease states due to excess production from bilirubin. In patients with biliary duct obstruction, urobilinogen may be reduced or absent from the urine. In neonates, urobilinogen is not present because of the absence of bacterial flora that reduce bilirubin to urobilinogen in the adult.

Test Principle.   The N-Multistix test is based on the well-known Ehrlich aldehyde reaction.[28,29] The reagent, p-dimethyl-amino-benzaldehyde, reacts with urobilinogen in a strongly acidic medium to produce a brown-orange color. The reaction is read in Ehrlich units/dl, where 1 U equals 2 μmole (1 mg) of urobilinogen. Comparison blocks from 0.1 to 12 Ehrlich units/dl are on the color chart, and values are read at 45 seconds.

The Chemstrip system is based on a test (principle of azo-coupling) developed by Kutter et al. The reagent area is impregnated with 4-methoxy-benzene-diazonium-tetra-fluoroborate which, in an acid medium, reacts with urobilinogen to form a red-azo dye. Values are read at 10 to 30 seconds.

Sensitivity. N-Multistix will detect urobilinogen concentrations in urine as low as 2 μmole/L (0.1 Ehrlich unit/dl).[24,28,29,49] Normally, 0.2 μmole/L to 2 μmole/L (0.1 to 1.0 U/dl) is present in a random specimen. Chemstrip sensitivity is approximately 8 μmole/L (0.4 mg/dl), and again most normal urines will demonstrate a positive color reaction (slight pink) up to 1.0 U/dl.

Interference factors, such as the presence of formalin preservative (concentrations greater than 400 μmole/L or 200 mg/dl) or nitrite (concentrations above 5 mg/dl), can reduce test sensitivity. This may produce false negative results due to a decrease in the color reaction (reported with Chemstrip). Urobilinogen is an unstable urinary constituent, and it is rapidly oxidized to nonreacting urobilin. Therefore, testing must be performed on a fresh specimen protected from light. The total absence of urobilinogen cannot be determined by this method.

Specificity. Chemstrip, unlike N-Multistix, is specific for urobilinogen.[28,29,49] It is not subject to the known interference factors of the Ehrlich test and, therefore, does not react with nonspecific diazo-positive substances such as p-amino-salicylic acid. However, false positive reactions may occur in patients on phenazopyridine drug therapy. In the N-Multistix test system azo drug metabolites may give an atypical golden color reaction. In this instance, the speed of the reaction should usually alert the test strip user of the possibility of a false positive reaction. Interfering substances are likely to react immediately, whereas color development due to the presence of elevated amounts of urobilinogen is usually gradual.[24]

CONFIRMATORY PROCEDURES

Other procedures should be used to further confirm and quantitate the positive chemical findings. This is because in some instances there are interferences or limitations that can cause false negative or false positive results with the colorimetric reagent strip systems used routinely to screen urine. The following is a discussion of three such confirmatory procedures.

Protein

Test Principle. Protein, denatured by the addition of acid, becomes less soluble and precipitates out of solution.[34,50] Organic acids have this capability at room temperature. The resulting turbidity is roughly proportional to the amount of protein in the specimen.

Reagent. Sulfosalicylic acid (SSA) solution is the reagent needed. Bumintest, a commercially available tablet test system, is convenient to use.[50] These tablets, containing SSA and sodium bicarbonate (an effervescent base) are dissolved in distilled water to prepare a 5 percent stable solution (store at room temperature).

Method. To urine, clarified by centrifugation, add an equal amount of sulfosalicylic acid reagent. Mix well. Observe the degree of turbidity compared to an aliquot of the original clarified specimen. Report results as negative, trace, or 1+ to 4+ based on comparison to prepared standards of known concentration.[50]

Sensitivity. Concentrations as low as 5 to 10 mg of protein/dl may be detected.[33,34,50] High levels of detergents in the urine specimen or a highly buffered alkaline urine may decrease the test sensitivity and give false negative results.

Specificity. The test is specific for albumin as well as globulins, Bence-Jones proteins, and glucoproteins.[13,24,33,34,50] The presence of x-ray contrast media and metabolites of the drug tolbutamide may cause false positive results.

Comments. Usually the specific gravity of urine containing contrast media is greater than 1.050, and unusual crystals are seen in the urine sediment.[13,24] A check with the ward will usually confirm that the patient has recently undergone a diagnostic procedure, such as an IVP (intravenous pyelogram). Another specimen should be requested, but remember that the effects of the radiocontrast dye can persist for several days and that the colorimetric reagent strip system is not affected. While the sulfosalicylic turbidimetric method will detect Bence-Jones protein in urine in most instances, the best method available at present is by protein electrophoresis where the appearance of a distinct homogeneous protein band in the globulin region is diagnostic.

Glucose and Other Reducing Substances

Test Principle. The test is based on the classic Benedict's copper reduction reaction.[51] Reducing substances if present in the urine specimen will react with the copper sulfate reagent, and the blue cupric sulfate is subsequently reduced to cuprous oxide. The resultant color change from blue through green to orange is proportional to the amount of reducing substance.

Reagent. Clinitest, a tablet test system, is composed of several dual-function reactive ingredients: copper sulfate, sodium hydroxide, sodium carbonate, and citric acid.[51] The

sodium hydroxide provides the alkaline pH necessary for the reaction. The combination of the sodium hydroxide, citric acid, and added water provides heat for the reaction. The sodium carbonate and citric acid are necessary to dissolve the tablet.

Method. The test consists of dispensing the specified number of drops of urine (2 or 5) into a test tube, adding 10 drops of water and then a reaction tablet. Fifteen seconds after the boiling reaction ceases, the test tube is gently shaken, and the color of the reaction mixture is compared to the color chart for quantitation of results. The color chart specific for the 2-drop or 5-drop method must be used.[51,52]

Sensitivity. The lower limit of detection is 13.9 mmole/L (250 mg/dl) of glucose, and the accuracy is reported to be plus or minus one color block.[51]

Specificity. The test is not specific only for glucose but will also react with any reducing sugar, such as galactose, fructose, lactose, maltose, or pentose.[13,24,38,51,53] Various drugs, such as ascorbic acid (a reducing substance) and nalidixic acid if present in high concentration, may cause false positive reactions as will homogentisic acid, which is excreted in high concentrations in the inherited disease, alkaptonuria. Creatinine and uric acid, which have no effect on the glucose oxidase reagent strip system, may also cause a false positive reaction with the copper reduction system.

Comments. With both the 5-drop standard method, which measures glucose concentrations up to 111 mmole/L (2 g/dl), and the 2-drop modified procedure, which extends the quantitation range up to 278 mmole/L (5 g/dl), it is very important to observe the solution color change while the boiling reaction occurs. This is because urine with large concentrations of sugar present can exhibit the so-called pass-through phenomenon in which there is a rapid color change to orange and then a reversal back to a brown color which can cause an underestimation of the amount of reducing substance actually present.

The presence of a high concentration of protein will extend the boiling reaction time and increase foam formation, which may interfere with visual comparison to the color chart. However, the addition of a drop of a surface active agent (octyl or caprylic alcohol) to the urine prior to adding the reagent tablet will prevent excessive foaming.[24]

Clinitest tablets contain acid and alkali which interact in the presence of water. Therefore, the tablets, which are stable if kept dry, must be protected even from ambient moisture. Tablets that have absorbed moisture turn a speckled blue color. One alternative for the bulk bottled tablets is to use tablets that are individually packaged in foil.

Bilirubin

Test Principle. The test is based on the diazotization coupling reaction.[54] If bilirubin is present in the urine, it will react to produce a blue or purple color, the intensity of which is proportional to the amount present.

Reagent. Ictotest, a tablet test system, contains the reactive ingredients *p*-nitro-benzenediazonium *p*-toluene-sulfonate, sulfosalicylic acid, and effervescent base.[54]

Method. Five drops of urine are dispensed onto an absorbent asbestos mat supplied with the kit. A reagent tablet is then placed onto the moistened area and two drops of water dispensed so it flows over the edges of the tablet. The color change of the mat around the tablet is observed (read at 30 seconds). A blue or purple color indicates bilirubin (ignore any pink or red color).[54]

Specificity. The test is specific for bilirubin, but pyridium drug metabolites may mask the reaction of small amounts of bilirubin and give a bright red-orange color.[24,54] If present in large amounts, phenothiazine metabolites (Chlorpromazine) may cause a false positive result.

Sensitivity. The level of detection is as low as 0.85 to 1.7 μmole/L (0.05 to 0.1 mgdl) bilirubin and is therefore more sensitive than the reagent strip system.[24,54] The product itself is particularly labile and must be protected from light, excessive heat, and moisture which can alter its reactivity. It is important also to examine only fresh urine specimens as bilirubin is rapidly decomposed if subject to light or heat.

Comments. Free and Free[3,24] have suggested a wash-through technique to distinguish color reactions due to drug metabolites. Basically duplicate tests are conducted except that 10 drops of water are added to one of the mats to wash away any drug after the urine has been absorbed. The test is then completed in the regular manner. The color reaction of the wash-through mat is compared to the other mat. If the color is significantly lightened or has disappeared, the reaction is probably due to a drug but not bilirubin (bilirubin will stay absorbed to the mat surface).

THE URINARY SEDIMENT IN HEALTH AND DISEASE

In recent years, especially in light of increased awareness of added health care cost without comparable patient benefits, there has been considerable debate on the value of the microscopic examination of urinary sediment and its diagnostic yield after a negative macroscopic analysis.[7–9,55–57] Schumann and associates,[11] after an extensive prospective/retrospective study, concluded that the routine microscopic examination of urine specimens from asymptomatic individuals, which are macroscopically normal, is time-consuming and unnecessary. Results of their study revealed that there was less than a 3 percent diagnostic yield, i.e., clinically significant positive findings in macroscopically negative specimens examined microscopically. However, Schreiner has said, "In our own clinical experience, no other single laboratory or diagnostic procedure of any kind has yielded such a high percentage of positive results such as the microscopic examination of urine."[58]*

In any case, the evaluation and subsequent clinical interpretation of the microscopic findings depend ultimately on the accurate recognition and quantitation of the formed elements, such as cells and casts, found during the examination of the urine sediment. This in turn requires technical expertise, time, and experience acquired through proper training and many hours at the microscope studying urinary sediments.

Unfortunately, urine microscopy itself is still an ill-defined technique. Whereas most tests performed in the modern clinical laboratory have been carefully controlled and standardized, there is no established standard method to perform the microscopic examination of urinary sediment. There are so many variables inherent in the current methods (variation in amount of urine centrifuged, time and speed of centrifugation, amount of sediment examined) that it is difficult if not impossible to obtain good precision and accuracy.

Consequently, several clinical investigators[1,59-61] have stressed that the microscopic examination of urine must be done using scientific techniques and that normal values must be established if urinalysis is to continue to be an important laboratory test. As Kesson has expressed it, "Attitudes towards routine microscopic examination as a diagnostic tool . . . are ambivalent. On one hand too much reliance is placed on techniques which are often unscientific or unspecified; on the other, the results of the examination are regarded as imprecise and therefore of little value."[60]†

Winkel et al[62] have evaluated the precision of routine urine microscopy for counting cells using a statistical technique known as "multifactorial experimental design." They examined the contribution of the technologist preparing the specimen and reading the sediment, the time elapsed between specimen receipt and processing of the urine, and the effect of the particular microscope used. They found that the significant variation in results obtained was due to variation in the preparation techniques of the sediment used by the different technologists. Their study demonstrated statistically that the examination of urine for cellular elements is more imprecise than is generally known and that the technique (urine sediment preparation) must be standardized.

Preparation of Urine for Microscopic Examination of Sediment

As mentioned previously there is no standard method as yet for the preparation of urine for microscopic analysis. The technique varies between clinical laboratories and sometimes even within the same laboratory. The single most important factor in the preparation of a urine specimen for sediment examination is consistency. A suggested procedure for the routine clinical laboratory is as follows[1,13,16,56]:

1. Thoroughly mix a fresh, midstream urine specimen to resuspend the sediment. Ideally the urine should be less than one hour old. If the urine cannot be processed immediately, it should be refrigerated and/or a preservative added to maintain the integrity of such formed elements as casts. However, if a preservative is used, the specimen should be first divided into two aliquots—one for chemical analysis, since some preservatives interfere with chemical tests, and another for sediment examination. A first morning specimen, because it is more concentrated, is also recommended.

2. Pour 10 ml of the specimen into a graduated, conical centrifuge tube.

3. Centrifuge the urine for 5 minutes at 400 × gravity. (It is not correct to ex-

*Copyright 1961 Ciba Pharmaceutical Company Division of Ciba-Geigy Corporation. Reprinted with permission from Clinical Symposia by George E. Schreiner, MD.

†Kesson AM, et al.: Microscopic examination of urine. Lancet 2:810, 1978. Permission from The Lancet, London.

press centrifugation speeds in rpm's only, unless the centrifuges used have the same rotating radius.)

4. Decant 9 ml of the supernate and resuspend the sediment in the remaining 1 ml using a pipette. This equals a tenfold concentration.

5. Place one drop of the resuspended sediment on a clean, labeled glass slide and coverslip (use 22 × 22 mm square coverglass). Avoid bubbles, do not add too much specimen, and do not allow the wet mount to dry before completing the examination. (A commercial system for standardized urinalysis, the Kova system,* is available. It provides a complete system which includes a graduated centrifuge tube, transfer pipette, stain, and a special plastic microscope slide with covered examination areas of exact depth.)

6. Examine the mount using the 10× objective and 10× ocular to obtain an overall view of the sediment. The area viewed in this way is a low power field. Scan the perimeter of the coverglass, since casts in particular have a tendency to localize along the edges. Read at least 10 low power fields and enumerate and average those elements (casts, crystals, and miscellaneous structures) reported per low power field. Identify and grade each cast type separately. Normal crystals can be reported as few, moderate, or many per low power field, but abnormal crystals should be quantified. Squamous epithelial cells are reported as few, moderate, or many per low power field.

7. Switch to the high power objective (44×) and count cells (RBC, WBC, and so on) seen in 10 fields. Report the average per high power field. Structures that can be identified correctly under high power, such as parasites or ova and bacteria, can be reported as few, moderate, or many. The type of cast is also identified under high

*ICL Scientific, Fountain Valley, California.

power. Remember to constantly adjust the fine focus of the microscope in order to examine several planes of the specimen. A reporting scale based on averaging the elements seen in 10 representative fields is shown in Table 5.3.

Microscopic Techniques Used in Urinary Sediment Examination

Brightfield Microscopy. The traditional method used to examine urine sediment routinely is conventional brightfield microscopy of an unstained, wet mount preparation which depends on amplitude modulation in the specimen to delineate detail.[63–65] Cellular elements are fairly easy to identify. However, formed elements such as casts, which are very important to recognize, are the most difficult to see because the cast matrix has a similar refractive index to the urine liquid medium itself, and hence they are barely visible.

In order to increase optical contrast, the microscopist usually lowers the substage condenser, stops down the condenser iris diaphragm and views the sediment under reduced light. With this method, visibility, particularly of casts, is increased somewhat. However, maximum specimen definition has been sacrificed, and it is still difficult for even an experienced examiner of urine sediment to distinguish between bacteria and amorphous crystals or to see nuclear detail necessary to distinguish white blood cells or renal tubular epithelial cells, for example.

To further facilitate the identification of cells and casts using brightfield microscopy, urinary sediments are sometimes stained with dyes. This enhances their light absorption characteristics and contrast in relation to the background illumination. Sternheimer[66] published a report on an improved supravital diagnostic staining method that is rapid yet simple enough to be used for routine urinalysis and screening procedures. The stain used is a mixture of a copperphthalocyanine dye, National fast blue, and pyronin B, a red xanthene dye. It is particularly useful in the differentiation of polymorphonuclear leukocytes from lympho-

TABLE 5.3. GRADING SYSTEM OF THE URINARY SEDIMENT

Constituent	Negative	Occasional	1+	2+	3+	4+
RBC/high-power field	0	Less than 4	4–8	8–30	Greater than 30, less than packed	Packed field
WBC/high-power field	0	Less than 5	5–20	20–50	Greater than 50, less than packed	Packed field
Casts/low-power field	0	Less than 1	1–5	4–10	10–30	Greater than 30
Abnormal crystals/ low-power field	0	Less than 1	1–5	4–10	10–30	Greater than 30

This grading system applies to a microscope field viewed with the usual 10× eyepiece and the 10× and 44× objectives lenses. The appropriate diameters of such a field under low and high power are 1.5 and 0.35 mm, respectively. A correction should be applied when a microscope with a different-sized field is used in order to maintain consistency in the reporting of results.
From Linne JJ, Ringsrund KM: Basic Laboratory Techniques for the Medical Laboratory Technician, 1970, p 259. Courtesy of McGraw-Hill Book Company.

cytes and renal tubular epithelial cells and the recognition of malignant cells. It also stains casts and their inclusions.

"A standardized brightfield microscopic examination of urine sediment is quite useful in mass screening, but for symptomatic patients and/or urine sediments that contain unidentifiable mononuclear cells, further investigations using special techniques are indicated."[61]* Therefore, Schumann et al[61,67,68] have recommended a combined cytocentrifugation/stain technique which they feel is diagnostically more sensitive and specific. Briefly, their technique involves centrifuging urine and using the resuspended sediment to prepare slides, which are then fixed and stained by the classic Papanicolaou technique. In addition to the preservation of cytologic elements and casts, the method also has several technical advantages including a standardized technique and a permanent slide preparation. Even urinary crystals can be identified.

Phase Contrast Microscopy. As mentioned under the discussion of the brightfield

*Schumann G, Henry JB: An improved technique for the evaluation of urine sediment. Lab Management 15:24, 1977.

examination of urinary sediment, details of formed elements such as casts and cells are difficult to distinguish. Therefore, some clinical laboratories today routinely use phase contrast microscopy to study unstained sediments.[10,64,65,69]

A phase contrast microscope is basically a brightfield microscope with two additional parts: an annular stop in the condenser matched to a phase-retarding ring or plate in the appropriate objective. Specimen details are made visible by optical staining, i.e., invisible phase differences are changed into visible amplitude or intensity differences which can be detected by the human eye. In the phase contrast method, the specimen requires essentially no preparation.

Differential Interference Contrast Microscopy. Interference contrast microscopy is another relatively new technique that has been used in urine sediment examination.[64,65,70,71] Its function is similar to that of phase contrast, i.e., to define detail in specimens lacking contrast in brightfield. Differential interference contrast provides the viewer with a relief image, giving a three-dimensional impression. Its main application has been to study the structural details of formed elements. Interference contrast microscopes are quite expensive, and therefore the method has not been used routinely.

Polarization Microscopy. A very useful additional microscopic technique frequently used is polarized light.[10,13,64,65] It is helpful particularly in the identification of certain crystals and doubly refractile oval fat bodies and fat droplets. While special polarizing microscopes with rotating specimen stages are available, any brightfield microscope can easily be adapted for polarized light examinations by the addition of two simple polarizing filters, an analyzer located usually in the ocular and a polarizer placed in the optical light path below the specimen in a filter holder in the condenser or positioned on top of the light source.

The basic principle underlying polarized light microscopy is that natural light oscillates at random in all directions or planes at right angles to the line of propagation. However, light, after passing through a polarizing filter, is oriented in one plane in the direction of the filter. If two such filters are oriented or positioned at right angles to each other, no light can pass through and the field is dark. However, if a birefringent or anisotropic specimen is placed between the crossed polarizers, it has the effect of uncrossing the filters, and a bright image of the specimen is seen.

Identification of Formed Elements in the Organized Urinary Sediment

"The primary objective of (the) microscopic examination of urine sediment is to define the cellular elements which have entered the urinary tract, to identify casts and the elements included in them as they (casts) are formed in the tubules (of the kidney) . . . a secondary objective is to identify crystals of metabolic or drug origin which may be of significance."[3]* The urinary sediment includes a great variety of solid elements, the

so-called formed elements, suspended in the urine. Certain constituents are normally found, but the presence of others is always abnormal. Therefore, it is important to learn to correctly identify and quantify both the normal and the abnormal constituents. Usually the normal formed elements are easy to recognize. Hence, care must be taken when examining the urine sediment that these normal elements do not mask detection of the abnormal constituents. The formed elements in the urinary sediment will often give the clinician valuable information about the kidneys and the urinary tract. In addition, the microscopic examination of the sediment can help to confirm the physicochemical findings. For instance, a positive chemical test for protein is often accompanied by the presence of casts in the sediment.

The various urinary sediment constituents may be classified into two broad categories: the organized sediment and the unorganized sediment.[16] The organized sediment refers to those structures that are of biologic origin, e.g., cells, casts, microorganisms. The unorganized sediment refers to the constituents of chemical origin, i.e., crystals and amorphous material. A miscellaneous group includes artifacts and contaminants in the urine (Table 5.4).

Cells. The examination of urinary sediment for cellular constituents is the most important part of the microscopic examination. Cells are estimated per field in most routine urinalyses, although a differential count and quantitative evaluation of granulocytes, mononuclear leukocytes, and renal epithelial cells have been reported,[72] and enumeration of cells has been done for many years by the Addis count.[73]

Red Blood Cells. Erythrocytes or red blood cells are one of the formed elements found in urine.[4,13,64,67] In a fresh urine specimen, they appear as pale, gray, smooth, anucleate, biconcave discs, measuring $7\ \mu$ in diameter. However, red blood cells rapidly undergo morphologic alteration in urine, and their

*Reprinted with permission from Free AH, Free HM: Urinalysis in Clinical Laboratory Practice. Copyright The Chemical Rubber Co, CRC Press, Inc.

TABLE 5.4. IDENTIFICATION OF SELECTED ELEMENTS FOUND IN URINARY SEDIMENT

Cell	Morphologic Features	Source	Differentiating Characteristics
Red blood cell (RBC)	Pale gray, biconcave disc in fresh unstained urine, faint colorless rings in old urine (hemoglobin dissolved out, membrane remains), 6-7 μ in diameter, may appear swollen and rounded in dilute urine or crenated and shrunken (with little spicules) in concentrated urine	Entire genitourinary tract	Lysed by 2% acetic acid, eosinophilic nonnucleated cells
White blood cell (WBC)	About 2× RBC (10-12 μ in diameter), spherical with characteristic cytoplasmic granulation and lobulated nucleus; cytoplasmic granules exhibit brownian movement when cells swell in hypotonic urine—glitter cells	Throughout genitourinary tract	Nuclei accentuated by acetic acid treatment, crystal violet/safranin stain—nuclei red-purple, cytoplasm violet to purple granularity

(Continued)

appearance is greatly influenced by the concentration of the urine. Notice the different sizes and shapes of the red blood cells in a urinary sediment, as shown in Figure 5.1 C.

In a dilute or hypotonic urine specimen (low specific gravity), the erythrocytes appear swollen and rounded. In old dilute urine with a specific gravity less than 1.005, they often appear as faint circles and are commonly referred to as shadow or ghost cells. This is because the cells have lysed to release their hemoglobin content, and all that remains is the colorless cell membrane.

In a hypertonic urine specimen (specific gravity of around 1.020 or greater), the red blood cells will appear crenated and shrunken in size and may possibly be confused with small white blood cells. However, the white blood cells are slightly larger, have a nucleus, and are granular in appearance. A drop of 2 percent acetic acid added to the mount will lyse the red blood cells and accentuate the nuclei of the white blood cells if differentiation needs to be confirmed.

Erythrocytes are often confused with other structures found in the sediment, particularly oil droplets and yeast cells. Yeast cells, however, are generally smaller than red blood cells, are ovoid in shape, show considerable size variation, and usually demonstrate budding (Figs. 5.1 F and 5.1 G). Acetic acid treatment can again be used to distinguish between the two. Erythrocytes are lysed in the acidified preparation, whereas the yeast cells will remain. Oil droplets of renal origin or as contaminants exhibit a great size variation and are more refractile than are red blood cells.

Red blood cells as well as white blood cells are found in even normal urine in small numbers. Exactly how these cells enter the urine and the line between physiologic or normal numbers and abnormal values is still under debate because of the nonstandardized methods used to prepare urine for sediment examination.[56] Freni et al[44] have drawn this level at about 2,000 RBC/ml, which corresponds in their laboratory to

TABLE 5.4 (Cont.)

Cell	Morphologic Features	Source	Differentiating Characteristics
Epithelial cells Renal tubular (RTE)	Granular cell with single, large, round or oval nucleus, cell slightly larger than WBC but usually less than 15 μ in diameter, nuclear to cytoplasmic ratio approximately 1:1	Renal parenchyma (tubules of nephron)	Not lysed by acetic acid, nucleus frequently eccentrically located
Squamous	Large flat cells (30-50 μ in diameter) with abundant cytoplasm and single, distinct, small, centrally located nucleus, margins often folded	Terminal third of urethra, in females line vagina also	Crystal violet/safranin stain—purple nucleus with cytoplasm pink to violet
Transitional	Cells with round or pear-shaped contours and round, centrally located nucleus, may have tail-like processes, 2-4× WBC diameter	Epithelium lining renal pelvis and calices, ureter, bladder and proximal two thirds of urethra	Crystal violet/safranin stain—dark blue nucleus with pale blue cytoplasm
Free fat droplets/ oval fat bodies	Free fat—spherical globules of varying size, yellowish brown, high refractive index; oval fat bodies—clusters of lipid-filled globules in RTE cells, cell outline frequently obscured	Lipids leaked from damaged glomeruli, free or absorbed by RTE cells, rare cases — exposed fatty marrow due to major skeletal trauma	Polarized light microscopy: anisotropic cholesterol lipids exhibit birefringence (maltese cross forms), fat stain positive (necessary to demonstrate presence of isotropic triglycerides)
Yeast	Typically ovoid, smooth, colorless, variable in size (3-5 μ), frequently budding or branching forms seen	Common skin or air contaminant, seen in some urinary tract infections	Not lysed by acetic acid, does not stain with eosin
Bacteria	Very small rods or cocci, occur singly or in chains	Contaminant or throughout genitourinary tract in infections	Gram stain (positive or negative), often motile

about 8 RBC/high-power field as performed by conventional urinalysis.

The presence of erythrocytes in the urine especially in a female can be due to contamination. However, the detection of true hematuria is an important laboratory finding. Elevated numbers of red blood cells may be found in the urine in diseases of the kidney and the lower urinary tract or associated with diseases that are not of renal origin, i.e., extrarenal.

White Blood Cells. White blood cells or leukocytes can usually be recognized by their granular appearance and characteristic nuclei.[4,13,64,67,74] They are spherical in shape and about 12 μ in diameter. These features can be seen in Figures 5.1 A and 5.1 B. As mentioned previously, in an unstained wet mount, nuclear detail can be enhanced by acidification.

The morphology of white blood cells is influenced by the concentration of the urine. In dilute or hypotonic urine, the cells swell and their internal cytoplasmic granules may exhibit brownian movement. These are the so-called glitter cells. At one time, this phenomenon was thought to be pathognomonic for pyelonephritis, but these cells are now known to occur in many other conditions. White blood cells are also rapidly lysed in hypotonic urine, and within two to three hours around 50 percent are destroyed.

Elevated numbers of leukocytes in the urine (pyuria) indicate inflammation and are associated with certain renal diseases and diseases of the urinary tract. While most laboratories still report WBC/high-power field seen in a centrifuged urine specimen, Musher and associates[75] have advocated the quantitative analysis of uncentrifuged urine specimens using a hemacytometer counting chamber for diagnosing urinary tract infections. They argue that the major source of error comes from the variability of the amount of urine centrifuged and the volume used to resuspend the sediment and that accurate quantitation is therefore not possible. Alwall,[59] however, in a reappraisal of the usual routine microscopic method to evaluate pyuria,

demonstrated that the determination of WBC/high-power field can be a reliable indicator if a standardized technique is used to prepare the urine for sediment examination.

The types of leukocytes present in the urine may be differentiated. For example, eosinophils[74] and plasma cells[76] have been reported in addition to neutrophils and mononuclear leukocytes.[72] Differentiation of urinary white cells is uncommon except in research or cytopathology laboratories.

Epithelial Cells. Squamous epithelial cells or pavement cells which line the structures that make up the lower genitourinary tract are usually of little clinical significance when found in the urine.[4,13,64,67,77] They often appear in specimens from female patients due to vaginal contamination. They are flat cells, large enough to be seen easily under low power. Squamous cells have abundant cytoplasm and a small, distinct, centrally located nucleus. They sometimes appear rolled up and might be mistaken for a cast. Their presence in large numbers is frequently a complicating factor in reading a urine sediment accurately. A squamous epithelial cell may be seen in the top center portion of Figure 5.1 R.

Transitional epithelial cells (two to four times the size of WBCs) which line the upper parts of the urinary tract are also present. They have a round, centrally located nucleus and are characteristically pear-shaped. They may have tail-like processes, in which case they are called "caudate cells." Their presence in small numbers (few) in urine reflects normal desquamation, but when they are seen in large numbers or sheets, a pathologic process may be indicated.

Renal tubular epithelial cells (RTE) which line the nephron tubules may also be seen in small numbers (occasional) in a normal urine sediment. They are slightly larger than white blood cells (approximately one-third larger) and have a single large nucleus frequently eccentrically located (Figs. 5.1 D and 5.1 E). Since they represent actual renal exfoliation, the presence of more than 15 in 10 high power fields suggests renal tubular damage and in the case of transplant patients is evidence for allograft rejection.[78]

Considerable difficulty exists in the accurate identification of renal tubular cells, particularly in distinguishing them from other mononuclear cells commonly found in urine using brightfield microscopy alone. Therefore, Schumann et al[67] have suggested the use of cytocentrifugation/stain techniques.

Oval Fat Bodies. Oval fat bodies are renal tubular cells that are filled with absorbed lipids or that have undergone degenerative changes.[79,80] (Note the refractile lipids in the tubular epithelial cells in Figure 5.1 E.) The use of polarized light microscopy is useful in the identification of the cholesterol esters in the fat. When viewed under polarized light, they exhibit the so-called maltese cross formation, i.e., shining crosses against a dark background. However, if the fat contains primarily triglycerides, special oil stains, such as Sudan III or oil red O are required (triglycerides are isotropic not birefringent and hence do not polarize).

Oval fat bodies are often associated with free-floating fat droplets in the urine. Fat is also sometimes seen incorporated into the matrix of casts. Lipiduria, the presence of lipids in urine, indicates a serious pathologic condition and is characteristic of the nephrotic syndrome. It may, however, occur in patients who have suffered major skeletal trauma.

Other Cells. Histiocytes,[67] exfoliated neoplastic cells,[81,82] platelets,[83] and viral inclusion cells[84] have also been identified in urine sediment. For routine screening the conventional microscopic examination is still valid, but for the accurate identification and evaluation of these type of cells, Schumann and others[61,67,68] have recommended the adoption of specialized techniques, such as the cytocentrifugation/Papanicolaou stain method.

Bacteria. Normal urine is sterile and does not contain any microorganisms. The presence of a few bacteria, due to contamination during collection, is found in most urine specimens, particularly if the specimen has been allowed to sit any length of time before processing, and therefore is not of clinical significance. However, the presence of elevated numbers of bacteria (more than 10^5/ml) in a clean-catch, midstream, or catherized urine specimen is highly suggestive of urinary tract infection.[10,48,75,85,86] This number corresponds to 10 or more bacteria per high power field. Bacteria may be seen as very small, faint bodies in the background of Figures 5.1 A and 5.1 B.

Significant bacteriuria is usually accomplished by pyuria (increased numbers of leukocytes). In an unstained sediment bacteria appear as small gray rods or cocci and, in some instances, may be misidentified as amorphous crystals. Bacteriuria should, therefore, be further studied by special staining and plating techniques (culture and sensitivity) to identify and quantify the causative organism.

Yeast. Yeast or fungi are not an unusual finding in urinary sediment.[4,67] They are usually of the *Candida* species (*Candida albicans*) and may be found in patients with urinary tract infections, vaginitis, or diabetes mellitus. Yeast, which is similar in appearance, may be confused with red blood cells particularly under low power. However, they have various distinguishing characteristics, such as variability in size, oval shape, and a higher refractive index than red blood cells. Branching mycelia or budding forms may be noted. Yeast are not lysed by acids and are slightly smaller (3 to 5 μ in diameter) than erythrocytes. Yeast cells, individual oval shapes and budding forms, are seen in profusion in Figures 5.1 F and 5.1 G. Generally, whenever yeast is found in the microscopic examination of the sediment, only a few cells are seen in any one field.

Parasites and Ova. The presence of animal parasites in urine usually indicates vaginal or fecal contamination.[13,64,67] The most frequently identified parasite in urine in North America is *Trichomonas vaginalis hominis.* In a

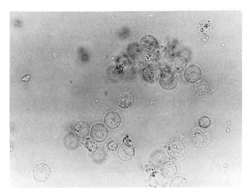

A. White blood cells. Brightfield. ×290.

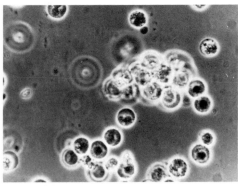

B. White blood cells. Phase contrast. ×290.

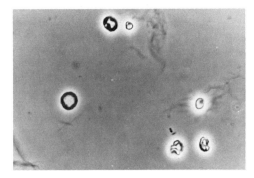

C. Red blood cells. Phase contrast. ×460.

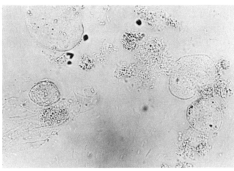

D. Degenerated epithelial cells—oval fat body. Brightfield. ×720.

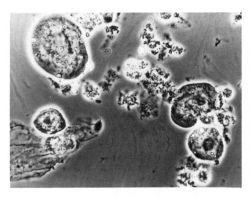

E. Degenerated epithelial cells—oval fat body. Phase contrast. ×720.

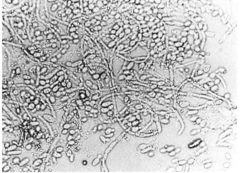

F. Yeast. Brightfield. ×320.

Figure 5.1. Urine sediment constituents (cells, parasites, casts). Several of the objects (in unstained sediment) are shown using brightfield and phase contrast microscopy to illustrate the enhancement of detail using phase. (Courtesy of Jose M. Trujillo, M.D., Department of Laboratory Medicine, The University of Texas M.D. Anderson Hospital at Houston. Object selection by Phyllis Sedgwick, B.S., MT(ASCP), photography by John Kuykendall.)

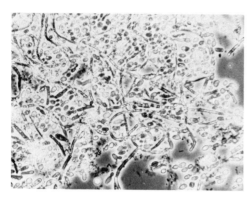

G. Yeast. Phase contrast. ×320.

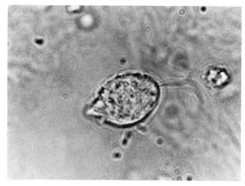

H. *Trichomonas vaginalis.* Brightfield. ×1115.

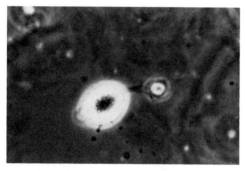

I. *Trichomonas vaginalis.* Phase contrast. ×1115.

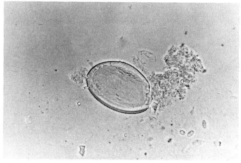

J. *Enterobius vermicularis* (pinworm) ovum. Brightfield. ×250.

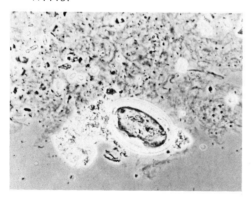

K. *Enterobius vermicularis* (pinworm) ovum. Phase contrast. ×250.

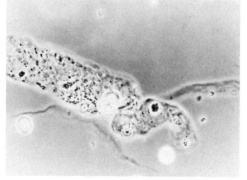

L. Mixed cast. Brightfield. ×450.

Fig. 5.1. *(Cont.)*

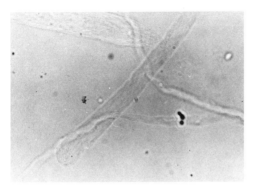

M. Finely granular cast. Brightfield. ×320.

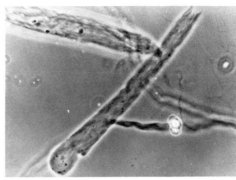

N. Finely granular cast. Phase contrast. ×320.

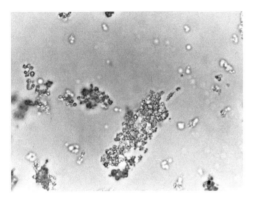

O. Pseudocast comprised of amorphous crystals. Brightfield. ×460.

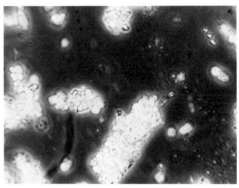

P. Pseudocast comprised of amorphous crystals. Phase contrast. ×460.

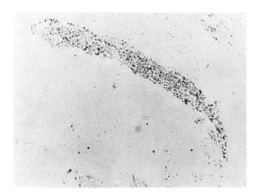

Q. Coarse granular cast. Brightfield. ×250.

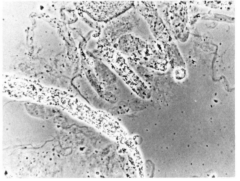

R. Coarse granular cast and epithelial cell. Phase contrast. ×250.

Fig. 5.1. (Cont.)

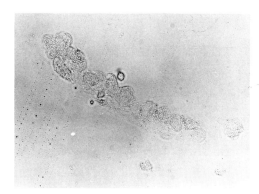

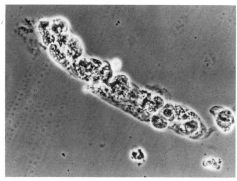

S. Renal tubular epithelial cell cast. Brightfield. ×275.

T. Renal tubular epithelial cell cast. Phase contrast. ×275.

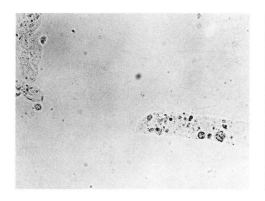

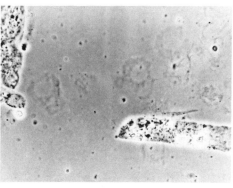

U. Red blood cell cast. Brightfield. ×250.

V. Red blood cell cast. Phase contrast. ×250.

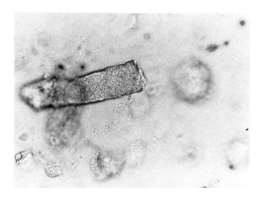

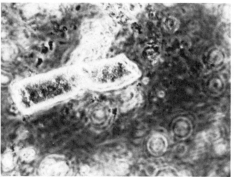

W.Waxy cast. Brightfield. ×290.

X. Waxy cast. Phase contrast. ×290.

Fig. 5.1. (*Cont.*)

fresh urine specimen, it is fairly easy to identify this protozoan, which has a characteristic pear shape and anterior flagella. A trichomonas organism with flagella in motion is shown in Figures 5.1 H and 5.1 I. However, if the trichomonads are not motile, they can easily be mistaken for epithelial or white blood cells. *Trichomonas* is most often found in urine specimens from females as a result of vaginal contamination. However, the parasite can also infect males.

Pinworm ova (eggs of *Enterobius vermicularis*) have also been seen in urine, usually from children, due to fecal contamination. A pinworm ovum is surrounded by a thick two-layered transparent capsule, and a coiled embryo may be visible inside. The egg has an ovoid shape and one side is characteristically flattened. An ovum of *E. vermicularis* is shown in Figures 5.1 J and 5.1 K.

Ova from other parasites that occur very rarely in urine include those of *Schistosoma haematobium* (Egyptian hematuria) which pass from the pelvic veins into the urinary bladder itself. Ova from the other species that cause schistosomiasis (*Schistosoma mansoni* and *Schistosoma japonicum*) more often rupture into the intestinal tract and are passed in the feces. Presence in the urine of ova is, therefore, due to fecal contamination. *Ascaris lumbricoides*, the roundworm species, has been found, as have ova from the hookworm species, *Ancylostoma duodenale* and *Necator americanus*.

Casts. As Schreiner has so aptly stated[58]:

> The imprint of a leaf . . . in the rock gives unmistakable information about the inhabitants of the globe thousands of years ago. Likewise, the appearance of a cast, its size, and its inclusions will offer incontrovertible evidence of the condition of at least one nephron of one kidney just prior to the passage of the urine. Red cells, white cells, bacteria or protein may be added to urine after its formation in the kidney. Casts, on the other hand, are formed only in the kidney. Therefore the contents of a cast are . . . indelibly labeled as originating in the kidney. . . . A cast provides

suggestive evidence of what has gone on before, and even what is likely to happen in the future.*

The absence of casts or the identification of the type of casts if present is, therefore, of special diagnostic importance.[13,64,67,68,71]

Casts, which are formed in the renal tubules from gelled mucoprotein, are cylindrical structures that have parallel sides. They are classified primarily on the basis of morphologic features and include hyaline, granular, cellular, waxy, fatty, and mixed (Table 5.5).

> The appearance of a particular urine cast is dependent upon three factors: 1. The initial composition of the cast (and) any cells or substances present in the lumen of the nephron at the time of glycoprotein gelation . . . (which) will be incorporated into the cast . . . 2. The portion of the nephron and its pathophysiologic status in which the cast was formed . . . (that) will determine the diameter and basic topographic features of the cast as well as whether it is straight or convoluted . . . (and) 3. The length of time the cast is retained in the kidney before being expelled.[87]†

Burton[88] has studied the effects of urinary pH, urine osmolality, and centrifugation time on the number of casts seen in urine sediment. The variables, osmolality and length of centrifugation, did not have any significant effect. However, he found an inverse relationship between the number of casts observed and the pH of the urine, i.e., a decrease in numbers of casts when the pH is elevated. Since the pH of urine rises with time due to growth of urea-splitting bacteria which produce ammonia, it is very important that

*Copyright 1961 Ciba Pharmaceutical Company Division of Ciba-Geigy Corporation. Reprinted with permission from Clinical Symposia by George E. Schreiner, MD.
†Cannon DC: The identification of pathogenesis of urine casts. Lab Med 10:8, 1979. Copyright The American Society of Clinical Pathologists, Denver.

TABLE 5.5. CLASSIFICATION OF CASTS IN THE URINARY SEDIMENT

Type of Cast	Morphologic Features/ Composition	Formation/Pathogenesis Due to	Recommended Type of Microscopy*
Hyaline	Homogeneous, transparent, cylindrical structures with parallel sides and blunt, rounded ends, low refractive index, composed primarily of uromucoid or Tamm-Horsfall mucoprotein, often contains cellular or granular inclusions	Stasis—diminished rate of urine flow, urinary pH (acidic), degree of proteinuria, high solute concentration (may be physiologic)	Ph, DIC
Cellular			
White cell	Semitransparent cylindrical structures filled with WBCs (multilobed nuclei) embedded in Tamm-Horsfall mucoprotein matrix	Inflammatory renal disease with exudation of WBCs into nephron	Ph, DIC
Red cell	Semitransparent cylindrical structures with RBCs in Tamm-Horsfall mucoprotein matrix, may appear brown in color (hemoglobin pigmentation)	Diseases involving renal parenchymaglomerular basement membrane injury, always pathologic and therefore presence is very diagnostically significant	BF, Ph, DIC
Renal tubular epithelial	Semitransparent cylindrical structures filled with renal tubular epithelial cells (single, large round or oval nucleus), Tamm-Horsfall mucoprotein matrix	Extensive sloughing of RTE cells following renal tubular damage	Ph, DIC
			(Continued)

NOTES:
1. The protein matrix of a cast (rarely) may also be composed of amyloid, Bence-Jones protein, or myoglobin.
2. With the exception of broad or renal failure casts which form in the larger collecting tubules, casts usually originate in the distal tubules of the kidney.
3. A mixed or hybrid cast is any combination of the above. It has two distinct portions.
4. Any cast may become bile stained due to absorption of bile pigment in the glomerular filtrate by the protein matrix of the cast.
5. A pseudocast is a group of closely packed RBCs or WBCs, crystals, mucus, or bacteria that resemble a true cast but are not embedded in a proteinaceous matrix.
*For unstained sediment. BF, brightfield; DIC, differential interference contrast; Ph, phase contrast; PL, polarized light.
Adapted from Haber MH: Urine Casts: Their Microscopy and Clinical Significance, 2nd ed, 1976, p 8. Courtesy of American Society of Clinical Pathologists.

TABLE 5.5 (Cont.)

Type of Cast	Morphologic Features/ Composition	Formation/Pathogenesis Due to	Recommended Type of Microscopy
Granular	Cylindrical structures with coarse or fine particles or granules embedded in Tamm-Horsfall mucoprotein matrix, relatively high refractive index	Usually degeneration of cellular casts, granules can be derived from aggregated plasma proteins[91]	BF, Ph, DIC
Waxy	Structures with homogeneous, smooth glassy appearance, opaque with cracked or serrated margins and irregular broken-off ends, high refractive index, Tamm-Horsfall mucoprotein matrix	Advanced progressive degeneration of cellular/granular casts, imply localized nephron obstruction due to severe renal dysfunction	BF, Ph, DIC
Fatty	Transparent cylinder filled with highly refractile lipid globules (oval fat bodies) or droplets in Tamm-Horsfall mucoprotein matrix, cholesterol lipids are birefringent and exhibit maltese cross forms	Autolytic changes in cellular casts, composed of lipid-laden renal tubular epithelial cells	BF, Ph, DIC, PL

urine be examined as soon as possible after collection, especially if casts are to be detected.

The appearance of casts in the urine (cylinduria) is not always indicative of renal disease. In fact, hyaline casts, the most frequently seen casts in the urine sediment, are observed in the urine of normal subjects, and their numbers are greatly increased after strenuous physical exercise.[89] Hence, hyaline casts are sometimes referred to as "physiologic" casts. The matrix of hyaline casts is predominantly Tamm-Horsfall glycoprotein,[31,90] a special material secreted only by the renal tubular epithelial cells. Hyaline casts are colorless, nonrefractile structures, which have a refractive index very similar to urine itself. Hence, using conventional brightfield microscopy on unstained sediment, they are very difficult to recognize. Hyaline casts typi-cally have rounded ends and often have inclusions.

Cellular casts refer to structures that have cells incorporated into a hyaline uromucoid cast matrix. Identification is usually uncomplicated, but when the cells begin to deteriorate due to autolytic action, identification becomes more difficult. For example, when leukocytes, primarily polymorphonuclear neutrophils, are incorporated, a white blood cell cast results. Red blood cell casts have red cells in the matrix. This type of cast is always pathologic and indicates injury to the glomerular basement membrane. If the red cells have degenerated, the casts are granular in appearance with a reddish brown color due to pigmentation by released hemoglobin. A red blood cell cast is shown in Figures 5.1 U and 5.1 V. A distinction between red blood cell casts (casts in which the red cell margins are distinct) and true blood casts (homogeneous casts in which outlines of the cells are not apparent) has been made. However, Cannon[87] feels that this division is arbitrary and recommends that only the terminology "red cell casts" be used.

Renal tubular epithelial cell casts are more difficult to identify and separate from white blood cell casts, particularly if the cells have started to deteriorate and nuclear structure is not discernible. The incorporated renal tubular cells, which have a single large nucleus, are typically arranged in two parallel rows. A renal tubular epithelial cast is shown in Figures 5.1 S and 5.1 T.

While many authorities believe that granular casts (casts with incorporated granules) are derived from cellular casts that have undergone progressive autolytic changes in their transit through the nephron, Rutecki and others[91] feel that this may not necessarily be the case in all instances. Their immunofluorescence investigation confirmed Tamm-Horsfall urinary mucoprotein as the primary cast matrix but showed that the cast granules in the patient specimens they studied were actually aggregated serum proteins. Finely granular and coarsely granular casts are seen in Figures 5.1 M and 5.1 N and 5.1 Q and 5.1 R, respectively.

Granular casts are occasionally seen in normal individuals, particularly in post-stress situations. However, increased numbers of granular casts, divided into coarse and fine granular based on size of the granules, are associated with renal disease.

Waxy casts because of their high refractive index and coloration (yellow-tan), characteristic broken-off ends, and cracked cell margins are easily recognized even in unstained sediments using brightfield microscopy. Brightfield and phase contrast views of a waxy cast are shown in Figures 5.1 W and 5.1 X. Whereas hyaline casts disintegrate rapidly in hypotonic and/or alkaline solutions, waxy casts are quite resistant. They are the final stage in the degeneration of cellular casts (coarsely granular → finely granular → waxy). Waxy casts are also the most frequently seen broad casts (casts with a diameter two to six times that of a regular cast). Their width indicates severe urinary stasis and cast formation in the large collecting tubules. Hence, their presence indicates a very poor prognosis.

Fatty casts have highly refractile fat droplets or globules embedded in a transparent hyaline matrix. The use of polarized light microscopy is particularly useful in the identification of cholesterol esters (this type of fat is doubly refractile and exhibits the characteristic maltese cross formation). However, fat stains are required to confirm the presence of isotropic, nonbirefringent triglycerides. Fatty casts are associated with free floating fat droplets and oval fat bodies.

Mixed casts, as the term implies, are combination casts with two distinct portions, such as cellular and granular. A mixed cast, coarsely granular with white cells, is shown in Figure 5.1 L. Urinary casts as well as cells in the urine can be stained by the absorption of pigments from bile, melanin, hemosiderin, and even some drugs present in the urine.

Pseudocasts refer to castlike structures that may be misidentified as true casts. They are comprised of aggregated groups of cells, bacteria, or crystals which however are not embedded in a mucoprotein matrix. Pseudocasts are shown in Figures 5.1 O and 5.1 P. Other structures commonly confused with casts by an inexperienced microscopist include mucous threads, rolled-up epithelial cells, hair and fibers, scratches on the coverglass, and even mycelia of fungi.

Identification of Formed Elements in the Unorganized Urinary Sediment

Crystals. The presence of crystals in urine (crystalluria) is usually of little clinical significance, and a variety of different kinds of crystals are commonly found in urine sediment.[12,13,64,67] It is important to learn to differentiate these normal crystals from those associated only with pathologic conditions, e.g., cystine crystals in cystinuria. In some instances, the appearance of the usually nonpathologic crystals may also be a significant finding (calcium oxalate crystals in oxalosis). The presence of amorphous crystals, in particular, can obscure or be confused with other elements of clinical importance.

Crystals are not usually present in freshly voided urine but form after the urine is allowed to stand. In effect, they are an artifact of collection where changes in pH, temperature, and other factors alter the solubility characteristics of the salts. The solutes precipitate out of the supersaturated solution, and crystal formation occurs. The type of crystal that is found depends primarily on pH, and certain types of urinary crystals are therefore associated with a urine of a particular pH.

Urine pH, morphology, color, refractile properties, and solubility characteristics of the crystals present are important in the identification of the particular crystal type. Brightfield microscopy can be used to identify most of the common crystalline forms, but the addition of polarized light capability is very helpful. Tables 5.6 and 5.7 give urine pH, morphology, and solubility characteristics associated with commonly encountered crystals.

Crystals Found in Normal Urine. Common crystals present in normal acid urine include uric acid crystals, amorphous urates, and calcium oxalate. Uric acid crystals are rather pleomorphic and occur in a variety of shapes, such as rhombic prisms, rosettes, and irregular plates. Rhombic crystals of uric acid are shown in Figures 5.2 E and 5.2 F. When examined under polarized light, they exhibit many interference colors. Uric acid crystals are stained by the absorption of urinary pigments and under brightfield illumination look yellow or brown. Urates appear in the urine primarily as amorphous crystals (very fine granules) also colored by urinary pigments. They are responsible for the pink sediment sometimes noted after centrifugation of the urine or in a specimen that has been refrigerated and the sediment has settled by gravity.

The most common form of calcium oxalate is small, colorless octahedrons, and because of their shape they are sometimes referred to as "envelope crystals" (Fig. 5.2 I). They ap-

pear also in the rarer hempseed form, a monohydrate of calcium oxalate.[92] Calcium oxalate crystals are also found in urine of neutral pH.

Common crystals found in normal alkaline urine include ammonium biurate (Fig. 5.2 K) and calcium carbonate (Fig. 5.2 H). Ammonium biurate crystals are small, yellow-brown crystals with irregular spines (thorn apple crystals). They can also occur without spines and then may be confused with yeast or leucine crystals. Calcium carbonate crystals are small, colorless crystals, dumbbell in shape. These small crystals in the presence of triple phosphate crystals are seen in Figure 5.2 H.

Amorphous phosphates, triple phosphates, and calcium phosphate crystals are found in either alkaline or neutral pH urine. Amorphous phosphates appear as colorless, granular masses and account for the white precipitate sometimes seen after centrifugation of the urine. Triple phosphate crystals (ammonium-magnesium phosphate) are commonly colorless prisms (so-called coffin lids). Prisms of triple phosphate crystals are seen in Figures 5.2 A and 5.2 B. Calcium hydrogen phosphates are less common crystals and are star-shaped or long, thin prisms or plates.

Abnormal Crystals Found in Urine. Abnormal crystals associated with liver and congenital metabolic diseases are usually found in urine with an acidic or neutral pH. They do not disappear if the urine is reheated to 37C as will most of the other normal crystals. Whereas crystals normally found in urinary sediment can be reported based solely on morphology, any abnormal crystals should be confirmed by special chemical tests before they are reported.

Bilirubin crystals, found in patients with bilirubinuria, can appear as rhombic plates, granules, or needles that are red-brown in color. They are birefringent under polarized light and may color uric acid crystals if present.

Cystine crystals,[93,94] which may be confused with uric acid crystals, appear as color-

TABLE 5.6. CRYSTALS FOUND IN NORMAL URINE

Urine pH	Morphology	Solubility Characteristics
ACID		
Calcium oxalate	Small, colorless octahedron common; dumbbell, ring form "envelope" crystal	Soluble in dilute HCL
Urates	1. Yellow, calcium, magnesium, and potassium, mostly amorphous	Soluble in alkali, soluble at 60C
	2. Potassium, small, spherical, brown	Soluble at 60C
	3. Sodium acid urate, colorless, needles or amorphous	Soluble at 60C
Uric Acid	Yellow, red-brown, large variety of crystals — rhombic, four-sided plates, rosettes. Colorless, smaller crystals. Pleomorphic	Soluble in alkali. Insoluble in alcohol, acids
NEUTRAL		
Calcium carbonate		
Calcium oxalate		
Phosphates: ammonium magnesium and calcium hydrogen*		
Urates: ammonium		
ALKALINE		
Calcium carbonate	Small, colorless dumbbells or spheres; rarely needles	Soluble in acetic acid with effervescence
Calcium oxalate (slight)		
Phosphates	Ammonium Magnesium	
Ammonium magnesium (triple phosphate)	Common form. Colorless, three to six-sided prisms, "coffin lid." Sometimes fern leaf	Soluble in dilute acetic acid
Calcium hydrogen	Less common. Star-shaped or long, thin prisms; needles or occasional plates	Soluble in dilute acetic acid
Urates	Ammonium, thorn apple, brown	Soluble at 60C with acetic acid; soluble strong alkali

*Also in acid urine—slight
Adapted from Bradley M, et al: Examination of urine. In Henry JB (ed): Todd-Sanford-Davidson Clinical Diagnosis and Management by Laboratory Methods, 16th ed. Philadelphia, Saunders, 1979, p 624. Used by permission.

less, highly refractile hexagonal plates (Fig. 5.2 J). They are seen in the rare congenital metabolic disorder known as cystinosis. Cholesterol crystals are also colorless plates but have the characteristic broken-off or notched corner. They are associated with some renal diseases.

The rare leucine and tyrosine crystals usually are found together in the urine in amino-aciduric diseases and indicate severe

TABLE 5.7. ABNORMAL CRYSTALS FOUND IN URINE*

Crystal	Morphology	Solubility Characteristics
Bilirubin	Reddish brown, amorphous needles, rhombic plates, or cubes, may color uric acid crystals	Soluble in alkali, acid, acetone, chloroform
Cholesterol	Rare, flat, colorless plates with corner notch	Very soluble in chloroform ether, hot alcohol
Cystine	Colorless, hexagonal, flat, rapidly destroyed by bacteria, may be confused with uric acid	Soluble in alkali, especially ammonia, and dilute hydrochloric acid, insoluble in boiling water, acetic acid, alcohol, ether
Hemosiderin	Clumps of golden brown granules	Blue with Prussian blue
Leucine	Yellow spheroids with striations, seen with tyrosine, probably not pure	Soluble in hot alcohol, alkali, slightly soluble in hot water, crystallizes out as hexagonal plates in pure form
Sulfonamides, sulfadiazine, acetylsulfadiazine	Dense, greenish globules, wheat sheaves, eccentric binding	Soluble in acetone
Tyrosine	Colorless or yellow, fine silky needles in sheaves or rosettes	Soluble in alkali, dilute mineral acid, relatively heat soluble, insoluble in alcohol, ether
Radiographic media (diatrizoate)	Colorless, thin, rhombic, some with notch	Soluble in 10% NaOH, insoluble in ether, chloroform

*All of these crystals are found in acid urine. Cholesterol, hemosiderin, and sulfonamides may also be present in neutral pH urine.

Adapted from Bradley M, et al. In Henry JB (ed): Todd-Sanford-Davidson Clinical Diagnosis and Management by Laboratory Methods, 16th ed, 1979, p 624. Courtesy of W.B. Saunders Co.

liver damage. Leucine crystals appear as highly refractile yellow spheroids with radial striations. Tyrosine crystals are colorless to pale yellow, fine silky needles in sheaves (Fig. 5.2 G).

Crystalline forms of various drugs have been noted in the urine, and their identification is primarily important in cases of drug toxicity. Sulfonamide crystals exhibit a great variety of shapes and colors and consequently may be misidentified as another type of crystal. One form of sulfa crystal is seen in Figures 5.2 C and 5.2 D. Their solubility in acetone is characteristic (uric acid crystals are not soluble). A tentative confirmatory test for sulfonamides is the lignin test.[95] One drop of urine is placed on a piece of newspaper and one drop of 25 percent hydrochloric acid is added; a positive reaction is yellow. Alfthan and Liewendahl[96] conducted an investigation of sulfonamide crystalluria and feel that the presence of sulfonamide crystals in urine sediment must be checked by examination of the specimen at 37C (the in vivo temperature) before a correct conclusion can be made.

Aspirin or salicylic acid[95] is one of the more common drugs associated with crystalluria. It is seen as prismatic or stellate crystals that are birefringent. The addition of 1 ml of 10 percent ferric chloride to acidified urine heated first to eliminate ketone bodies can be used to confirm the identification (a purple color indicates a positive reaction).

Radiographic (x-ray contrast media) dye has been detected in the urine sediment. In addition to gross turbidity and a markedly

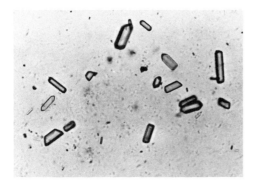

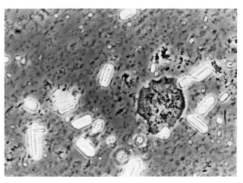

A. Triple phosphate crystals. Brightfield. ×350.

B. Triple phosphate crystals. Phase contrast. ×350.

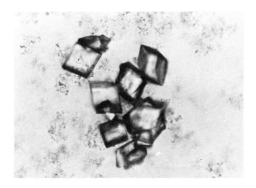

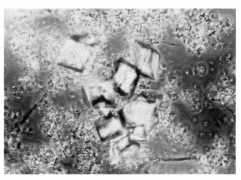

C. Sulfa crystals and amorphous material. Brightfield. ×200.

D. Sulfa crystals and amorphous material. Phase contrast. ×200.

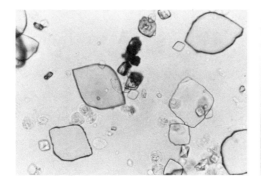

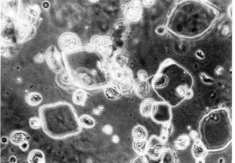

E. Uric acid crystals. Brightfield. ×200.

F. Uric acid crystals. Phase contrast. ×200.

Figure 5.2. Urine sediment constituents (crystals). (Courtesy of Jose M. Trujillo, M.D., Department of Laboratory Medicine, The University of Texas M.D. Anderson Hospital at Houston. Object selection by Phyllis Sedgwick, B.S., MT(ASCP), photography by John Kuykendall.)

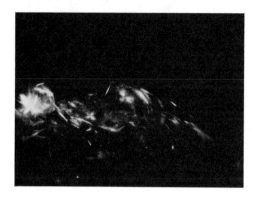

G. Tyrosine crystals. Polarized light. ×200.

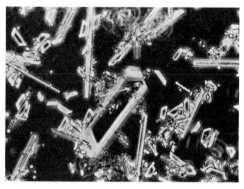

H. Calcium carbonate and triple phosphate crystals. Phase contrast. ×200.

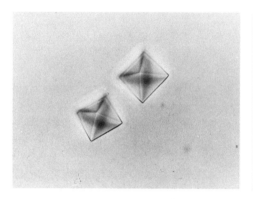

I. Calcium oxalate. Brightfield. ×290.

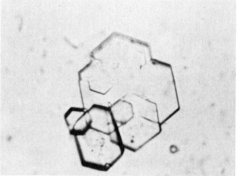

J. Cystine crystals. Brightfield. ×300.

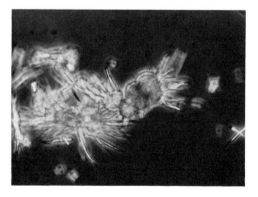

K. Ammonium biurate. Polarized light ×440.

Fig. 5.2. (*Cont.*)

elevated specific gravity, these pleomorphic crystals can easily mask important urinary sediment constituents.

Hemochromatosis is a disease in which excessive deposition of iron-containing pigments occurs in many organs of the body due to the increased absorption of dietary iron. In the kidneys, deposition of hemosiderin occurs in the renal tubular epithelial cells of the distal tubules, which are subsequently exfoliated. If these hemosiderin-laden cells disintegrate, hemosiderin pigment is released into the urine. In brightfield microscopy of an unstained sediment, they appear as coarse granules, golden-brown in color.

Artifacts and Contaminants. A variety of foreign materials added before or after collection may be seen in urinary sediment.[13,64,67] Their presence is usually not of any importance except that they may obscure significant clinical findings and even be misidentified as other elements. Artifacts range from the organic (plant particles, starch granules, oil droplets) to the inorganic (glass fragments and contrast media). Photomicrographs of artifacts and contaminants are shown in Figure 5.3.

Vaginal contaminants, mucus and cells, are frequently found and, in rare instances, fecal contaminants. Mucous threads, formed by the precipitation of mucoprotein in cooled urine, are found in nearly all specimens. They may be mistaken for casts by the inexperienced microscopist but are longer, less regular, and wavy in shape with tapered ends. Fibrin threads, on the other hand, are important. They are the result of urinary tract bleeding and are seen in cases of acute glomerulonephritis.

Spermatozoa, easily recognized particularly if motile by their oval bodies and long, thin, delicate tails, are frequently found in urine of males (Figs. 5.3 M and 5.3 N). They may also be seen in the urine of females after coitus. Their presence is usually not reported except in special instances.

The list of artifacts and contaminants found in urine is almost endless (Table 5.8).

Again, the necessity for a properly collected and processed specimen to ensure optimum conditions for analysis cannot be overstressed.

CONCLUSION

As Race and White have said[4]:

> Most laboratory procedures are performed to verify or disprove a diagnostic hypothesis previously gained by evaluation of a patient's history and physical findings. . . . Screening has been justified . . . when the procedure is used in the detection of a disease entity that . . . 1) occurs with a relatively high incidence in the general population; 2) has a silent symptomatology during the early stages or . . . manifestations as to preclude clinical recognition; 3) characteristically produces sequelae that are of serious consequences; or 4) is used in screening for drugs . . . (one laboratory procedure that meets these criteria is) a routine urinalysis for evidences of local renal pathology, generalized metabolic disturbances, or drugs.*

Medical laboratory personnel should remember that every laboratory test including urinalysis begins with and ends with the patient (Fig. 5.4, page 109). The ultimate goal of the clinical laboratory is, therefore, to provide rapid and accurate test results no matter how routine the test is considered.

Table 5.9 (page 110–11) summarizes the correlation of the physiochemical and microscopic findings of urine in selected clinical conditions. Indeed, routine urinalysis is an extremely important procedure for the early detection and diagnosis of certain disease states or to rule out a particular disorder. Negative as well as positive findings are, therefore, equally important in urinalysis.

*Race G, White MG: Basic Urinalysis, 1979, p 5. Courtesy of Harper & Row.

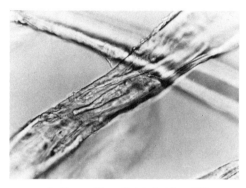

A. Paper fiber. Brightfield. ×290.

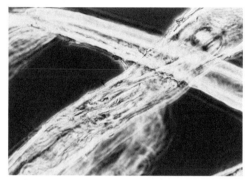

B. Paper fiber. Phase contrast. ×290.

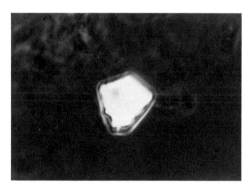

C. Plastic fragment. Brightfield. ×290.

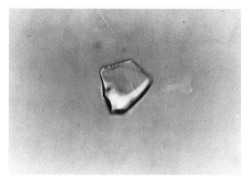

D. Plastic fragment. Phase contrast. ×290.

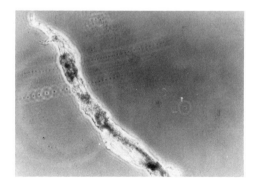

E. Cotton fiber. Brightfield. ×290.

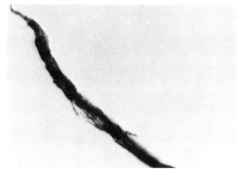

F. Cotton fiber. Phase contrast. ×290.

Figure 5.3. Common artifacts found in urine. (Courtesy of Jose M. Trujillo, M.D., Department of Laboratory Medicine, The University of Texas M.D. Anderson Hospital at Houston. Object selection by Phyllis Sedgwick, B.S., MT(ASCP), photography by John Kuykendall.)

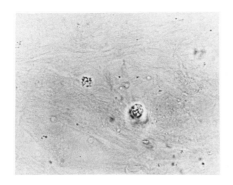

G. Mucous threads. Brightfield. ×460.

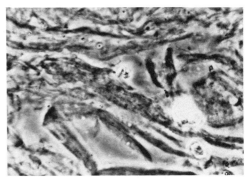

H. Mucous threads. Phase contrast. ×460.

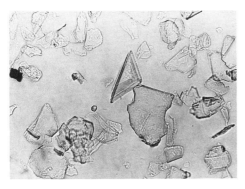

I. Talc. Brightfield. ×320.

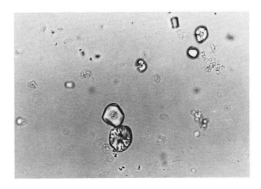

J. Starch. Brightfield. ×290.

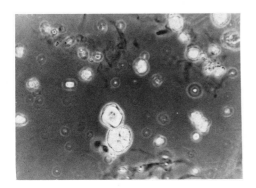

K. Starch. Phase contrast. ×290.

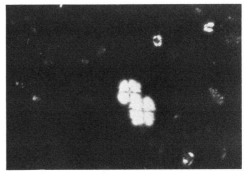

L. Starch. Polarized light. ×290.

Fig. 5.3. (*Cont.*)

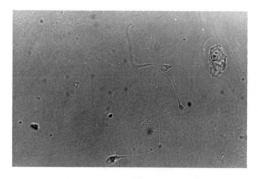

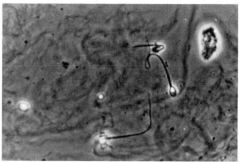

M. Spermatozoa. Brightfield. ×460.   **N.** Spermatozoa. Phase contrast. ×460.

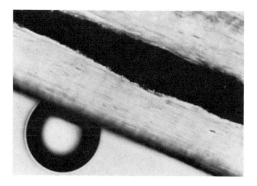

O. Hair. Brightfield. ×290.

Figure 5.3. (*Cont.*)

TABLE 5.8. ARTIFACTS IN MICROSCOPIC EXAMINATION OF URINARY SEDIMENT*

Artifact	Origin	Identification
Cotton, wool threads	Clothing	Refractile, flat ribbon shape
Hair	Human body	Hollow shaft
Paper fibers	Toilet paper	Refractile
Glass, plastic fragments	Urine container or pipettes	Sharp edges, refractile
Oil droplets	Catheter lubricant	No stain with Sudan IV
Starch	Food, surgeon's gloves, body powder	Stains with 3% iodine, will not dissolve in chloroform, confused with cholesterol, forms maltese cross with polarized light
Talc	Body powder	Irregular, sharp edges, refractile
Debris	Unclean slides	Refractile or black
Air bubbles	Faulty mounting	Round, refractile, vary in size
Meat, vegetable fibers	Fecal contamination	Striated bodies with blunt edges
Plant cells	Food	Refractile
Pollen	Air, container	Round, oval with smooth or serrated edges

*Some of the common artifacts encountered in urinary sediment examination are shown in Figure 5.4.

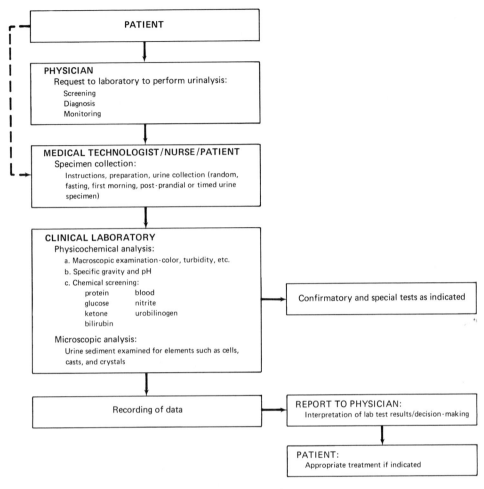

Figure 5.4. Routine urinalysis review.

CASES ILLUSTRATING DIAGNOSTIC PROBLEMS IN URINALYSIS

Chyluria*

Characteristic	Finding
†Color:	milky, pink
†Appearance:	moderately turbid
Specific gravity:	1.024
pH:	7

Characteristic	Finding
†Protein:	1+
Glucose:	negative
Ketone:	negative
Bilirubin:	negative
†Blood:	small
Urobilinogen:	normal
†WBC/hpf:	1+
†RBC/hpf:	1+
Casts:	none
†Other:	positive for lipids

*Klousia JW, et al: Chyluria—a case report. J Urol 117:393, 1977. © Williams & Wilkins Co., 1977.   †Abnormal values.

TABLE 5.9 CHARACTERISTIC PHYSICOCHEMICAL/MICROSCOPIC URINARY OBSERVATIONS/FINDINGS IN SELECTED DISEASE STATES

Physical Observations/ Findings	Chemical Findings	Microscopic Observations/ Findings	Disease State
Color: red-brown Turbidity: ↑ Specific gravity: ↑	Protein + Blood +	Cells: WBC, RBC, RTE Casts: hyaline, granular, RBC, waxy	Acute glomerulonephritis AGN
Urine volume: ↓ Turbidity: ↑ Odor: ↑ pH: ↑	Protein + Blood + Nitrite +	Cells: WBC and clumps, RBC, RTE Casts: cellular (WBC) Other: bacteria	Acute pyelonephritis
Specific gravity: ↓ Urine volume: ↓	Protein + Blood +	Cells: RTE (degenerated) WBC, RBC Casts: granular, RTE, waxy, broad	Acute tubular necrosis (ATN) or lower nephrosis
Specific gravity: ↓ (concentrating defect)	Protein ± Blood ±	Crystals: colorless, hexagonal plates (nonpolarizing)	Cystinosis
Specific gravity: N/↑ Odor: sweet	Protein ± Glucose + Ketone ±	Yeast sometimes present, in late stages of the disease, urinary microscopic findings similar to nephrosyndrome may be seen	Diabetes mellitus
Color: darker	Glucose + Ketone ± Blood + Bilirubin and urobilinogen + if liver involvement advanced	Cells: pigment-laden RTE (Prussian blue/iron reaction +) Casts: RTE cellular, granular Other: coarse, golden-brown hemosiderin granules free in sediment	Hemochromatosis

(Continued)

This urine specimen was from a Vietnamese immigrant admitted to the hospital for examination of transient unexplained anemia and weight loss.[98] Aside from urinary complaints (passage of pink urine on several occasions over a number of years) the woman had been in excellent health. Physical examination was unremarkable. The other admitting laboratory studies were as follows:

- Blood chemistry: Routine blood analyses were within normal limits.
- Hematology: All studies were within normal limits, except the differential revealed an eosinophil count of 23 percent (marked increase).
- Stool: Examination was positive for ova and parasites identified as *Strongyloides*.
- Additional studies: A lymphangiogram showed abnormal renal lymphatics (associated with the right kidney) and obstruction of lymphatic flow.

The patient was put on drug therapy for the parasitic infection. This case is an example of chyluria due to parasitic infestation.

TABLE 5.9 (Cont.)

Physical Observations/ Findings	Chemical Findings	Microscopic Observations/ Findings	Disease State
Turbidity: ↑	Protein + Blood ±	Casts: cellular, granular, fatty, waxy Other: oval fat bodies and free-floating fat droplets (birefringent) RTE cells with lipid inclusions	Nephrotic syndrome
Specific gravity: ↓ (concentrating defect)	Protein ± Blood +	Sickled RBC have been noted in some cases	Sickle cell syndromes
Turbidity: ↑	Protein +	Cells: RBC, WBC, RTE Casts: many types— cellular and inclusion	Systemic lupus erythematosus
Urine volume: ↓	Protein + Blood +	Cells: WBC, RBC, RTE Casts: hyaline, granular, and RTE	Thrombotic thrombo-cytopenic purpura (TTP)

N, normal; RBC, red blood cells; RTE, renal tubular epithelial cells; WBC, white blood cells; ↑, increased/above normal; ↓, decreased/below normal; +, positive; ±, positive/negative or trace.

Is It Blood?*

Characteristic	Finding
†Color:	yellow-brown
Appearance:	slightly turbid
Specific gravity:	1.024
pH:	7
†Protein:	trace
Glucose:	negative
Ketone:	negative
Bilirubin:	negative
†Blood:	4+
Urobilinogen:	normal
WBC/hpf:	occasional
RBC/hpf:	occasional
Casts:	none noted

*Said R: Contamination of urine. JAMA 242:748, 1979. Copyright 1979 American Medical Association.

†Abnormal values.

This specimen (voided spontaneously) was from a 7-year-old child a few hours after an appendectomy had been performed.[99] Physical examination at that time showed that the patient was recovering well from the surgery and did not have any complaints of muscular pain or weakness.

Requested laboratory studies for blood urea nitrogen, serum creatinine, bilirubin, and haptoglobin were within normal limits, but the serum creatinine phosphokinase which was slightly elevated. The tentative diagnosis given at this point was rhabdomyolysis (disintegration of muscle tissue associated with the excretion of myoglobin in the urine) of unknown etiology. The serum was clear without discoloration, and the urine was pigmented.

The patient was administered fluids intravenously to maintain diuresis, and over a 12-hour period the urine gradually became clear and the reagent test strip became negative for blood. When the creatinine phosphokinase returned to an almost normal level, the patient was discharged. The elevated CPK was thought to be due to muscle injury during surgery.

It was later suspected that the unusual urine color might be due to contamination of the urine with the antiseptic used for the preoperative abdominal skin preparation. The staff decided to test this hypothesis and mixed povidone-iodine solution with a sample of the patient's urine. The urine spiked with the antiseptic matched the originally tested specimen and also gave a strong positive reaction for blood.

Systemic Lupus Erythematosus

Characteristic	Finding
Color:	yellow
Appearance:	slightly turbid
Specific gravity:	1.020
pH:	6
*Protein:	3+
Glucose:	negative
Ketone:	negative
Bilirubin:	negative
*Blood:	small
Urobilinogen:	normal
WBC/hpf:	occasional
*RBC/hpf:	2+
*Casts:	cellular 1+
	fatty 1+
*Other:	oval fat bodies 2+
	(maltese cross
	under polarized
	light)

*Abnormal values.

This specimen is from a 26-year-old white female with a three-year history of systemic lupus erythematosus (SLE) admitted to the hospital due to edema of the legs and a weight gain of 9.07 kg (20 pounds) in the last week. Renal involvement is frequently a sequela of SLE.

Leukemia

Characteristic	Finding
Color:	yellow
Appearance:	cloudy
Specific gravity:	1.024
pH:	5.0
Protein:	3+
Glucose:	negative
Ketone:	negative
Bilirubin:	negative
Blood:	negative
Urobilinogen:	normal
WBC/hpf:	occasional
RBC/hpf:	rare
Casts:	none
Other:	degenerated epithelial cells 1+, bacteria 4+, uric acid crystals 4+

This urine specimen was from a 13-year-old white female with generalized weakness for several months prior to admission to the hospital. The history revealed progressive pancytopenia with fever. The bone marrow biopsy indicated many multiple odd forms. She had 2.88 by 10^{12}/L red blood cells (2.88 by 10^6 cells/mm^3) of blood and 9.0 by 10^9/L (9 by 10^3/mm^3) platelets in the same volume.

The postmortem findings were:

1. Respiratory failure secondary to pulmonary edema.
2. Acute monocytic leukemia in relapse with blastic crisis.
3. Acute urine acid overload secondary to lysis of leukemia cells from chemotherapy.
4. Acidosis on basis of above conditions.
5. Oliguria secondary to uric acid nephropathy.

This case serves to illustrate the relationship of pathology of the blood to ensuing renal disease.

Review Questions

Choose the best response for each question.

1. Urine color and urine concentration commonly vary together. T or F
2. The normal yellow color of urine is due primarily to urobilin and uroerythrin. T or F
3. A turbid urine specimen always indicates a pathologic condition. T or F
4. The incidence of turbidity of urine increases following refrigeration. T or F
5. Major solutes found in normal urine include:
   A. Calcium
   B. Urea
   C. Creatinine
   D. All of the above
   E. Only A and C above
6. Patients with diabetes insipidus are unable to excrete a concentrated urine because they have a deficiency of a hormone (ADH) secreted by the adrenal glands. T or F
7. For each of the terms in Column A select the appropriate definition in Column B.

Column A—Term
A. Anuria
B. Oliguria
C. Polyuria

Column B—Definition
1. Decreased urine output below normal
2. Increased urine output above normal
3. Little or no urine output

8. For the methods used to measure urine specific gravity listed in Column A, select the appropriate advantages/inadequacies in Column B.

Column A—Method
A. Refractometry
B. Urinometry

Column B— Advantages/Inadequacies
1. Only 1 to 2 drops urine needed
2. Minimum 15 ml urine needed
3. Temperature compensated
4. Temperature correction necessary
5. Not necessary to correct for elevated amounts of glucose and protein
6. Necessary to correct for glucosuria and/or proteinuria

9. The presence of a nonelectrolyte solute contributes more to the osmolality of a urine specimen than does an electrolyte. T or F
10. Water reabsorption occurs in the proximal segment of the renal tubules. T or F
11. The recommended method available today to detect Bence-Jones protein in urine is:
    A. Sulfosalicylic acid precipitation
    B. Heat and acetic acid
    C. Chemical reagent strip
    D. Thermal differential solubility
    E. Protein electrophoresis
12. The pH of urine even in the presence of disease is not different from the normal range but, if used in conjunction with other test findings, can still be useful to the clinician. T or F
13. The colorimetric reagent strip test for protein is most sensitive toward:
    A. Globulins
    B. Bence-Jones protein
    C. Albumin
    D. Dipeptides
    E. Amino acids
14. Residues of strong oxidizing agents can cause false positive reactions with the glucose oxidase test. T or F
15. High ascorbic acid levels may cause false negative reactions with the glucose oxidase test because the specificity of the reaction is affected. T or F
16. Match the chemical constituent listed with the test principle below.

Constituent

A. Protein
B. Glucose
C. pH
D. Blood
E. Bilirubin
F. Ketone
G. Urobilinogen

Principle

1. Double dye indicator
2. Based on perioxidase-like activity
3. Error of indicators
4. Double-sequential enzymatic reaction
5. Diazo reaction
6. Ehrlich aldehyde reaction
7. Legal's method (nitroprusside)

17. The specificity in urine testing refers to the ability of a test to detect only the analyte under determination, whereas sensitivity refers to the detection of the lowest clinically significant level of the tested substance. T or F

18. A positive chemical test for blood but a negative microscopic analysis for red blood cells could be explained by:
    A. A urine that has a low specific gravity (a hypotonic solution) in which the cells lyse
    B. Presence of myoglobin
    C. Collection of urine in a container that has been washed with a strong oxidizing agent
    D. All of the above
    E. Only A and B
    F. Only A and C

19. Match the following disorders with the chemical and microscopic findings for blood.

Disorder

A. Hematuria
B. Hemoglobinuria
C. Myoglobinuria

Chemical/Microscopic Findings for Blood

1. Both chemical test and microscopic examination positive
2. Both chemical test and microscopic examination negative
3. Chemical test positive but microscopic examination negative
4. Chemical test negative but microscopic examination positive

20. Ketonuria can occur even in normal individuals. T or F

21. The ketone bodies detected by Legal's nitroprusside method include:
    A. Acetone
    B. Acetoacetic acid
    C. β-Hydroxybutyric acid
    D. A and B only
    E. All of the above

22. In hemolytic anemias, there is increased formation of bilirubin with elevated blood levels as well as urine levels. T or F

23. Urobilinogen is normally present in urine. T or F

24. The Ictotest for bilirubin is more sensitive than the reagent strip systems. T or F

25. Bacteria must be incubated in the bladder for four to six hours to allow the conversion of nitrate to nitrite to occur. T or F

26. Variables inherent in the preparation of urine sediment include:
    A. Amount of urine centrifuged
    B. Time and speed of centrifugation
    C. Amount of sediment examined
    D. All of the above
    E. Only A and C above

27. The single most important factor in the preparation of urine for sediment examination is consistency. T or F

28. The traditional method used to examine urine sediment has been bright-field microscopy. However, many laboratories have adapted the following method for routine sediment examination:
    A. Differential interference contrast microscopy
    B. Phase contrast microscopy
    C. Darkfield microscopy
    D. Immunofluorescence

29. Polarized light microscopy is particularly useful in the identification of iso-

tropic material. T or F

30. Differential interference contrast microscopy provides the viewer with a three-dimensional image and therefore is excellent for studying structural details of formed elements. T or F

31. Erythrocytes appear crenated or shrunken if the urine is:
    A. Hypotonic
    B. Isotonic
    C. Hypertonic

32. Red blood cells swell in hypotonic urine and shrink in hypertonic. T or F

33. The best test for the presence of intact red blood cells in urine is microscopic examination of the urine sediment. T or F

34. Presence of erythrocytes in the urine is always indicative of a disease of renal origin. T or F

35. The line between physiologic or normal values and abnormal values of cells in urine is well defined. T or F

36. Pyuria refers to elevated numbers of leukocytes in the urine. T or F

37. Glitter cells are pathognomonic for pyelonephritis. T or F

38. All fat found in urine is birefringent or doubly refractile. T or F

39. Isotropic or nonbirefringent fat is best identified by a fat stain such as Sudan III. T or F

40. Other cells that have been identified in urine include:
    A. Histiocytes
    B. Exfoliated neoplastic cells
    C. Platelets
    D. All of the above
    E. Only A and B above

41. Normal urine is sterile and does not contain any microorganisms if collected under sterile conditions. T or F

42. Yeast found in urine is usually of the *Candida* species. T or F

43. The most frequently identified parasite found in urine in North America is:
    A. *Trichomonas vaginalis*
    B. *Schistosoma haematobium*
    C. *Enterobius vermicularis*

44. Yeast have all of the following characteristics except:
    A. 3-5 μ in diameter
    B. Oval shape
    C. Variable in size
    D. Lysed with acetic acid
    E. High refractive index

45. According to Burton's study, the variable that has the most significant effect on the number of casts seen in the urine is:
    A. Length of centrifugation
    B. Urine Osmolality
    C. Urine pH

46. The number of casts preserved decreases as the urine pH decreases. T or F

47. The pH of urine usually rises after collection due to the growth of urea-splitting bacteria which produce ammonia. T or F

48. The appearance of casts in the urinary sediment is always pathologic. T or F

49. Casts are classified primarily on the basis of morphologic features. T or F

50. Waxy casts are the end stage in the degeneration of cellular casts. T or F

51. Waxy casts in contrast to hyaline casts are more resistant and do not disintegrate as rapidly in hypotonic and/or alkaline solutions. T or F

52. Leucine crystals are usually found together in urine with:
    A. Uric acid
    B. Cystine
    C. Cholesterol
    D. Tyrosine
    E. Only B and D above

53. Match the crystal with the pH in which it is usually found.

Crystal	Urine pH Where Found
A. Calcium oxalate	1. Acid
B. Uric acid	2. Alkaline
C. Triple phosphate	
D. Bilirubin	
E. Tyrosine	

54. For each crystal in Column A, select the appropriate description in Column B.

Crystal
A. Uric acid
B. Calcium oxalate
C. Leucine
D. Cholesterol
E. Triple phosphate
F. Ammonium urate

Description
1. Thorn apple, brown
2. Coffin lid
3. Envelope
4. Pleomorphic
5. Notched corner
6. Yellow spheroids

55. Contaminants and artifacts in urine range from the organic to the inorganic. T or F
(See Appendix for answers.)

Case Studies

Case Study 1

Characteristic	Finding
Color:	yellow
*Appearance:	very turbid
Specific gravity:	1.019
pH:	6
*Protein:	1+
Glucose:	negative
Ketone:	negative
Bilirubin:	negative
Blood:	small
Urobilinogen:	normal
*WBC/hpf:	3+ and clumps
*RBC/hpf:	1+
*Casts:	1+ (WBC)
*Other:	renal tubular epithelial cells, bacteria—many motile, nitrite rx. positive

*Abnormal results.

This specimen was from a 14-year-old boy who came to his physician with a fever of 40.6C, shaking chills, and pain on the right costovertebral angle of one day's duration. On physical examination, mild tenderness in the region of the right kidney was noted. The diagnosis was acute pyelonephritis, and appropriate therapy was started.

Questions
1. Is there a relationship between the turbidity and any other finding reported on this urinalysis? If so, what is it?
2. Is there a relationship between the specific gravity result and that of any other finding? If so, what is it?
3. Is there a relationship between the color of the urine and the diagnosis? If so, discuss.

Answers
1. The presence of elevated numbers of cells (in this case white blood cells and red blood cells) can impart turbidity to urine. Recall, however, that the appearance of urine by itself is usually of limited diagnostic significance.
2. The presence of abnormal amounts of dissolved substances in urine can falsely elevate specific gravity. Recall that it is necessary to correct the specific gravity by subtracting 0.003 for each g/dl of protein. Osmolality values, however, do not need to be corrected. In this case, the concentration of protein is equivalent to 30 mg/dl, and no correction of specific gravity is necessary.
3. In this case, the color of the urine has no diagnostic significance. The color of urine is affected by such factors as concentration, presence of food pigments, and various constituents, such as blood and bile pigments.

Case Study 2

Characteristic	Finding
Color:	yellow
Appearance:	clear

Characteristic	Finding
Specific gravity:	1.010
pH:	6.5
*Protein:	1+
*Glucose:	2+
*Ketone:	small
Bilirubin:	negative
Blood:	negative
Urobilinogen:	normal
*WBC/hpf:	1+
RBC/hpf:	rare
*Casts:	cellular casts occasional

*Abnormal results.

This specimen is from a 32-year-old female who noted an increase in appetite and thirst over the past six months although she only gained 5 pounds. The patient also had complaints of polyuria but no associated dysuria. She has a family history of diabetes.

Questions

1. The presence of what particular chemical constituent is suggestive of diabetes?
2. The reagent strip system for glucose utilizes what reaction?
3. Is a positive reaction for ketones an unusual finding in patients with glycosuria? Discuss.
4. What other tests done routinely may be abnormal in diabetic patients other than those discussed above?

Answers

1. The presence of glucose in the urine is suggestive of diabetes. Diabetes mellitus, a disorder of carbohydrate metabolism, is caused by a lack of insulin. The disease is manifested by the accelerated conversion of amino acids to glucose. Hyperglycemia leads to excretion of glucose in the urine (glycosuria) and to polyuria.
2. The reagent strip methodology is based on a double-sequential reaction, the specific glucose/peroxidase enzymatic method.
3. Uncontrolled diabetes is often accompanied by the overproduction of ketone bodies, the products of incomplete fat metabolism. The presence of ketonemia in the blood leads to excretion of ketone bodies in the urine (ketonuria).
4. Other tests in the routine urinalysis that may be abnormal in the urine of long-term diabetics are (1) protein and (2) specific gravity, when the glucose is increased in addition to ketones. (3) In addition, yeast or bacterial infections are not uncommon, and these organisms may be seen in the microscopic examination.

Case Study 3

Characteristic	Finding
Color:	yellow
Appearance:	clear
Specific gravity:	1.015
pH:	6.5
Protein:	negative
Glucose:	negative
Ketone:	negative
Bilirubin:	negative
Blood:	negative
Urobilinogen:	normal
WBC/hpf:	occasional
RBC/hpf:	rare
Casts:	none
Other:	Clinitest positive

This specimen is from a 2-year-old female who was admitted to the hospital because of failure to grow and occasional episodes of vomiting. Slight hepatosplenomegaly was noted upon physical examination.

Questions

1. Identify the abnormal test result(s).
2. What conditions could explain a positive Clinitest and a negative strip test for glucose?
3. Is the age of the patient of any importance in this case study? Why?

Answers

1. All results are normal except for the positive Clinitest performed to detect

the presence of other reducing substances not detected by the enzymatic specific glucose oxidase test.

2. The conditions that can explain a positive Clinitest and a negative glucose oxidase test are:
   (a) the presence of a reducing substance other than glucose, e.g., lactose, and
   (b) the presence of a large concentration of ascorbic acid or other reducing substance which can cause a negative glucose oxidase but a falsely positive Clinitest. Recall that ascorbic acid can inhibit the enzyme reaction.
3. Patients who are young children or infants generally have both the reagent strip (glucose oxidase) test performed and the Clinitest (reducing substances) test performed upon routine examination because several of the inherited metabolic diseases may be detected by the presence of reducing substances in the urine.

Case Study 4

Characteristic	Finding
Color:	yellow
Appearance:	slightly turbid
Specific gravity:	1.015
pH:	6
Protein:	negative
Glucose:	negative
Ketone:	negative
Bilirubin:	negative
Blood:	negative
Urobilinogen:	normal
WBC/hpf:	occasional
RBC/hpf:	rare
Casts:	none
Other:	rare ovum noted with thick capsule and flattened side

This urine specimen was from a 4-year-old girl who had been complaining of periodic abdominal pain of several days duration. Physical examination revealed a well-developed afebrile child with no defined abdominal tenderness. Possible appendicitis was considered, but all routine blood chemistries and hematologic studies were within normal limits. Urinalysis was negative except for the presence of a rare ovum.

Questions

1. What is the most likely parasite represented by this ovum?
2. What is the usual route of entry into the urine?
3. Is a confirmatory test required? Name one.

Answers

1. The most likely parasite with this characteristic ovum is pinworm or *Enterobius vermicularis*.
2. The usual route of entry of parasites and ova into the urine is fecal or vaginal contamination.
3. When ova and/or parasites are noted in the urine sediment, further confirmatory tests are required. In this case a Scotch tape examination for ova and parasites was requested, and microscopic examination confirmed infestation by *Enterobius vermicularis*.

Case Study 5

Characteristic	Finding
Color:	yellow
Appearance:	cloudy
Specific gravity:	1.011
pH:	9.0
Protein:	3+
Glucose:	negative
Ketone:	negative
Bilirubin:	negative
Blood:	2+
Urobilinogen:	normal
WBC/hpf:	rare
RBC/hpf:	3+
Casts:	none
Other:	bacteria 1+, calcium carbonate crystals few

This urine specimen is from a 64-year-old male who 14 months previously had a cystectomy and urethrectomy followed by radiation therapy. These measures were taken following a diagnosis of transitional cell carcinoma of the bladder. At the time the urinalysis was performed, the patient had a blood urea nitrogen of 36.4 mg/dl (13 mmole/L) and a creatinine of 2.2 mg/dl (194 μmole/L), both of which are higher than normal. His blood cell count and differential count were within normal limits except that his white blood cell count was slightly decreased.

Questions

1. Is the presence of calcium carbonate crystals indicative of disease.
2. Are these crystals to be expected in a urine with this pH?
3. What is the relationship, if any, among the protein, blood, red blood cell numbers, and the patient's condition?

Answers

1. The presence of calcium carbonate crystals is not indicative of disease, since these crystals may be found in normal alkaline urine.
2. Yes, these crystals would be found in urine with a pH of 9. Although this pH may indicate a renal tubular defect in the ability to acidify urine, the presence of the alkaline pH and of the crystals does not specifically indicate the origin of the problem.
3. The presence of red blood cells in the urine is common in patients who have malignancies of the kidney or urinary tract. The leaking of blood into the urine may be accompanied by blood serum that contains an elevated concentration of protein (approximately 70 g/L)—thus the association among red blood cells, the positive chemical test for blood, and a positive chemical test for proteinuria.

Case Study 6

Characteristic	Finding
Color:	yellow-brown
Appearance:	cloudy

Specific gravity:	1.011
pH:	9
Protein:	trace
Glucose:	trace
Ketone:	negative
Bilirubin:	positive
Blood:	negative
Urobilinogen:	8 Ehrlich units
WBC/hpf:	rare
RBC/hpf:	rare
Casts:	none
Other:	deep yellow, fine needle-like crystals, some in sheaves, mucus and bacteria

This urine specimen is from a 49-year-old male who was referred to the hospital for an evaluation of a liver tumor. He is employed at a chemical plant which manufactures fluorocarbons and alkaline caustic soda. He smokes two cigars and drinks two mixed drinks each day. He has no history of hepatitis or liver disease, although one of his parents had liver cancer. His blood count showed him to be slightly anemic but otherwise was within normal limits.

Questions

1. What are the crystals seen in the urinary sediment?
2. What is a confirmatory test for these crystals?
3. What other results obtained on the routine urinalysis are consistent with the finding of these crystals?

Answers

1. These crystals are tyrosine crystals. Although the description could be confused with sulfa crystals, the pH of the urine would not be consistent with sulfa crystal formation. The patient has a liver tumor, and tyrosine crystals are found in the urine of some patients who have liver disease.
2. The confirmatory test for tyrosine crystals is a color reaction given by the crystals with Millon's reagent (Hoffman's

test) or Morner's reagent.[97] Millon's reagent is 1 part by weight mercury, 2 parts by weight nitric acid, and 2 parts by volume water. To about 3 ml of urine add 4 drops of Millon's reagent and heat. Tyrosine will give a red color due to the presence of the hydroxyphenol group. Morner's reagent is 1 volume of formalin, 45 volumes of distilled water, and 55 volumes of concentrated sulfuric acid. This reagent requires a greater concentration of tyrosine to give a green color when it is heated with urine in a 3:1 vol/vol mixture.

3. Other results that are consistent with tyrosine crystals in urine are those results related to the presence of liver disease—urine color (yellow-brown) and the positive chemical tests for bilirubin and urobilinogen.

REFERENCES

1. Haber MH: A Primer of Microscopic Urinalysis, Fountain Valley, Calif., ICL Scientific, 1978.
2. Hayashi Y: The value of qualitative tests of the urine. Cited in Young DS: Urinalysis: diagnostic role, usefulness of tests and inherent problems. Ann Biol Clin 36:228, 1978.
3. Free AH, Free HM: Urinalysis in Clinical Laboratory Practice. Cleveland, CRC Press, 1975.
4. Race GJ, White MG: Basic Urinalysis. New York, Harper & Row, 1979.
5. Young DS: Urinalysis: diagnostic role, usefulness of tests and inherent problems. Ann Biol Clin 36:228, 1978.
6. Bradley GM: Urinary screening tests in the infant and young child. Med Clin North Am 55:1457, 1971.
7. Fraser CG, Smith BC, Peake MJ: Effectiveness of an outpatient urine screening program. Clin Chem 23:2216, 1977.
8. O'Kell RT: Microscopic urinalysis as a screening procedure. Am J Clin Pathol 72:1041, 1979.
9. Tammes AR: Macroscopic urinalysis as a screening procedure. Am J Clin Pathol 72:1040, 1979.
10. Brody LH, Salladay JR, Armbruster K: Urinalysis and the urinary sediment. Med Clin North Am 55:243, 1971.
11. Schumann G, Greenberg NF: Usefulness of macroscopic urinalysis as a screening procedure. A preliminary report. Am J Clin Pathol 71:452, 1979.
12. Hyde TA, Mellor LD, Raphael SS: The kidney. In Raphael SS (senior author): Lynch's Medical Laboratory Technology, 3rd ed. Philadelphia, Saunders, 1976, pp 144–177.
13. Bradley M, Schumann GB, Ward PJ: Examination of urine. In Henry JB (ed): Todd-Sanford-Davidson Clinical Diagnosis and Management by Laboratory Methods, 16th ed. Philadelphia, Saunders, 1979, pp 559–643.
14. Wolf AV: Renal concentration tests—osmotic pressure, specific gravity, refraction and electrical conductivity compared. Am J Med 46:837, 1969.
15. Wolf AV: Urinary concentrative properties. Am J Med 32:329, 1962.
16. Linne JJ, Ringsrud KM: Basic Laboratory Techniques for the Medical Laboratory Technician. New York, McGraw-Hill, 1970.
17. Juel R, Steinrauf MA: Refractometry. In Hicks R, Schenken JR, Steinrauf MA (eds): Laboratory Instrumentation, 2nd ed. Hagerstown, Md., Harper & Row, 1980, pp 128–138.
18. Steinrauf MA: Osmometry. In Hicks R, Schenken JR, Steinrauf MA (eds): Laboratory Instrumentation, 2nd ed. Hagerstown, Md., Harper & Row, 1980, pp 117–127.
19. Wilson DM: Urinalysis and other tests of renal function. Minn Med 58:9, 1975.
20. Gardner KD: Uromancy 1971: tricks with sticks. N Engl J Med 285:1026, 1971.
21. Modern Urine Chemistry. Elkhart, Ind., Ames Division, Miles Laboratories, Inc., 1979.
22. Smith BC, Peake MJ, Fraser CG: Urinalysis by use of multitest reagent strips: two dipsticks compared. Clin Chem 23:2337, 1977.
23. Urinalysis with Chemstrip. Indianapolis, Ind., Bio-Dynamics/bmc, Division of Mannheim Boehringer, 1978.
24. Free AH, Free HM: Rapid convenience urine tests: their use and misuse. Lab Med 9: 9, 1978.
25. Brereton DM, Sontrop ME, Fraser CG: Timing of urinalysis reactions when reagent strips are used. Clin Chem 24: 1420, 1978.
26. Peele JD, Gadsden RH, Crews R: Evaluation of Ames' Clinitek. Clin Chem 23:2238, 1977.
27. Peele JD, Gadsden RH, Crews R: Semiautomated vs. visual reading of urinalysis dipsticks. Clin Chem 23:2242, 1977.
28. Product Information: Chemstrip, Biodynamics/bmc, Division of Boehringer Mannheim, Indianapolis, Ind., 1978.
29. Product Information: N-Multistix, Ames Division, Miles Laboratories, Inc., Elkhart, Ind., revised 1979.
30. James GP, Bee DE, Fuller JB: Accuracy and precision of urinary pH determinations using two commercially available dipsticks. Am J Clin Pathol 70:368, 1978.
31. Hoyer JR, Seiler MW: Pathophysiology of

Tamm-Horsfall protein. Kidney Int 16:279, 1979.

32. Bowie L, Smith S, Gochman N: Characteristics of binding between reagent-strip indicators and urinary proteins. Clin Chem 23:128, 1977.

33. Gyure WL: Comparison of several methods for semiquantitative determination of urinary protein. Clin Chem 23:876, 1977.

34. Pesce AJ: Methods used for the analysis of proteins in the urine. Nephron 13:93, 1974.

35. Free HM, Free AH: Studies with a urine test for semiquantitative enzymatic glucose and ketone. Clin Chem 17:649, 1971.

36. Dyerberg J, Pedersen L, Aagaard O: Evaluation of a dipstick test for glucose in urine. Clin Chem 22:205, 1976.

37. Free AH, Free HM: Influence of ascorbic acid on urinary glucose tests. Clin Chem 19:662, 1973.

38. Free AH, Free HM: Urine sugar testing—state of the art. Lab Med 6:23, 27, 45, 1975.

39. Free AH, Free HM: Influence of diet on urine ketone excretion. Clin Chem 19:653, 1973.

40. Couch RD: Routine screening for urinary bilirubin in hospitalized patients. Am J Clin Pathol 53:194, 1970.

41. Ivy JH, Hurley JW: Routine urine bilirubin determinations. JAMA 176:689, 1961.

42. Bates HM: Microhematuria is an important laboratory finding. Lab Management 17:31, 1979.

43. Fairbanks V: Hemoglobin, hemoglobin derivatives and myoglobin. In Tietz NW (ed): Fundamentals of Clinical Chemistry, 2nd ed. Philadelphia, Saunders, 1976, pp. 401–454.

44. Freni SC, Heederik GJ, Hol C: Centrifugation techniques and reagent strips in the assessment of microhaematuria. J Clin Pathol 30:336, 1977.

45. Blondheim SH, Margoliash E, Shafur E: A simple test for myohemoglobinuria (myoglobinuria). JAMA 167:453, 1958.

46. Free AH, Free HM: Identification and significance of nitrate and nitrite in urine. Clin Chem 18:697, 1972.

47. James GP, Paul KL, Fuller JB: Urinary nitrite and urinary tract infection. Am J Clin Pathol 70:671, 1978.

48. Kory M, Waife SO (eds): Kidney and Urinary Tract Infections. Indianapolis, Ind., Lilly Research Laboratories, 1971.

49. Hager CB, Free AH: Urine urobilinogen as a component of routine urinalysis. Am J Med Technol 36:227, 1970.

50. Product Information: Bumitest, Ames Division, Miles Laboratories, Inc., Elkhart, Ind., revised 1974.

51. Product Information: Clinitest, Ames Division, Miles Laboratories, Inc., Elkhart, Ind., revised 1978.

52. Belmonte MM, Sarkozy E, Harpur ER: Urine sugar determination by the two-drop clinitest method. Diabetes 16:557, 1967.

53. Potter JL: Simultaneous testing for glucose and total reducing substance in routine urinalysis. Clin Chem 26:172, 1980.

54. Product Information: Ictotest, Ames Division, Miles Laboratories, Inc., Elkhart, Ind., revised 1978.

55. Donauer RM: The value of microscopic examination of urinary sediment. JAMA 240:2044, 1978.

56. Heimann GA, Frohlich M, Bernstein M: Physician's response to abnormal results of routine urinalysis. Can Med Assoc J 115:1094, 1976.

57. Pai SH: Microscopic examination of urine sediment. JAMA 241:1574, 1979.

58. Schreiner GE: The urinary sediment. Ciba Clin Sympo 13:35, 1961.

59. Alwall N: Pyuria: deposit in high-power microscopic field—WBC/hpf vs WBC/mm^3 in counting chamber. Acta Med Scand 194:537, 1973.

60. Kesson AM, Talbott JA, Gyory AZ: Microscopic examination of urine. Lancet, 2:809, 1978.

61. Schumann GB, Henry JB: An improved technique for the evaluation of urine sediment. Lab Management 15:18, 1977.

62. Winkel P, Statland BE, Jorgensen K: Urine microscopy, an ill-defined method, examined by a multifactorial technique. Clin Chem 20:436, 1974.

63. Schumann GB, Greenberg NF: Does brightfield microscopy really analyze urine sediment? Lab Med 9:23, 1978.

64. Urine Under the Microscope, Nutley, N.J. Rocom, Division of Hoffman-La Roche, Inc., 1975.

65. Wilson MB: The Science and Art of Basic Microscopy. Houston, American Society for Medical Technology, 1976.

66. Sternheimer R: A supravital cytodiagnostic stain for urinary sediments. JAMA 231:826, 1975.

67. Schumann GB: Urine Sediment Examination. Baltimore, Md., Williams & Wilkins, 1980.

68. Schumann GB, Harris S, Henry JB: An improved technic for examining urinary casts and a review of their significance. Am J Clin Pathol 69:18, 1978.

69. Brody LH, Webster MC, Kark RM: Identification of elements of urinary sediment with phase-contrast microscopy. JAMA 206:1977, 1968.

70. Haber MH: Interference contrast microscopy for identification of urinary sediments. Am J Clin Pathol 57:316, 1972.

71. Haber MH: Urine Casts: Their Microscopy and Clinical Significance, 2nd ed. Chicago,

American Society of Clinical Pathologists, 1976.

72. Wahlin A: Differential count and quantitative estimation of granulocytes, mononuclear leukocytes and renal epithelial cells in urine. Ups J Med Sci 83:109, 1978.

73. Addis T: The number of formed elements in the urinary sediment of normal individuals. J Clin Invest 2:409, 1926.

74. Helgason S, Lindqvist B: Eosinophiluria. Scand J Urol Nephrol 6:257, 1972.

75. Musher DM, Thorsteinsson SB, Airola VM: Quantitative urinalysis—diagnosing urinary tract infection in men. JAMA 236:2069, 1976.

76. Riggs SA, Minuth AN, Nottebohm GA, Rossen RD, Suki WN: Plasma cells in urine—occurrence in multiple myeloma. Arch Intern Med 135:1245, 1975.

77. Kern WH: Epithelial cells in urine sediments. Am J Clin Pathol 56:67, 1971.

78. Schumann GB, Burleson RL, Henry JB, Jones DB: Urinary cytodiagnosis of acute renal allograft rejection using the cytocentrifuge. Am J Clin Pathol 67:134, 1977.

79. Hudson JB, Dennis AJ, Gerhardt RE: Urinary lipid and the Maltese cross. N Engl J Med 299:586, 1978.

80. Zimmer JG, Dewey R, Waterhouse C, Terry R: The origin and nature of anisotropic urinary lipids in the nephrotic syndrome. Ann Intern Med 54:205, 1961.

81. Sherer JF, Smith V: Examination of the unstained urinary sediment for malignant cells of urothelial origin. J Urol 111:386, 1974.

82. Holmquist ND: Detection of urinary cancer with urinalysis sediment. J Urol 123:188, 1979.

83. Sutor AH, Ketelson UP, Schindera F: Platelets in the urine: further evidence. Thromb Haemostas. 36:647, 1976.

84. Kurtzman NA, Rogers PW: A Handbook of Urinalysis and Urinary Sediment. Springfield, Ill., Thomas, 1974.

85. Greenhill A, Gruskin AB: Laboratory evaluation of renal function. Pediatr Clin North Am 23:662, 1976.

86. Robins DG, Rogers KB, White RHR, Osman MS: Urine microscopy as an aid to detection of bacteriuria. Lancet 1:476, 1975.

87. Cannon DC: The identification and pathogenesis of urine casts. Lab Med 10:8, 1979.

88. Burton JR, Rowe JW, Hill RN: Quantitation of casts in urine sediment. Ann Intern Med 83:518, 1975.

89. Haber MH, Lindner LE, Ciofalo LN: Urinary casts after stress. Lab Med 10:351, 1979.

90. McQueen EG, Sydney MB: Composition of urinary casts. Lancet 1:397, 1966.

91. Rutecki GJ, Goldsmith C, Schreiner GE: Characterization of proteins in urinary casts. N Engl J Med 284:1049, 1971.

92. Colando K: Urinalysis problem. Am J Med Tech 45:146, 1979.

93. Berman LB: Urinary hexagons. JAMA 229:827, 1974.

94. Middleton JE: A simple safe nitroprusside test using Ketostix reagent strips for detecting cystine and homocystine in urine. J Clin Pathol 23:90, 1971.

95. Monte-Verde D, Nosanchuk JS, Rudy MA, Ziemba R, Anuskiewcz K: Unknown crystals in the urine. Lab Med 10:299, 1979.

96. Alfthan OS, Liewendahl K: Investigation of sulfonamide crystalluria in man. Scand J Urol Nephrol 6:40, 1972.

97. Oser BL (ed): Hawks Physiological Chemistry, 14th ed. New York, McGraw-Hill, 1965, pp 1153–1205.

98. Klousia JW, McClennan BL, Semerjian HS: Chyluria: a case report and brief literature review. J Urol 117:393, 1977.

99. Said R: Contamination of urine with povidone-iodine. JAMA 242:748, 1979.

Linda P. Crum

CHAPTER 6

Screening Tests for Metabolic and Other Disorders

Objectives

It is expected that the information presented in this chapter will enable the reader to:

1. Identify the metabolic defect of each of the various disorders discussed.
2. Identify the principal abnormal urinary constituents of the disorders.
3. Identify the clinical symptoms of the disorders.
4. Determine the appropriate laboratory test(s) to aid in the diagnosis of the disorders.
5. Determine a specific disorder based on the clinical and/or laboratory findings.

This chapter is designed to give the reader an overview of some of the inherited metabolic disorders that can be partially or wholly diagnosed in the urinalysis laboratory. Many of the metabolic disorders described are very rare. The exact genetic and metabolic defects are known for some of the disorders and only suggested for the other disorders.

Also included in this chapter are four topics (urinary fat, sulfa, melanin, and myoglobin) which may or may not have a genetic defect involved.

AMINOACIDURIAS

Pathologic aminoaciduria can be classified into four major types:

1. Overflow aminoaciduria occurs when the amount of amino acid in the plasma exceeds the amount the kidney is able to reabsorb. Hence the amino acid overflows into the urine.
2. Competition or combined aminoaciduria occurs when more than one amino acid shares a common transport system. The increased amount of one amino acid in the plasma inhibits the binding and reabsorption of the other amino acids in the groups. Therefore, one amino acid is increased in the urine because of the overflow mechanism while the others have an increased renal clearance because of competitive inhibition.
3. Specific renal aminoaciduria occurs when impaired binding of an amino acid or group of related amino acids is caused by a mutation of the renal tubular reactive site or carrier.
4. Generalized renal aminoaciduria occurs when there is an impairment in the active tubular reabsorption of amino acids. Other substances, such as glucose, protein, and phosphorus, may also be involved. The following disorders of amino acid metabolism are discussed in this chapter: phenylketonuria, tyrosinosis, tyrosinemia, alcap-

tonuria, maple syrup urine disease, cystinosis, and cystinuria. Other aminoacidurias include severe liver disease in which metabolism of all amino acids is impaired, resulting in a generalized aminoaciduria. Wilson's disease and infantile galactosemia are other examples of generalized aminoacidurias. Additional information about these disorders can be found in Chapter 7.

PHENYLKETONURIA

Classic phenylketonuria (PKU) is one type of abnormality of phenylalanine metabolism. The phenylketonuric patient has inherited a single autosomal recessive gene from each parent. Both sexes are affected equally. The metabolic defect is the absence of phenylalanine hydroxylase activity in the liver. This defect prevents the normal oxidation of dietary phenylalanine to tyrosine.

Biochemical and Clinical Features

Amino acids have highly individual metabolic pathways. Normally phenylalanine is metabolized to tyrosine. However, in phenylketonuria this metabolic pathway is not open due to the lack of phenylalanine hydroxylase. Thus phenylalanine takes a secondary pathway. The secondary pathway is a common nonspecific pathway of amino acid degradation through keto, lactic, and acetic acids. It is through these secondary pathways that the metabolites of phenylketonuria are formed (Fig. 6.1).

These normal metabolites are found in abnormal amounts of phenylketonuria. Due to the inactivity of phenylalanine hydroxylase in the liver, the normal oxidation of dietary phenylalanine is stopped. This deficiency of phenylalanine hydroxylase occurs not only as an inherited condition but also in premature infants who eventually synthesize the enzyme. This one defect causes several amino acids to be found in abnormal amounts. There is an accumulation of phenylalanine in the blood, the level of which is directly related to the amount of dietary phenylalanine. The high level of phenylalanine inhibits the

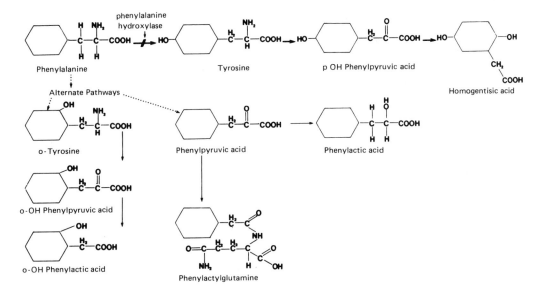

Figure 6.1. Pathways of phenylalanine metabolism.

transport of tyrosine and other amino acids. There is inhibited absorption of these amino acids by the intestine. Thus the plasma levels of tyrosine and other amino acids except phenylalanine are lower than normal. A reduction of dietary phenylalanine will restore the plasma level of these other amino acids to normal. Plasma serotonin levels are also depressed in phenylketonuria.

The phenylketonuric patient appears normal at birth. If the infant is allowed to eat a normal diet, severe mental retardation will occur in many cases. Most untreated patients have an IQ below 20, and the rest usually have an IQ below 50.[1] The mechanism by which the brain is damaged to produce mental retardation is unknown. Life expectancy of the untreated phenylketonuric is reduced. Most of these patients are found in institutions, and approximately 75 percent will die by 30 years of age.[2] The adult phenylketonuric usually shows such abnormal behavior as agitation, aggression, and hyperactivity.[25]

Another clinical finding is the reduction of pigmentation. According to such studies, a majority of phenylketonurics have blond hair and blue eyes. In almost all cases the pigmentation compared to the other unaffected family members is less. This reduction in pigmentation can be attributed to the depressed tyrosine levels, which in turn inhibit melanin formation.

Skin lesions or eczema are fairly common in the phenylketonuric. However, this is not a universal finding, and the relationship with phenylketonuria is questionable.

Phenylketonuric patients have a musty or mousy odor which is due to the metabolite phenylacetic acid in the sweat and urine.

Laboratory Findings. Plasma phenylalanine levels are normal at birth in the phenylketonuric infant. Within a matter of days after the ingestion of dietary L-phenylalanine, the phenylalanine plasma level begins to rise, reaching sustained levels of over 1 nm. Phenylalanine metabolites begin to appear in the urine in abnormal amounts. These metabolites include phenylpyruvic acid, phenyllactic acid, phenylacetic acid and its glutamine conjugate, and o-hydroxyphenylacetic acid.

Phenylpyruvic acid when combined with ferric chloride yields an olive green color.[3] If this method is used as a basis for screening, one fourth to one half of the phenylketonuric individuals will be overlooked in the newborn period. Phenylpyruvic acid is relatively unstable, and its excretion can be delayed during the newborn period due to transient phenylalanine aminotransferase deficiency.

Ferric chloride also reacts with a large number of substances, some of which are excreted in other inborn errors of metabolism, e.g., hereditary tyrosinemia.[4] Another method used for screening is one that detects keto acids in urine. The reagent is 2,4-dinitrophenylhydrazine, which reacts with the increased phenylpyruvic acid excreted in phenylketonuria.[5] This reagent also reacts with a number of other urinary substances, e.g., acetone and acetoacetic acid. Acetest* enables the distinction among acetone, diacetic acid, and the α-keto acids because it reacts with the first two but not with the last.[6]

Thin-layer chromatography can also be used to detect phenylketonuria.[7–10] This technique is the preferred screening test for aminoaciduria. It can be carried out on an early morning specimen. Preservation is usually accomplished by the addition of thymol. Although two-dimensional chromatography is used, the rapid and simple one-dimensional chromatography is adequate in most cases to detect an abnormality and to indicate within a group of amino acids where the abnormality exists. Thin-layer plates coated with cellulose are spotted with 5 μl of urine at one end. After the spot has dried, the plate is slowly and evenly placed in a developing tank that has a layer of butanol/acetic acid solvent in the bottom in a volume sufficient to contact the cellulose but not the spot where the urine was applied. After the solvent has traveled up the plate to about 8 cm from the bottom, the plate is removed and placed in an oven at 60C for about 15 minutes to remove the solvent. The plates are sprayed with a ninhydrin solution, heated, and observed for the development of a pink to purple color at the location of the amino acids. A pattern of urinary amino acids obtained by one-dimensional chromatography is shown in Figure 6.2.

Blood screening to detect increased phenylalanine levels is recommended for detection of phenylketonuria. The screening for hyperphenylalaninemia should be around the second week of life before mental retardation begins. Sometimes an initial screening is performed before the infant is discharged from the hospital. The increase of blood phenylalanine depends on dietary intake and may also be sex dependent. Female patients may have a slower rise in blood phenylalanine. Thus by means of a follow-up screening at the second week after birth to test for the disorder, these patients will have a greater chance for identification.

A widely used method for detection is the Guthrie bacterial inhibition assay (GBIA). It is based upon the counteraction of phenylalanine in the specimen of a metabolic antagonist in an agar plate containing spores of *Bacillus subtilis*. When the phenylalanine in the specimen reaches an abnormally high level, bacterial growth occurs.

To develop a PKU screening program, the Maternal and Child Health Service of the United States Department of Health and Human Services suggests the following criteria[11]:

1. The test should be efficient, simple, and economic.
2. The laboratory must have adequate facilities to process sufficient samples to maintain skill in recognizing abnormal results. A quality control program is necessary.
3. Blood samples should be obtained before the infant is discharged from the hospital and again at a few weeks of age.
4. Positive cases obtained by the screening method must be checked by a specific confirmatory test.
5. Procedures should be developed to refer the phenylketonuric infant to an evaluation and treatment center.

Treatment. Treatment should begin before the infant is one month old. Since phenylalanine is an essential amino acid, it must be provided in the diet. The amount of

---

*Ames Division, Miles Laboratories, Inc., Elkhart, Indiana.

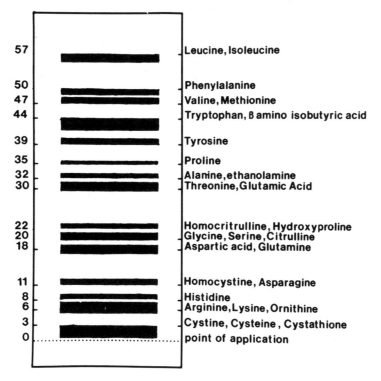

57	Leucine, Isoleucine
50	Phenylalanine
47	Valine, Methionine
44	Tryptophan, ß amino isobutyric acid
39	Tyrosine
35	Proline
32	Alanine, ethanolamine
30	Threonine, Glutamic Acid
22	Homocritrulline, Hydroxyproline
20	Glycine, Serine, Citrulline
18	Aspartic acid, Glutamine
11	Homocystine, Asparagine
8	Histidine
6	Arginine, Lysine, Ornithine
3	Cystine, Cysteine, Cystathione
0	point of application

Figure 6.2. One-dimensional chromatography of amino acids (diagram of typical pattern).

phenylalanine provided in the diet must meet but not exceed the nutritional requirements, which for infants is approximately 50 to 70 mg/kg. This requirement will decrease to approximately 20 mg/kg by 3 years of age when the child is not growing as rapidly.[2] The age at which an individual may be removed from the low phenylalanine diet has not been firmly established.

ALCAPTONURIA

The Metabolic Defect

Alcaptonuria is a rare metabolic disorder. It is inherited as a simple autosomal recessive trait. The specific metabolic defect is the absence of the enzyme homogentisic acid oxidase. This defect results in the accumulation of homogentisic acid which is excreted in the urine.

Homogentisic acid is a normal intermediate of phenylalanine and tyrosine metabolism (Fig. 6.1). Normally, homogentisic acid is metabolized to maleylacetoacetic acid, which is metabolized to fumarylacetoacetic acid and finally to fumaric acid and acetoacetic acid. The products of homogentisic acid metabolism are shown in Figure 6.3.

Homogentisic acid oxidase activity occurs mostly in the liver, and less activity occurs in the kidney. Other tissues of the body have no significant activity. The absence of homogentisic acid oxidase prevents the complete metabolism of tyrosine and phenylalanine. The amount of homogentisic acid excreted in the urine is directly related to the dietary intake of these two amino acids.

Clinical Findings. During childhood, the only symptom of alcaptonuria is the darkening of the urine upon standing at an alkaline

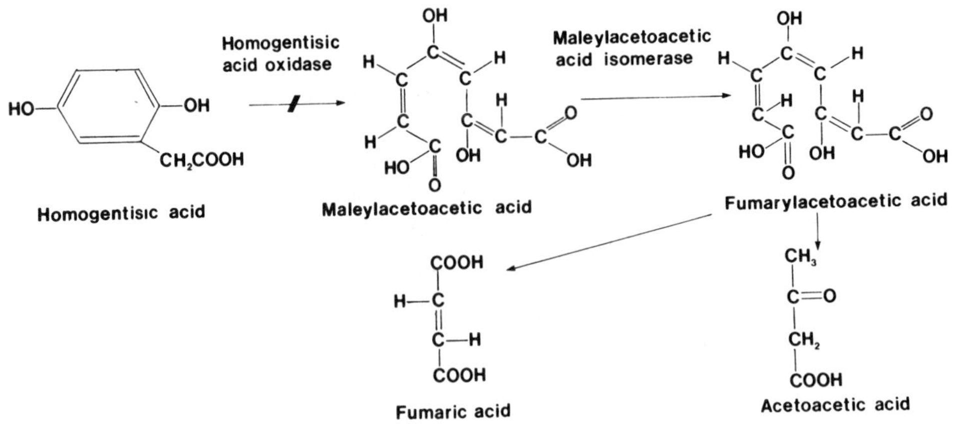

Figure 6.3. Products of homogentisic acid metabolism.

pH. If the urine remains at an acid pH or contains high level of ascorbic acid which protects homogentisic acid from being oxidized, the disease may go unnoticed until later years when other clinical symptoms appear.

When the alcaptonuric patient reaches 20 to 30 years of age, a pigmentation of connective tissue begins to become noticeable. A slight gray to bluish black pigmentation of the sclerae or ears is generally the earliest external change.[12] Microscopically, the pigment is ochre in color. Thus the pigmentation condition is named "ochronosis." The pigment may appear in the perspiration, and the skin in the axillary and genital regions may have a brownish discoloration.

In contrast, the pigmentation of the connective tissues in the elderly alcaptonuric patient is striking. The dense pigmentation is coal black in such areas as the costal, laryngeal, and tracheal cartilage. Pigmentation throughout the body is seen at operation or during postmortem.

The exact chemical structure of the pigment deposited in ochronosis has not been established. It shares many chemical characteristics with melanin. In fact, there is no stain to differentiate the two pigments.[12]

Another clinical finding in the older alcaptonuric patient is arthritis. While the incidence of alcaptonuria is approximately equal in males and females, arthritis appears at an earlier age and is more severe in males. How-

ever, nearly all alcaptonuric patients develop arthritis at an older age.

Other clinical findings that occur in alcaptonuric patients with higher frequency than in the general population include heart disease, ruptured intervertebral disks, prostatitis, and renal stones.[11]

Laboratory Findings. The urine of the alcaptonuric patient will darken upon standing if the pH of that urine is alkaline. The darkening is due to the oxidation of homogentisic acid, and, therefore, it begins at the surface of the urine and moves downward. As mentioned earlier, two factors will inhibit or slow down the oxidation process. If the urine remains at an acid pH or contains a reducing substance such as ascorbic acid, the oxidation process may be delayed several hours and even go unnoticed since urine is disposed of rather quickly. Other substances that may also darken the urine but can be easily distinguished from homogentisic acid include bile, porphyrin, myoglobin, and hemoglobin.

Homogentisic acid is a reducing substance and will react and darken with the alkaline Benedict's reagent found in Clinitest* to yield a yellow-orange precipitate in a muddy brown solution. Ferric chloride added to the urine of the alcaptonuric patient will yield a

*Ames Division, Miles Laboratories, Inc., Elkhart, Indiana.

purple-black or dark blue color. A saturated silver nitrate and ammonia solution produces a black color with homogentisic acid. However, ascorbic acid will also produce a black color with the silver nitrate solution.

A simple and useful screening test used in our laboratories is the development of photographic film in the presence of homogentisic acid and sodium hydroxide.[13,14] Such a test can be performed in full light, and results of a semiquantitative adaptation are shown in Figure 6.4. Paper and thin-layer chromatography can also be used. The thin-layer chromatographic method uses urine that has been processed through a cation exchange urine. The development of a thin-layer plate of silica gel G is made using a hexane-ethyl acetate-acetic acid solvent.[15] The plate is examined for a reacting band in the urine at the position of the reference standard after color has been developed with ammonium molybdate. Caution must be exercised in interpreting these tests because of the nonspecific reactions that can be given by a variety of substances that have similar molecular structures. Some, e.g., L-dopa and gentisic acid, result from medications. Aspirin is often responsible, and patients who have arthritis and some alcaptonuric symptoms are the most likely candidates for the tests.

A specific test that allows the quantitation of homogentisic acid employs purified homogentisic acid oxidase from rat liver.[16] The homogentisic acid in the urine is converted to maleylacetoacetic acid, the absorption of which can be measured at 330 nm. The procedure is simple if one can obtain the enzyme commercially.

TYROSINOSIS AND TYROSINEMIA

The normal catabolic pathway of tyrosine metabolism leads to the end products, fumarate and acetoacetate. Disorders of tyrosine metabolism have been reported along various steps of the pathway (Figs. 6.1 and 6.3).

The first step in tyrosine metabolism is the transamination of tyrosine to the keto acid,

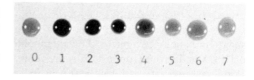

Figure 6.4. Photographic paper test for homogentisic acid. O, normal urine; 1, with 2 mg/ml homogentisic acid (HA); 2, with 1 mg/ml HA; 3, with 0.5 mg/ml HA; 4, with 0.1 mg/ml HA; 5, with .05 mg/ml HA; 6, with 0.025 mg/ml HA; 7, with 0.0025 mg/ml HA.

p-hydroxyphenylpyruvic acid (p-HPPA). Disorders of transamination include the Oregon type of tyrosinemia in which there is a deficiency in the soluble (cytosol) form of tyrosine aminotransferase. Tyrosinosis, described by Grace Medes in 1932, may also be a disorder of transamination, although she reported the disorder as a deficiency in p-hydroxyphenylpyruvic acid oxidase activity.[17] The second step in tyrosine metabolism is the oxidation of p-HPPA to homogentisic acid by the enzyme p-hydroxyphenylpyruvic acid oxidase. Hereditary tyrosinemia and transient neonatal tyrosinemia are two disorders which are attributed to either a primary or a secondary impairment in this oxidase step.

Alcaptonuria is a classic disorder of the third step of tyrosine metabolism where a homogentisic acid oxidase deficiency prevents the conversion of homogentisic acid to 4-maleylacetoacetic acid.

Tyrosinosis

There has been only one case of tyrosinosis reported. The patient, suffering from myasthenia gravis, was found to excrete p-HPPA in the urine. Medes attributed the disorder to a deficiency in p-HPPA oxidase activity.

Although Medes reported that tyrosinosis was caused by a deficiency in p-HPPA oxidase, current understanding of tyrosine metabolism sheds some doubt on this theory. p-HPPA was the only metabolite excreted in tyrosinosis except when a high diet of tyrosine was fed. During a high tyrosine diet, 3,4-dihydroxyphenylalanine (dopa) was excreted. In other conditions, i.e., tyrosinemia, p-hydroxyphenylactic acid (p-HPLA) is the major metabolite excreted. The metabolite p-HPLA is derived from p-HPPA via reduction in an alternate pathway by the lactic dehydrogenase of muscle. In view of the difference in the tyrosyluria found in tyrosinosis from that found in tyrosinemia, it has been postulated that the metabolic effect of tyrosinosis occurs higher in the pathway.

Tyrosinemia

Discussion of tyrosinemia in this chapter will be limited to transient neonatal tyrosinemia and hereditary tyrosinemia. Transient neonatal tyrosinemia is the most common disorder of amino acid metabolism. Over 100 cases of hereditary tyrosinemia have been reported. This condition is pathologic.

Transient Neonatal Tyrosinemia

Transient neonatal tyrosinemia occurs more often in premature newborn infants than in full-term infants. Males are more affected by the disorder than females. Partial impairment of p-HPPA oxidase in the immature liver of infants causes the enzyme activity to be insufficient to oxidize the p-HPPA formed from the infant's high dietary intake of tyrosine. The high dietary intake of tyrosine and a low dietary intake of ascorbic acid can further inhibit the enzyme's activity.

Clinical and Laboratory Findings. There is no liver damage involved with transient tyrosinemia. Although some premature infants have shown signs of dull motor activity and lethargy, the condition is considered harmless in most cases. A reduction of phenylalanine and tyrosine intake or an increase in ascorbic acid intake is effective in reducing the tyrosinemia. The condition peaks after one week of life in the majority of cases.

Tyrosinemia and tyrosyluria both occur in this condition. The excessive urinary excretion of tyrosine, p-HPPA, and p-HPLA can be demonstrated using paper or thin-layer chromatography. Tyrosine crystals may be observed in the urine. A simple, nonspecific test for tyrosine is the nitrosonaphthol test.[18]

The nitrosonaphthol reagent, nitric acid, and sodium nitrate are mixed with the urine which will give an orange-red color if tyrosine is present in large amount. Millon's reaction can be used as a screening test for tyrosine in urine. The tyrosine and other phenolic compounds react with mercuric salts in strong acid to produce an orange-red color.[19]

Hereditary Tyrosinemia

Hereditary tyrosinemia is a pathologic condition that can take an acute or chronic course. The acute form of the condition appears early in life (about one month) and ends in death by liver failure at about three to eight months of life if untreated. The chronic form appears later and may have acute episodes.

The metabolic defect is a severe deficiency in the synthesis of p-HPPA oxidase in the liver of patients who have hereditary tyrosinemia. However, enzyme determinations have not been performed on undamaged liver tissue from these patients so it is not known if the enzyme deficiency exists prior to liver damage. Other biochemical abnormalities exist in the condition. Hypermethioninemia can be demonstrated, particularly in the acute form of the condition. δ-Amino-levulinic acid and catecholamines are formed and excreted in excessive amounts.

There is some question as to whether the metabolic defect is simply a p-HPPA oxidase deficiency. Further investigations of this disorder hopefully will clear up the controversy.

Clinical and Laboratory Findings. Clinical features of hereditary tyrosinemia include rickets, vomiting, diarrhea, edema, ascites, abdominal enlargement, and hepatosplenomegaly. Mental retardation has been reported in some cases. A characteristic cabbagelike odor, which may be due to a metabolite of methionine, has been reported.

There is damage to the renal tubules in this disorder which causes impairment in the reabsorption of phosphorus, glucose, protein, and amino acids. These substances will therefore be excreted in increased amounts in the urine. The generalized aminoaciduria is characteristic of the disorder. Tyrosine is the predominant amino acid excreted.

Others include, in decreasing order, proline, threonine, alanine, glycine, phenylalanine, α-aminobutyric acid, isoleucine, serine, leucine, aspartic acid, methionine, and ethanolamine.

Liver damage causes the coagulation factors to be decreased. As the patient goes into liver failure, serum protein levels will fall and serum bilirubin will increase.

Because of a deficiency in p-HPPA oxidase activity, p-HPPA is metabolized along an alternate pathway, forming p-HPLA which is excreted in increased amounts in the urine.

Treatment. Restriction of dietary intake of phenylalanine and tyrosine is successful in counteracting the renal tubular lesions. The abnormally increased urine values of phosphorus, glucose, protein, and amino acids return to normal. The special diet is not as successful in improving the liver damage.

BRANCHED-CHAIN KETONURIA (MAPLE SYRUP URINE DISEASE)

Maple syrup urine disease (MSUD) is one abnormality of branched-chain amino acid metabolism. Other abnormalities are hypervalinemia and isovaleric acidemia. This discussion is limited to maple syrup urine disease.

Maple syrup urine disease is a rare disease occurring when there is a deficiency in the oxidative decarboxylation of the three branched-chain amino acids, leucine, isoleucine, and valine. The term branched-chain is used to describe these three amino acids because each contains a methyl group which diverges from the main carbon chain. Classic MSUD and three variant forms have been described. The variant forms have been tentatively classified as "intermittent" MSUD, "mild" MSUD, and "thiamine-responsive" MSUD. The different forms of maple syrup urine disease are sometimes difficult to separate on a clinical basis because environmental conditions seem to play a role in determining the clinical phenotype. However, there seems to be enough of a difference in enzyme activ-

ity found in each variant to separate them. A comparison of enzyme activity will be made in the discussion of the disease. All three keto acids are affected in each variant.

Classic Maple Syrup Urine Disease

There have been only about 50 cases of classic MSUD reported in the literature. Only a handful of the variant forms have been reported.

The Metabolic Defect. Catabolism of the amino acids, leucine, isoleucine, and valine, is a complex process. The first step involves transamination where valine, leucine, and isoleucine are converted to the corresponding α-keto acids, α-ketoisovaleric acid, α-ketoisocaptroic acid, and α-keto-β-methylvaleric acid. Transamination occurs normally in maple syrup urine disease. It is at the next step, oxidative decarboxylation, where the defect occurs. Oxidative decarboxylation is carried out by a multienzyme complex. Each step of the decarboxylation process is carried out by a component of the enzyme complex. It is not clear if the metabolic defect in MSUD is the result of a defect in one enzyme or three specific enzymes. One possible explanation is that one gene controls the action of the enzymes or the decarboxylase portion of the enzyme complex.

Clinical and Laboratory Findings. The infant with maple syrup urine disease appears normal at birth, but by one week of life the child will usually show symptoms of the disease. The accumulation of the keto acids occurs early, causing vomiting, lethargy, and convulsions. The urine has the distinct odor of maple syrup or burned sugar. The child with MSUD usually dies of infection during the first year of life.

Blood or plasma may be used for the analysis of valine, leucine, and isoleucine. These amino acids will be elevated due to the normal reverse transamination of keto acids. Methods used to detect the elevation include thin-layer chromatography,[20] column chromatography,[21] and microbiologic assay.[22] The positions of valine, leucine, and isoleucine on a one-dimensional development by their layer chromatography are shown in Figure 6.2. These bands are broader and more highly stained in maple sugar urine disease.

Qualitative values of increased urinary keto acids can be determined by adding 2,4-dinitrophenylhydrazine in a hydrochloric acid solution. A yellow precipitate indicates a positive test.[5] Further extraction with ether and then with sodium bicarbonate causes the yellow 2,4-dinitrophenylhydrazines of keto acids to develop a deep red color in the water phase when an equal volume of sodium hydroxide is added.

The identification of the keto acids can be made by using thin-layer chromatography[8] and gas-phase chromatography.[23] The latter method allows the keto acids to be quantitated, as does spectrophotometry.

The branched-chain keto acids are not normally present in urine in significant amounts. However, in MSUD the keto acids will be found in increased amounts in urine and blood.

Metabolism of the amino acids within the leukocytes will demonstrate the metabolic defect in maple syrup urine disease. Decarboxylase activity can be assessed by incubating the leukocytes with leucine-1-^{14}C, and subsequently measuring the liberated $^{14}CO_2$. Levels of the decarboxylase activity in classic MSUD are less than 5 percent of normal.

Treatment. Removal of branched-chain amino acids from the diet is very difficult, since all proteins with good biologic value contain them. A semisynthetic diet using a gelatin base to which other amino acids have been added has been used with success. A diet free of branched-chain amino acids must be started in the first weeks of life and strictly adhered to if brain damage, mental retardation, and even death are to be prevented.

Variants of Maple Syrup Urine Disease

There are three variants: (1) intermittent MSUD, (2) mild MSUD, and (3) thiamine-responsive MSUD.

The intermittent form of the disease may not become apparent until late infancy or childhood, usually when the patient is under stress, such as an intercurrent illness. A sudden increase in protein intake can also trigger the disorder. Attacks of the intermittent form are just as severe as the classic form and must be treated accordingly. Decarboxylase activity in these individuals is 10 to 20 percent of normal between episodes. The plasma concentration of the branched-chain amino acids is normal except during episodes when the concentration may be 10 times the normal value. Ketoaciduria in these individuals is intermittent. Mental retardation occurs in some patients.

The main features of mild MSUD are that the branched-chain amino acids are present continuously in plasma at 5 to 15 times the normal amount and that ketoaciduria is constant. The decarboxylase activity in leukocytes is 15 to 25 percent of normal. Mental retardation is common in mild MSUD also. There is a fine line of distinction between intermittent and mild MSUD, since environmental conditions may be a factor in determining the phenotype.

Patients with thiamine-responsive MSUD have shown branched-chain amino acid plasma levels of three times normal. Ketoaciduria is variable. Partial decarboxylase activity of approximately 25 percent of normal occurs when the plasma branched-chain amino acid level is within the physiologic range. When the branched-chain amino acid level is 5 to 10 times normal during intercurrent illness, the decarboxylase activity is near normal. Thiamine administration of about 10 times (10 mg per day) the recommended amount produces amelioration of the disorder.

CYSTINOSIS AND THE FANCONI SYNDROME

The Fanconi syndrome consists of nephrotic-glycosuric dwarfism with hypophosphalemic rickets. The syndrome, described by Fanconi in 1936, is found in a variety of primary hereditary and acquired disorders. Cystinosis is the most common disorder in children who exhibit the Fanconi syndrome. Other disorders discussed in this chapter that cause the Fanconi syndrome include tyrosinemia, Wilson's disease, and galactosemia.

Cystinosis

Cystinosis is inherited as an autosomal recessive trait, although the exact genetic defect is unknown. There are three forms of the disorder which suggests genetic heterogeneity. The most severe form is the nephropathic form which appears in infancy. These patients usually die before puberty. The juvenile form appears during the second decade of life and is intermediate in its severity. The benign form appears in adults in whom the kidney is not harmed.

Clinical Findings. Children with nephropathic cystinosis begin to show symptoms of the disorder in the first year of life. The renal tubular defect impairs water reabsorption, resulting in polyuria and polydipsia. Acidosis is common. Rickets develops due to the loss of phosphate and does not respond to vitamin D therapy. The child's failure to thrive is evidenced by very poor growth, usually in the third percentile in height and weight.

Cystine crystals are deposited in the body tissues, bone marrow, and conjunctiva of the eye. Other crystalline deposits are found in the cornea of the eye. These deposits are found consistently in all three types of cystinosis and are usually the only clinical sign of the adult form of the disease. The mechanism responsible for the crystalline deposits is unknown.

The kidney undergoes tubular and glomerular damage in nephropathic and juvenile forms of cystinosis. The damage is attributed to the deposition of cystine crystals. The proximal tubules undergo atrophy and produce the swan-neck deformity which is characteristic of cystinosis. The normal epithelial cells of the tubules are replaced by simple cuboidal epithelium. The junction between the cortex and the medulla of the kidney is obscure. The weight of the kidney is much less than normal.

Laboratory Findings. There is increased urinary excretion of glucose, amino acids, phosphate, and potassium. The aminoaciduria is of a generalized type, with some 10 different amino acids being present. Cystine is not excreted in greater proportions than the other amino acids, and cystine calculus formation has been reported in only one individual with cystinosis. Proteinuria is common. Due to the increased amount of ammonium ion and bicarbonate excreted, the pH of the urine is alkaline. Cystine crystals may not be seen in the urine as cystine becomes soluble at an alkaline pH.

Blood changes include metabolic acidosis with a decrease in CO_2. Serum phosphorus and potassium are decreased. Alkaline phosphatase and the erythrocyte sedimentation rate are increased. Early in the disease, the blood urea nitrogen and creatinine are usually normal. Cystine crystals can be seen in the bone marrow. Since cystine is very soluble in formalin, alcohol is the preservative of choice for all tissue to be examined for cystine crystals.

CYSTINURIA

Cystinuria is the most common disorder involving an inborn error of metabolism. It is inherited as an autosomal recessive trait. The incidence for the homozygous state has been estimated to be from 1 in 7,000 to 1 in 20,000 persons.

The Metabolic Defect

The specific defect is in the epithelial cells of the intestine and proximal renal tubules. The defective cells impair the transport of the amino acids cystine, lysine, arginine, and ornithine. These four amino acids are transported by a common process in the intestine and kidney. However, there are two other separate transport mechanisms, one for cystine and the other for the dibasic amino acids, lysine, arginine, and ornithine. The separate transport systems are a probable explanation for the difference in single family members, some who excrete only cystine in the urine and others who excrete only the dibasic amino acids.

Genetics and Clinical Findings. The genetics of cystinuria are complex. The disorder is inherited as an autosomal recessive trait, but because of allelic mutations three genetically distinct types of cystinuria have been described. The types are designated as Type I, Type II, and Type III. The homozygous individuals can be differentiated and placed into one of the three types by in vitro studies of the intestinal transport system.[24] Differences in urinary amino acid excretions are not helpful in differentiating the homozygous individuals but do correlate well with the heterozygous individuals. However, Type I heterozygotes do not exhibit aminoaciduria and, therefore, cannot be differentiated from normal individuals on the basis of amino acid excretion.

Cystine calculi formation is common in patients with cystinuria. Cystine is least soluble in the pH range of 4.5 to 7, which is the most common pH range of urine. Calculi formation is a constant threat, particularly at night when the concentration of the urine increases. Men and women are affected equally in calculi formation, but men are more severely affected due to the longer urethra. Calculi formation appears most often during the third and fourth decades of life. Calculi formation predisposes the patient to urinary tract obstruction and infection.

Laboratory Findings. The disorder is characterized by the urinary excretion of four amino acids, cystine, lysine, arginine, and ornithine. Cystine is the least soluble of the four and crystallizes in the pH range of 4.5 to 7. The other amino acids are very soluble and remain in solution. A microscopic examination of the urine sediment will reveal the hexagonal crystals of cystine as shown in Figure 5.3 J.

The cyanide-nitroprusside test can be used to screen individuals for cystinuria.[25] In this test cystine is reduced to cysteine, which combines with sodium nitroprusside to form a magenta red color complex. A weak positive may be seen in heterozygous individuals of Types II and III. A false positive reaction may be obtained with acetonuria and homocystinuria. To confirm the presence of cystinuria, the characteristic aminoaciduria can be demonstrated with thin-layer chromatography[9,10] or automated column chromatography.[2]

Treatment. Dietary restriction of protein has been helpful in some cases of cystinuria. However, the most helpful measures have been to increase the fluid intake so that calculi do not form easily. It is important that a high fluid intake be maintained during the night as well as during the day.

Raising urine pH to above 7.5 will make cystine more soluble. However, an around-the-clock therapy of sodium bicarbonate has the danger of causing calcium salts to precipitate.

Administration of D-penicillamine will cause urinary cystine levels to fall. However, long-term therapy can cause allergic reactions, destruction of vitamin B_6 and subsequent deficiency, impairment of wound healing, an increase in the ratio of soluble to insoluble collagen, and proteinuria which may progress to the nephrotic syndrome.

5-HYDROXY INDOLEACETIC ACID (5-HIAA)

5-Hydroxy indoleacetic acid is a metabolite of serotonin (5-hydroxytryptamine). Serotonin is metabolized in the argentaffin cells of the intestine from tryptophan and subsequently is found in blood platelets.

The pathway for the synthesis of serotonin from tryptophan is shown in Figure 6.5. Abnormal amounts of urinary 5-hydroxy indoleacetic acid are found in malignant, inherited, and benign conditions. Malignant tumors of the argentaffin cells cause excessive production of serotonin, thereby increasing the amount of 5-hydroxy indoleacetic

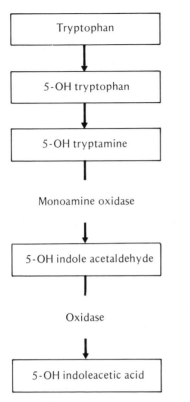

Figure 6.5. Synthetic pathway of 5-OH indole acetic acid.

acid excreted in the urine. Increased values of 5-hydroxy indoleacetic acid have been reported in the CSF of hyperactive patients.

The presence of serotonin in fruits, such as bananas, tomatoes, pineapples, and avocados, causes increased 5-hydroxy indoleacetic acid in the urine when these fruits are eaten. For this reason they should be eliminated from the diet prior to urinalysis for 5-hydroxy indoleacetic acid. Patients should also refrain from taking any drugs prior to testing. Phenothiazines and acetanilid drugs interfere with the analysis of 5-hydroxy indoleacetic acid.

Phenylketonuria is an inherited disorder in which tryptophan metabolism is altered. The alteration causes only a slight decrease in urine 5-hydroxy indoleacetic acid.

A random urine specimen may be screened for excess 5-hydroxy indoleacetic acid with

nitrous acid and 1-nitroso-2-naphthol.[26] The development of a purple color is specific for 5-hydroxy indoles. Urine from patients with malignant tumors of the argentaffin cells will show a black color with the screening test due to the extremely high level of 5-hydroxy indoleacetic acid. A quantitative method should be used to confirm the screening method.

PORPHYRIA AND PORPHYRINURIA

Porphyrins are intermediate products in the biosynthesis of heme. Porphyrins serve as metal chelates which enable iron to be used for a number of biochemical functions. For example, iron plays a role in the decomposition of hydrogen peroxide. The catalase activity of chelated iron is many times that of inorganic iron.

Physical and Clinical Characteristics of Porphyrins

The excretory route varies with the porphyrins and is related to the water solubility of the various porphyrins. Uroporphyrin, δ-aminolevulinic acid (ALA) which is the aliphatic precursor of porphyrins, and porphobilinogen (PBG) which is the monopyrrole precursor of porphyrins are very water soluble. These substances are mainly excreted in the urine. Coproporphyrin is less water soluble and is eliminated mainly through the bile but somewhat eliminated in the urine as coproporphyrinogen. Protoporphyrin is the least water soluble and is normall excreted exclusively in the bile.

The porphyrins share an absorption spectrum in the near ultraviolet and visible region. The Soret band, characteristic of all porphyrins, has an intense absorption near 400 nm. This absorption band can reveal the intense red fluorescence of the free porphyrins present in the teeth and bone marrow of patients with congenital erythropoietic porphyria.

When porphyrins are present in alkaline solution or organic solvents, they impart a red or brown color, whereas they impart a red-purple color in acid solution. One of the characteristic laboratory findings is a port wine or red-brown urine specimen when the porphyrins are present in large amounts.

Metabolic Disorders

Heme is synthesized via δ-aminolevulinic acid, porphobilinogen, uroporphyrinogens, coproporphyrinogens and protoporphyrinogens to result in protoporphyrin IX that chelates iron.

Metabolic defects in heme biosynthesis cause porphyrin disorders. There are many porphyrin disorders. Some are genetically determined, others are acquired. The genetically determined porphyrin disorders are known as "porphyria," whereas the porphyrin disorders acquired as a result of lead poisoning or chronic alcoholism are known as "porphyrinuria."

The porphyrin disorders can be further classified into three general groups, erythropoietic, hepatic, and erythrohepatic. Three groups and examples of disease in abnormalities within each group are shown in Table 6.1.

Laboratory Findings. Identification of the various porphyrins and porphyrin precursors is essential in diagnosing the specific

TABLE 6.1. DISORDERS OF PORPHYRIN METABOLISM

Erythropoietic Disorders
  Congenital erythropoietic porphyria
  Erythropoietic coproporphyria

Hepatic Disorders
  Acute intermittent porphyria
  Variegate porphyria
  Hereditary coproporphyria
  Porphyria cutanea tarda and acquired
    symptomatic porphyria from chronic
    alcoholism, liver disease, estrogen therapy,
    iron overload, hexachlorobenzene
    poisoning, hepatoma

Erythrohepatic Disorders
  Protoporphyria
  Porphyrinuria from lead intoxication

porphyrias. Screening, confirmatory, and quantitative tests are available.

The two porphyrin precursors, ALA and PBG, which are commonly increased in the hepatic porphyrias, can be detected by screening for urinary PBG with the Watson-Schwartz test.[27] In this test, porphobilinogen combines with dimethylaminobenzaldehyde (Ehrlich's reagent) to give a magenta-red color. False positive results with the Watson-Schwartz test can occur with urobilinogen and other substances, such as methyl red, melanogen, pyridium, and beets. The Hoesch test[28] eliminates the positive urobilinogen reaction. The other substances mentioned above are pink-red in the presence of the strong acid of the Ehrlich's reagent. Positive urine samples should, therefore, be checked by the addition of 22 percent HCl to a control sample, and butanol extraction should be employed. A diagram of the Watson-Schwartz test is shown in Figure 6.6.

A summary of the usual findings of the porphyrin disorders is shown in Table 6.2. The clinical symptoms and the type of porphyrin or porphyrin precursor found in the urine, feces, and red blood cells are used to differentiate the various porphyrin disorders.

The pH of the urine to be tested for ALA and PBG should be maintained between 6 and 7. Tests for ALA and PBG should be performed on fresh urine specimens.

Porphobilinogen easily forms porphyrins and other pigments upon being exposed to light. The change in porphobilinogen (a colorless compound) to porphyrin will cause the urine to become red upon standing. Delayed testing can cause the Watson-Schwartz test to become negative even though PGB levels remain within the test limits. The reason for this phenomenon is unknown.

Screening tests for porphyrins are based on the red fluorescent characteristic of all free porphyrins. Following separation of coproporphyrin by its extraction into an organic solvent, diethyl ether, at acid pH and from that solvent into hydrochloric acid, the red fluorescence is observed with an ultraviolet light.[29] The uroporphyrin is then extracted

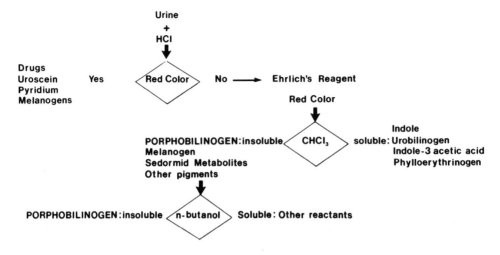

Figure 6.6. The Watson-Schwartz test for porphobilinogen.

from the urine into ethylacetate and from the ethylacetate into hydrochloric acid and also observed by ultraviolet light. Another test uses 0.5 g of talc to absorb the porphyrins from 10 ml of urine at pH 4. Following centrifugation and decantation, the talc is observed for the characteristic brick-red fluorescence of the porphyrins in ultraviolet light (~366 nm).[30] This test becomes definitely positive when the concentration is 0.5 mg/L or greater. The test described by Castrow utilizes a prepurification step, absorption on an ion exchange resin (AG 1 × −8) followed by elution and fluorescence.[31] Columns for this procedure are commercially available from Bio-Rad laboratories.

MUCOPOLYSACCHARIDES

Acid mucopolysaccharides or glycosoaminoglycans (GAGs) are the major compounds present in the ground substance of connective tissue. These compounds are long polysaccharide chains of alternating hexamosamine and uronic acid groups, except for keratan sulfate that has galactose in place of the uronic acid. Acid mucopolysaccharides have been found to participate in several body functions. For example, dermatan sul-

fate has antithrombin and lipemia clearing activity, and heparin has similar activities.

Clinical Findings. The glycosaminoglycans of medical interest are hyaluronic acid (HA), chondroitin-4-sulfate (ch-4-S), chondroitin-6-sulfate (ch-6-S), dermatan sulfate (DS), keratan sulfate (KS), heparan sulfate (hs), and heparin (H). Elevated levels of these substances have been found in rheumatoid arthritis, lupus erythematosus, and leukemia, but most of the investigations regarding the synthesis, metabolism, and analysis have been made on urine of patients who had inherited defects in mucopolysaccharide degradation or metabolism. The inherited defects are called mucopolysaccharidoses and include the following syndromes: Hurler's, Hunters, Sanfillipo's, Morquio's, Scheie's, Maroteaux-Lamy, and β-galactosidase deficiency. Much of the clinical investigation has been focused on relating the quantities and specific types of mucopolysaccharides that are excreted in the urine to the clinical features that are seen. These features include grotesque facies, dwarfism, skeletal malformations, mental retardation, cardiopulmonary defects, hepatosplenomegaly, corneal clouding, and hearing loss.[32]

TABLE 6.2. USUAL FINDINGS IN THE PORPHYRINURIAS

	Congenital Erythropoietic Porphyria	Erythropoietic Coproporphyria	Acute Intermittent Porphyria	Variegate Prophyria (Acute)	Hereditary Coproporphyria (Acute)	Cutanea Tarda and Acquired Porphyrias	Protoporphyria	Lead Intoxication
Urine								
ALA	N	N	++	++	++	N-+	N	+
PBG	N	N	++	++	++	N-	N	N-+
URO	+++	N	+	++	+	+++	N	N
COPRO	++	N	N-+	++	++	++-+++	N	+
Feces								
URO	++	N-+	N-++	N-+	?	++	N-+	N
COPRO	+++	N-+	N-++	++	+++	+-++	N-+	N
PROTO	N	N	N-++	++	N-+	N-+	N-++	N
RBC								
URO	+++	+	N	N	N	N	N	N
COPRO	++	++	N	N	N	N	N-+	N-+
PROTO	+	+	N	N	N	N	++	+
Clinical symptoms								
Photosensitivity	++	±	-	±	±	±	++	-
Skin lesions	++	-	-	+	±	+	N-+	-
Appearance of urine	Red	N	N	Red	Red	N	N	N
Anemia	+	-	-	-	-	-	±	+
Other	Red fluorescence of teeth		Psychosis, acute abdominal pain, peripheral neuropathy, can be precipitated by drugs, barbiturates	Peripheral neuropathy	Latent cases are frequent		Latent cases are frequent	

ALA, Δ-aminolevulinic acid; COPRO, coproporphyrin; N, normal; PBG, porphobilinogen; PROTO, protoporphyrin; URO, uroporphyrin; +, increased; ++, marked increase.

Metabolic Defect. The defect in the muco-polysaccharidoses was demonstrated by Fratantoni, Hall, and Neufeld in 1968 to be impaired degradation of mucopolysac-charides.[33] This was later shown to be due in each syndrome or disease to the deficiency of one or more lysosomal enzymes.[34] The prin-cipal enzymes that are deficient in each type of mucopolysaccharidoses are given in Table 6.3. These defects result in the increased uri-nary excretion of dermatan sulfate, heparan sulfate, keratan sulfate, and chondroitin-4- and chondroitin-6-sulfates.

Laboratory Studies. Screening tests com-monly used, all performed on either a ran-dom or 24-hour urine collection, are:

1. Precipitation by quaternary am-monium salts or albumin,
2. Electrophoretic demonstration of MPS, and
3. Thin-layer chromatography.

The high molecular weight compounds are precipitable by quaternary ammonium salts.[35] This has become the basis for a very useful screening test for mucopolysaccha-rides. The quaternary ammonium salt used by Pennock in the development of a reliable screening test is cetylpyridinium chloride (CPC).[36] Concentration, temperature, and pH can affect the precipitation of MPS in this method. However, the pH is controlled by using a buffer. The turbidity that results is compared visually with a standard solution of either chondroitin sulfate or hyaluronic acid. Renuart uses cetyltrimethyl ammonium bromide in a similar screening test.[37]

False positives with Pennock's method have been reported to be 3.6 percent of 1,000 chil-dren tested.[38] A 1 percent false positive in 2,000 urine specimens has been reported for the test designed by Renuart. The quaternary ammonium salt precipitation methods will detect all mucopolysaccharidoses with the possible exception of older patients who have Morquio's disease.[32]

Albumin solutions also form turbid solu-tions with glycosaminoglycans. This is the basis of a test used by Dorfman that is dis-cussed by Thomas and Howell.[6] It has largely been replaced by the quaternary ammonium salt turbidity tests.

Another type of screening test is based on the metachromasia that occurs when a basic dye, such as alcian blue or toluidine blue, is in contact with the anionic glycosaminogly-cans.[39] The blue color of the dye becomes pink when paper impregnated with the blue dye has a drop of urine containing a large concentration of glycosaminoglycans placed upon it. MPS* strips are commercially avail-able.

*Ames Division, Miles Laboratories, Inc., Elkhart, Indiana.

TABLE 6.3. GLYCOSAMINOGLYCAN URINARY EXCRETION AND ENZYME DEFICIENCIES IN MUCOPOLYSACCHARIDOSES

Mucopolysaccharidosis	Major Glycosaminoglycan Excreted	Deficient Enzyme
Hurler's syndrome	Dermatan sulfate/heparan sulfate (2–4:1)	α-L-iduronidase
Hunter's syndrome	Dermatan sulfate/heparan sulfate (1:1)	L-sulfoiduronate sulfatase
Scheie's syndrome	Dermatan sulfate/heparan sulfate (2–4:1)	α-L-iduronidase
Sanfillipo's syndrome	Heparan sulfate	Heparan sulfate sulfamidase
Morquio's syndrome	Keratan sulfate/chondroitin sulfate	N-acetylgalactosamine-6-sulfatase
Maroteaux-Lamy syndrome	Dermatan sulfate	N-acetylgalactosamine-4-sulfatase

Electrophoresis of glycosaminoglycans on cellulose acetate membranes in barium acetate buffer results in the separation and identity of some but not all of the types that may be present.[40] The GAGs are precipitated and removed from the urine by the addition of quaternary ammonium salt or calcium salts and centrifugation. The GAGs are then applied to the cellulose acetate membrane, and in the barium acetate buffer system, the electric current carries heparan sulfate, dermatan sulfate, and chondroitin sulfate into three distinct bands. A typical separation is shown in Figure 6.7. Chondroitin sulfate is not separated from keratin sulfate, nor is hyaluronic acid separated from dermatan sulfate by this method. However, as one can see from Table 6.3, the ratio of dermatan sulfate to heparan sulfate is important in the distinction of the type of mucopolysaccharidosis, and this ratio can be evaluated by electrophoresis.

Thin-layer chromatography may also be used to separate and identify the urinary GAGs.[41] Calcium salts of GAGs are separated on the thin-layer plate by their different mobilities in graded alcohol. The mobility of keratan sulfate is the greatest, followed by ch-6-S, ch-4-S, HS, and DS.

The excretion patterns of GAGs in the mucopolysaccharidoses are given in Table 6.3. Sly discusses the heterogeneity of molecular weights of GAGs and distribution patterns in some patients and points to the exceptional patients whose laboratory tests do not place them in any one of the idealized patterns.[32]

Quantitative methods for the measurement of GAGs are discussed in Chapter 7.

FAT

Fat can be found in the urine of patients who have sustained a bone-crush injury or who have fatty degeneration of the kidney. Whenever urine is to be examined for fat, two points in specimen collection must be followed. First, the specimen container must be a fat-free, non-waxed carton. Second, the bladder must be emptied completely and the entire specimen submitted. The fat tends to

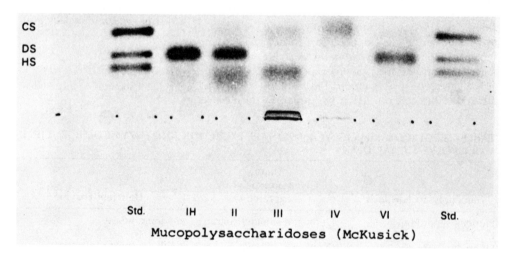

Figure 6.7. Electrophoretic separation of urinary glycosaminoglycans (0.1M barium acetate for 3 hours at 7.5 V/cm). Standard markers: CS, chondroitin sulfate; DS, dermatan sulfate; HS, heparan sulfate. IH, II, III, IV, VI, are McKusick's classification for Hurler, Hunter, Sanfillipo, Morquio, and Maroteaux-Lamy syndromes. (From Whiteman P: Acid glycosaminoglycan excretion in the mucopolysaccharidoses. In Holton JB, Ireland JT (eds): Inborn Errors of Skin, Hair and Connective Tissue, 1975, p 259. Courtesy of MTP Press, Lancaster, England.)

float on top of the urine in the bladder and is the last to be voided.

Fat will stain bright orange with oil red O or Sudan III. The portion of the centrifuged urine specimen to be tested should be taken from the top of the supernatant. A positive human fat control can be obtained from a bone marrow specimen, which can be preserved in 10 percent formalin.

SULFONAMIDES

The sulfonamide drugs that are manufactured today are very soluble and do not crystallize as easily as sulfa drugs of the past. However, patients who do not drink sufficient fluids while taking sulfonamide may pass sulfa crystals in the urine. Sulfa will crystallize in the acid or neutral urine. The crystals appear as yellow-brown wheat sheaves, as greenish globules with radial striations, or as cubes.

To confirm the presence of a sulfonamide in the urine, the lignin test can be performed. Sulfonamides, which are aniline derivatives, will produce a bright yellow color on a product such as newspaper, which has a high wood fiber or lignin content, when hydrochloric acid is added.

Sulfonamides may be quantitated by diazotization with N-(1-naphthyl)-ethylenediamine to produce a red-purple color.[42]

MELANIN

The conversion of the amino acid tyrosine to melanin is catalyzed by the enzyme tyrosinase. The biosynthesis of melanin takes place in specialized cells called "melanocytes." Melanocytes can be found in the skin (hair bulbs, dermis, and dermoepidermal junction), mucous membranes, nervous system, and eye (uveal tract and retinal pigment epithelium). Except for the melanocytes located in the hair bulbs and retinal pigment epithelium, all melanocytes have the ability to form malignant melanomas. Patients who have malignant melanomas will excrete a precursor of melanin into the urine. The pre-

cursor, 5,6-dihydroxyindole, will polymerize to form the dark pigment, melanin, which causes the urine specimen to become black.

Two screening tests can be performed to test the urine specimen for melanin. In one test, ferric chloride is added to the urine and causes a gray precipitate that turns black if melanin is present.[43] In the other test (Thormählen), sodium nitroprusside combines with melanin in an alkaline solution to form a red color.[44] Acetone and creatinine will cause a false positive test. Melanin can be differentiated with the addition of glacial acetic acid. Melanin will cause a green, blue, or black color depending on the amount present. A purple color denotes the presence of acetone, and an amber color is caused by creatinine.

MYOGLOBIN

Myoglobin consists of one protein molecule bound to one heme molecule and has a molecular weight of 17,000 (the molecular weight of hemoglobin is 60,000). Myoglobin is found in the muscle tissue and combines reversibly with oxygen to supply the muscle with oxygen during activity. Whenever there is injury to the muscle, such as crushing injuries sustained in accidents or beatings, myoglobin is released from the muscle and is quickly cleared to appear in the urine. Myoglobin also appears in the urine following extensive muscular activity, myocardial infarction, and participation in contact sports. Patients with muscular dystrophy will display myoglobinuria. The muscle tissue of dystrophy patients shows a marked decrease in the quantity of myoglobin. However, the myoglobin's quantitative characteristics remain the same as in normal muscle tissue.

The appearance of the urine specimen which contains myoglobin is light brown to black in color. The volume is usually small (less than 5 ml) because the presence of myoglobin reduces the urine output.

Hemoglobin and myoglobin will both give a positive test for hemoglobin or blood with the commercial reagent strips. After obtaining a positive reaction with the reagent strip, a screening test using ammonium sulfate can be performed.[45] Urine and ammonium sulfate are mixed and filtered. Myoglobin remains in solution with the addition of ammonium sulfate, and the filtrate will remain brown-black. Hemoglobin is precipitated by ammonium sulfate and remains on the filter, yielding a clear filtrate. Spectrophotometric methods can be used to confirm the presence of myoglobin.[46] Electrophoresis can be used if the patient does not have hemoglobin C.[47] Hemoglobin C and myoglobin have the same electrophoretic mobility and cannot be distinguished. Ultrafiltration can also be used because hemoglobin is a larger molecule than myoglobin.[48] Urine specimens containing myoglobin can be preserved by adjusting the pH to 7.5 with sodium hydroxide and refrigerating. The specimen should *not* be frozen.

SCREENING PROGRAMS

The development of a screening program for metabolic disorders requires consideration of medical effectiveness (can the result be used by the physician to help the patient?), the sensitivity and specificity of the tests, the confirmatory tests that are available, the cost to the patient or public, and the relationships of screening tests for more than one disorder in terms of the type and volume of specimen that is required and the maximum information that can be derived. Discussion of screening programs in a historical context can be found in a publication of The National Academy of Sciences,[49] along with detailed descriptions of most of the techniques. A discussion of structural guidelines for a metabolic disorder screening program is available in a book by Shih.[50]

Review Questions

One or more responses may be correct.
1. A red colored compound produced by mixing urine, sodium acetate, and para dimethyl amino benzaldehyde is insoluble in chloroform and butanol. This reaction is likely due to the presence of:
   A. Uroporphyrin
   B. Porphobilinogen
   C. Urobilinogen
   D. Delta aminolevulinic acid
   E. Protoporphyrin
2. Extraction of urine acidified with acetic acid by shaking with ether results in a red fluorescence in the ether extract alone. Which of the following is present?
   A. Uroporphyrin
   B. Delta aminolevulinic acid
   C. Porphobilinogen
   D. Protoporphyrin
   E. Coproporphyrin
3. A disease that causes large amounts of branched chain amino acids (valine, leucine, and isoleucine) to be excreted in the urine is:
   A. Hurler's
   B. Cystinuria
   C. Maple sugar urine disease
   D. Porphyria
   E. Alkaptonuria
4. Phenylketonuria is caused by a functional absence of which enzyme?
   A. *p*-Hydroxyphenylpyruvic oxidase
   B. Tyrosinase
   C. Phenylalanine oxidase
   D. Phenylalanine hydroxylase
   E. Homogentisic acid oxidase
5. The disease phenylketonuria (PKU) is characterized by which of the following laboratory results?
   A. Elevated serum phenylalanine and tyrosine and elevated urine phenylketones
   B. Elevated serum phenylalanine and elevated urine homogentisic acid
   C. Decreased activity of parahydroxyphenylpyruvic acid oxidase and an accumulation of phenylpyruvic acid in urine
   D. Elevated serum phenylalanine, decreased serum tyrosine and ac-

cumulation of phenylpyruvic acid in urine

E. A positive ferric chloride test and a positive ammoniacal silver nitrate test

6. The increased excretion of copro-porphyrins may be due to which of the following conditions?
A. Liver damage
B. Infection
C. Accelerated erythropoiesis
D. Lead intoxication

7. Which of the following is/are charac-teristic(s) of *all* porphyrins?
A. Function as prosthetic group in proteins
B. Insoluble in aqueous solution
C. Chelate iron to form heme
D. Exhibit strong red fluorescence when excited at 400 nm

8. A thin-layer chromatogram of a urine specimen when developed with nin-hydrin gives a purple band of abnor-mal amount near the origin, the sodium cyanide-nitroprusside test performed on the urine gives a magenta color. These results are most likely due to:
A. Phenylalaninuria
B. Tyrosinuria
C. Histidinuria
D. Cystinuria

9. Alkaptonuria may be demonstrated by which of the following?
A. Deficient enzyme, homogentisic acid oxidase
B. A positive reducing test on urine, e.g., Clinitest
C. An increased urinary excretion of homogentisic acid
D. An accumulation of maleylaceto acetic acid in the blood

10. Hereditary tyrosinemia results in which of the following?
A. Liver damage
B. Damaged renal tubules
C. Excessive urinary excretion of tyrosine
D. Excessive excretion of several amino acids

11. The ketoacid metabolites of which of the following amino acids are ex-creted in increased amounts in maple syrup urine disease?
A. Cystine
B. Leucine
C. Phenylalanine
D. Valine

12. Urinary ketoacids can be determined by their reaction with which of the following reagents?
A. 1-Nitroso-2-naphthol
B. Sodium nitroprusside
C. Para dimethyl amino benzalde-hyde
D. 2, 4-Dinitrophenylhydrazine

13. Persons being tested for urinary 5-hydroxytryptamine(5HT) must eliminate which of the following items from their diet because of their con-tent of 5 HT?
A. Bananas
B. Peaches
C. Tomatoes
D. Oranges

14. Glycosaminoglycans of medical im-portance include which of the follow-ing?
A. Hyaluronic acid
B. Chondroitin-4-sulfate
C. Chondroitin-6-sulfate
D. Dermatan sulfate

15. An increase in mucopolysaccharide excretion in the urine can be de-monstrated by which of the following?
A. Precipitation upon addition of quaternary ammonium salts
B. Electrophoresis and staining with alcian blue
C. Thin layer chromatography and staining with toluidine blue
D. Precipitation with 1-nitroso-2-naphthol

16. Sulfonamides will give a red-purple color in a screening test that employs which of the following?
A. Lignin
B. P-Dimethyl amino benzaldehyde
C. Sudan III
D. N-(1-naphthyl)-ene diamine

17. Screening tests for melaninuria are:
    A. Ferric chloride (gray precipitate)
    B. A dark color of the urine upon standing
    C. Sodium nitroprusside (red in alkali)
    D. Sudan III (red color)

(See Appendix for answers.)

Case Studies

Case Study 1

A 3-year-old female with a history of poor growth since birth and chronic acidosis failed to respond to treatment prescribed by her family physician. The physician referred her to a large pediatric clinic. Upon physical examination she was found to have the height of a one-year-old. Her limbs were very thin, and she showed signs of rickets, which was confirmed by x-ray. Other abnormal clinical findings included polydipsia and polyuria. A urine specimen gave the following results:

Characteristic	Finding
Color:	yellow
Character:	cloudy
Specific gravity:	1.009
pH:	7.5
Protein:	100 mg/dl
Glucose:	0.5% (0.5 g/dl)
Acetone:	trace
Blood:	negative
Bilirubin:	negative
Urobilinogen:	0.1 EU
Nitrate:	negative

Microscopic examination was essentially normal

Other laboratory data:
Serum creatinine: 2.1 mg/dl
BUN: 60 mg/dl
Fasting blood glucose: normal
Two-hour postprandial: normal

Questions

1. Which of the following laboratory test(s) or clinical findings would be helpful in diagnosing the child's condition:
   A. Urinary phosphorus level
   B. Examination of bone marrow
   C. Analysis of urinary amino acids
   D. Eye examination
   E. Thyroid hormones
2. Of the laboratory tests chosen in the previous question, list the test(s) and their expected results.
3. The laboratory data and clinical findings are consistent with which of the following diseases:
   A. Fanconi syndrome
   B. Cystinuria
   C. Cystinosis
   D. Tyrosinemia
4. Name three major differences between cystinosis and cystinuria that can be demonstrated in the laboratory.

Answers

1. A,B,C,D
2.
   A. Urinary phosphorus level—increased
   B. Examination of bone marrow—presence of cystine crystals
   C. Analysis of urinary amino acids—generalized aminoaciduria involving 10 amino acids.
   D. Eye examination—crystalline deposits in the conjunctiva
3. C
4.
   A. Aminoaciduria of cystinuria is limited to cystine, lysine, arginine, and ornithine, whereas aminoaciduria of cystinosis is generalized.
   B. Cystine stone formation is found in cystinuria but extremely rare in cystinosis
   C. Deposits of cystine crystals in body tissue including bone marrow occur in cystinosis, not in cystinuria

Case Study 2

A 35-year-old male was seen by his physician. His chief complaints were acute abdominal pain, constipation, nausea, and weight loss. There were no other abnormalities found on physical examination. A medical history revealed that the patient had recently begun to take a barbiturate. An examination of the patient's urine was normal except that the specimen turned red upon standing. The Watson-Schwartz test was positive for porphobilinogen. The patient's symptoms disappeared when the barbiturate was discontinued.

Question
1. What is the most likely type of porphyria described in the patient?

Answer
1. Acute intermittent porphyria. The patient showed no photosensitivity as seen in other types of porphyrias.

Case Study 3
A two-week-old infant was admitted to the emergency room with vomiting, lethargy, and convulsions. Blood and urine specimens were sent to the laboratory. The technologist noticed that the urine had the peculiar odor of maple syrup.

Questions
1. What abnormal amino acids would be expected to be present in the serum?
2. At what step in the catabolism of the amino acids does the metabolic defect occur?

Answers
1. Valine, leucine, and isoleucine
2. The oxidative decarboxylation of the α-keto acids

Case Study 4
A two-month-old infant was brought to the physician's office. His symptoms included vomiting, diarrhea, edema, and enlargement of the abdomen, spleen, and liver. A urine sample gave the following results:

Characteristic	Finding
Color:	yellow
Character:	cloudy
Specific gravity:	1.010
pH:	7.0

Protein:	100 mg/dl
Glucose:	0.5%
Ketone:	negative
Blood:	negative
Bilirubin:	negative
Urobilinogen:	0.1 EU
Nitrate:	negative

Other laboratory tests:
Urinary phosphorus: increased

Questions
1. What additional tests would be helpful in diagnosing the disease?
2. What are the expected results of the additional tests?
3. Which of the following diseases is most consistent with the clinical and laboratory findings?
   A. Cystinosis
   B. Cystinuria
   C. Transient normal tyrosinemia
   D. Hereditary tyrosinemia
   E. Fanconi syndrome
4. What is the deficient enzyme of the above disease?
5. Which of the following parts of the kidney is damaged in this disease?
   A. Glomerulus
   B. Renal tubules
   C. Cortex
   D. Medulla

Answers
1.
   A. Analysis of urinary amino acids
   B. Eye examination for crystalline deposits
   C. Examination of bone marrow for crystalline deposits
2.
   A. Urinary amino aciduria of a generalized type with tyrosine predominating
   B. Eye examination and bone marrow examination—no crystalline deposits seen
3. D
4. p-Hydroxyphenylpyruvic acid oxidase
5. B

REFERENCES

1. Grant G, Kachmar JF: Amino acids and related metabolites. In Tietz N (ed): Fundamentals of Clinical Chemistry. Philadelphia, Saunders, 1976, p 390.
2. Knox WE: Phenylketonuria. In Stanbury JB, Wyngaarden JB, Frederickson DS (eds): The Metabolic Basis of Inherited Disease, 3rd ed. New York, McGraw-Hill, 1972, pp 266–296.
3. Renaurt AW: Screening for inborn errors of metabolism associated with mental deficiency or neurological disorders or both. N Engl J Med 274:384, 1966.
4. Gentz J, Jagenburg R, Zetterstrom R: Tyrosinemia. An inborn error of tyrosine metabolism with cirrhosis of the liver and multiple renal tubular defects (de-Toni-Debre-Franconi syndrome). J Pediatr 66:670, 1965.
5. Penrose L, Quastel JH: Metabolic studies in phenylketonuria. Biochem J 31:266, 1937.
6. Thomas H, Howell RR: Selected Screening Test for Genetic Metabolic Diseases. Chicago, Year Book, 1974, p 20.
7. Menkes JH: Maple syrup disease. Isolation and identification of organic acids in urine. Pediatrics 23:348, 1959.
8. Dancis J, Hutzler J, Levitz M: Thin-layer chromatography and spectrophotometry of α-keto acid hydrazones. Biochem Biophys Acta 78:85, 1963.
9. Saifer A: Rapid screening methods for the detection of inherited and acquired aminoacidopathies. In Bodansky O, Latner AL (eds): Advances in Clinical Chemistry. New York, Academic, 1971, vol 14, pp 145–218.
10. Kelly S: Biochemical Methods in Medical Genetics. Springfield, Ill., Thomas, 1974, pp 17–25.
11. Recommended Guidelines for PKU Programs for the Newborn. US Dept of Health, Education and Welfare, Maternal and Child Health Service, Washington D.C., US Govt Printing Office, 1971.
12. LaDu BN: Alcaptonuria. In Stanbury JB, Wyngaarden JB, Frederickson DS (eds): New York, McGraw-Hill, 1972, pp 308–325.
13. Fischberg EH: The instantaneous diagnosis of alkaptonuria on a single drop of urine. JAMA 119:882, 1942.
14. Sommerfelt SC, Wynstroot E: Detection and rough estimation of homogentisic acid in urine. Scand J Clin Lab Invest 9:196, 1957.
15. Ibbott F: Amino acids and related substances. In Henry RJ, Cannon DC, Winkelman JW (eds): Clinical Chemistry Principles and Technics, 2nd ed. New York, Harper & Row, 1974, pp 625–626.
16. Seegmiller JE, Zannoni VG, Laster L, LaDu BN: An enzymatic spectrophotometric method for the determination of homogentisic acid in plasma and urine. J Biol Chem 236:774, 1961.
17. Medes G: A new error of tyrosine metabolism: Tyrosinosis. The intermediary metabolism of tyrosine and phenylalanine. Biochem J 26:917, 1932.
18. Bradley M, Schumann GB, Ward PC: Examination of the urine. In Henry JB (ed): Clinical Diagnosis by Laboratory Methods and Management, 16th ed. Philadelphia, Saunders, 1979, p 607.
19. Grant G, Kachmar JF: Amino acids and related metabolites. In Tietz N (ed): Fundamentals of Clinical Chemistry. Philadelphia, Saunders, 1976, pp 396–397.
20. Gerritsen T, Niederwieser A: Amino acids. In Curtius HC, Roth M (eds): Clinical Chemistry Principles and Methods. New York, Walter de Gruyter, 1974, vol II, pp. 1076–1077.
21. Ibbott F: Amino acids and related substances. In Henry RJ, Cannon DC, Winkelman JW (eds): Clinical Chemistry Principles and Technics, 2nd ed. New York, Harper & Row, 1974, pp 582–589.
22. Meister A: Biochemistry of the Amino Acids. New York, Academic, 1965, vol I, pp 256–258.
23. Horning EC, Horning MG: Human metabolic profiles obtained by GC and GC/MS. J Chromatogr Sci 9:129, 1971.
24. Thier SO, Segal S: Cystinuria. In Stanbury JB, Wyngaarden JB, Frederickson DS (eds): New York, McGraw-Hill, 1972, pp 1504–1519.
25. Brand E, Harris MM, Biloon S: Cystinuria: The excretion of cystine complex which decomposes in the urine with the liberation of free cystine. J Biol Chem 86:315, 1930.
26. Sjoerdsma A, Weissbach H, Udenfriend S: Simple test for diagnosis of metastatic carcinoid (argentaffinoma). JAMA 159:397, 1955.
27. Labbe R: Porphyrins and related compounds. In Tietz N (ed): Fundamentals of Clinical Chemistry. Philadelphia, Saunders, 1976, p 462.
28. Lamon J, With TK, Redeker AG: The Hoesch test: bedside screening for urinary porphobilinogen in patients with suspected porphyria. Clin Chem 20:1438–1440, 1974
29. Labbe R: Porphyrins and related compounds. In Tietz N (ed): Fundamentals of Clinical Chemistry. Philadelphia, Saunders, 1976, p 467.
30. Doss MO: Porphyrins and porphyria precursors. In Curtius HC, Roth M (eds): Clinical Biochemistry Principles and Methods. New York, Walter de Gruyter, 1974, vol II, p 1336.
31. Castrow FF II, Mullins JF, Mills GG: Newer screening test for porphyria. J Invest Dermatol 50:340, 1968.
32. Sly WS: The mucopolysaccharidoses. In Bondy PK, Rosenberg LE (eds): Metabolic

Control and Disease, 8th ed. Philadelphia, Saunders, 1980, pp 545–581.

33. Fratantoni JC, Hall CW, Neufeld EF: The defect in Hurler's and Hunter's syndromes: faulty degradation of mucopolysaccharides. Proc Soc Natl Acad Sci 60:699, 1968.

34. Neufeld EF, Lim TW, Shapiro LJ: Inherited disorders of lysosomal metabolism. Annu Rev Biochem 44:357, 1975.

35. Di Ferrante N, Neri G, Neri ME, Hoosett WE III: Measurement of urinary glycosaminoglycans with quaternary ammonium salts—an extension of the method. Connect Tissue Res 1:93, 1972.

36. Pennock CA: A review and selection of simple laboratory methods used for the study of glycosaminoglycan excretion and the diagnosis of the mucopolysaccharidoses. J Clin Pathol 29:111, 1976.

37. Renuart AH: Screening for inborn errors of metabolism associated with mental deficiency or neurological disorders or both. N Engl J Med 274:384, 1966.

38. Valdivieso F, Martinez Valverde A, Matres M, Ugarte M: Early diagnosis of hypermucopolysacchariduria. Clin Chim Acta 44:357, 1973.

39. Berry HK, Spinanger J: A paper spot test useful in study of Hurler's syndrome. J Lab Clin Med 55:136, 1960.

40. Wessler E: Analytical and preparative separation of acid glycosaminoglycans by electrophoresis in barium acetate. Anal Biochem 26:439, 1968.

41. Humbel R, Charmoles NA: Sequential thin-layer chromatography of urinary glycosaminoglycans. Clin Chim Acta 40:290, 1972.

42. Bratton AC, Marshall EK Jr: A new coupling component for sulfanilamide determination. J Biol Chem 128:537, 1939.

43. Bradley M, Schumann G, Ward PC: Examination of the urine. In Henry JB (ed): Clinical Diagnosis by Laboratory Methods and Management, 16th ed. Philadelphia, Saunders, 1979, p 497.

44. Beeler MF, Henry JB: Melanogenuria—evaluation of several commonly used laboratory procedures. JAMA 176:52, 1961.

45. Blondheim SH, Margoliash E, Shafir EA: A simple test for myohemoglobinuria (myoglobinuria). JAMA 167:453, 1958.

46. Glauser SC, Wagner H, Glauser EM: A rapid simple accurate test for differentiating hemoglobinuria from myoglobinuria. Am J Med Sci 264:135, 1972.

47. Boulton FE, Huntsman RG: The detection of myoglobin in urine and its distinction from normal and hemoglobin variants. J Clin Pathol 24:816, 1971.

48. Farmer TA Jr, Hammack WJ, Frommeyer WB Jr: Idiopathic recurrent rhabdomyolysis associated with myoglobinuria: report of a case. N Engl J Med 264:60, 1961.

49. Committee for the Study of Inborn Errors of Metabolism, Division of Medical Sciences, Assembly of Life Sciences, National Research Council: Genetic Screening Programs, Principles and Research, Washington, D.C., National Academy of Sciences, 1975.

50. Shih VE: Laboratory Techniques for the Detection of Hereditary Metabolic Disorders. Cleveland, CRC Press, 1973.

Doris L. Ross

	CHAPTER 7

Special Tests

Objectives

After studying this chapter, the student should be able to:

1. Identify the reasons for or against reporting the results of quantitative urine analysis by mass per volume and unit mass of analyte per unit mass of creatinine.
2. Compare the specifications of the Benedict's, o-toluidine, and glucose oxidase methods for quantitative measurement of urinary glucose.
3. Describe an enzymic method for urinary glucose determination.
4. Identify the normal urinary excretion of glucose.
5. Relate fructosuria, galactosuria, pentosuria, and lactosuria to their associated clinical conditions.
6. Define and characterize mucopolysaccharides.
7. Differentiate between Sanfillipo and Hurler syndromes based upon the mucopolysaccharide excreted and the enzyme deficiency.
8. List the reagents and techniques used to analyze quantitatively the mucopolysaccharides in urine.
9. Identify three mucolipidoses that are investigated by examining urine.
10. Identify the diseases or conditions that result in (a) overflow amioaciduria or (b) renal tubular defect.
11. Identify the three chemicals that react with urinary amino acids and are used in their quantitative measurement.
12. Describe the method for the quantitative analysis of each amino acid in urine.
13. Identify the two sources of protein in the urine.
14. Discuss the problems present in the determination of total urinary protein by the turbidity produced by organic acids.
15. Relate Coomassie blue, Ponceau S, Lowry's reagent, and absorbance of 280 nm and 210 nm to the characteristics of proteins that are utilized in their determination by these techniques.

16. List seven methods used to separate, identify, or quantitate urinary protein or fraction or individual entities.

17. Distinguish between a normal urinary protein electrophoretic pattern and one obtained on urine in renal tubular damage or glomerulonephritis.

18. Contrast and compare the results of agar gel and acrylamide gel electrophoresis with that performed on cellulose acetate.

19. Describe the Laurell or rocket immunoelectrophoresis method for the quantitation of urinary proteins.

20. Compare and contrast nephelometric, radial immunodiffusions, and radioimmunoassay methods for the quantitation of urinary proteins.

21. Recognize the causes and circumstances for the occurrence of proteinuria.

22. Compare and contrast glomerular, tubular, and overflow proteinuria with particular emphasis on the proteins excreted.

23. Identify two well-defined proteins that originate in the kidney.

24. Distinguish the usefulness of the determinations of alanine aminopeptidase, β-glucuronidase, lysozyme, lactate dehydrogenase, and glutamyltransferase.

25. Identify a critical point in the collection of a urine specimen for alkaloids and heavy metals.

26. Identify three factors that affect drug concentration in the urine.

27. List four immunoassay methods for drug determinations.

Through the years the analysis of urine has given physicians information to use in arriving at a diagnosis or in reaching a decision regarding the treatment of a patient's illness. The majority of tests performed on urine have been made to evaluate functions other than those of the kidney. The historical use of urine was based on (1) the availability of large quantities of fluid from which low concentrations of some analytes could be extracted, (2) the limitations of the available analytic methods at the time, and (3) the natural (noninvasive) means of obtaining the specimen.

The advances made each year in the sensitivity and selectivity of analytic methods have enabled laboratories to use blood more frequently as the source of information about the body's function. This is particularly true in the case of hormones and other substances against which antibodies can be raised. There is little doubt that this replacement of urine chemistry with blood chemistry will continue.

At the same time we can anticipate a growing interest in the chemical and cellular constituents in urine that are related to renal disease.

The quantitative analysis of a urinary constituent has several factors that must be considered. The volume of urine excreted within a given period of time fluctuates so that the unit of mass per volume has little meaning. The use of a timed urine overcomes this problem, and the excretion of an analyte can be recorded in mass per time, e.g., g/24 hours (d). Most quantitative urine analyses are made on 24-hour specimens. There is, however, a problem accompanying the use of timed specimens. In some cases the collection may not be complete, and therefore the mass per time is an incorrect report. To overcome this error, the creatinine concentration of the urine is determined at the same time as the determination of the analyte. The analyte is then reported as mass of analyte per mass of creatinine. Creatinine is excreted in constant amounts, and the report of an analyte in a ratio to creatinine excretion is useful in overcoming problems in timed volume collections. It has been shown that the total creatinine content of the first morning specimen is independent of dietary change.[1] Some variability in creatinine excretion by normal subjects under controlled conditions has been reported.[2] In spite of this, other investigators have found that reporting analytes in a ratio to creatinine in the first morning urine specimen is a useful method.[3–5]

DEFINITIVE TESTS FOR CARBOHYDRATES AND MUCOPOLYSACCHARIDES IN URINE

The quantitation of urinary carbohydrates and mucopolysaccharides is generally not a major activity in the laboratory of a general hospital. However, for some patients these tests can be of great help in establishing a diagnosis or in following the response to treatment. Most of these investigations will be made in regard to the excretion of monosaccharides or polysaccharides and mucopolysaccharides in metabolic diseases, many of which are inherited. Diabetes is included in this broad group. Several simple screening tests for these diseases are discussed in Chapters 5 and 6. In some instances, the quantitative determination of specific carbohydrates and mucopolysaccharides is useful.

Normal urine contains several sugars that are listed in Table 7.1.[6] Only a few of these are of interest to the clinical laboratory and will be discussed: glucose, lactose, fructose, galactose, pentoses, and also the mucopolysaccharides containing chondroitin-4-sulfate, chondroitin-6-sulfate, hyaluronic acid, dermatan sulfate, heparan sulfate, and keratan sulfate.

Glucose
Early colorimetric tests were based on the chemical reactions of reactive groups of carbohydrates, e.g., the reducing action of the enediol group of glucose, mannose, and fructose. This reducing property was utilized to assay these urinary sugars with alkaline copper salt solutions, e.g., Benedict's reagent,[7] and yellow ferricyanide.[8] However, these have been largely replaced by a method that employs o-toluidine, an aromatic amine, that condenses with aldoses in acid to give a blue-green compound, the Shiff base of n-glucosylamine.[9]

Glucose exists in several forms in solution. These forms are illustrated in Figure 7.1. The enediol is the reactive part of the glucose molecule that is easily oxidized. In solution α-D-glucopyranose undergoes mutarotation

TABLE 7.1. CARBOHYDRATES AND MUCOPOLYSACCHARIDES IN NORMAL URINE

	Mg/dl	MM/L	Mg/24 hours	Reference
Glucose	5.2	0.289	52	6
Lactose	9.5	0.277	23	6
Fructose	2.1	0.117	60	15
Galactose	10.0	0.56	14	17
Pentoses			255	6
Xylose	2.8	0.185	49	6
Arabinose	6.9	0.459	38	6
L-xyloketose			4	6
Sucrose	2.2	0.064		6
Mucopolysaccharides (as hexuronic acid)				
Females			11.3	28
Males			13.3	28

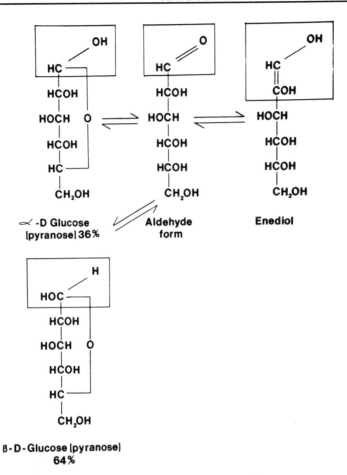

Figure 7.1. Forms of glucose in solution.

to β-D-glucopyranose, which at equilibrium is 36 percent α and 64 percent β.

The most specific methods for determining glucose are those employing enzymes, either glucose oxidase (which has a high specificity for β-D-glucose) or hexokinase. The glucose oxidase method usually requires the removal of interfering substances, such as uric acid, by adsorption on charcoal or Lloyd's reagent[10] or by an ion exchange resin.[11] The glucose oxidase reaction may be monitored in two ways: (1) a polarographic oxygen analyzer,[12] such as that used in the Beckman glucose analyzer, or (2) a colorimetric reaction involving the hydrogen peroxide that is formed. The polarographic measure-

ment does not require the precaution against interfering substances that the colorimetric tests require. Substances that have been used to react with the hydrogen peroxide are a second enzyme peroxidase and a chromogenic oxygen acceptor, e.g., o-toluidine, o-anisidine, or an iodide. The normal 24-hour urine excretion determined by o-toluidine is 0 to 1.375 mmole (0 to 0.25 g). Enzymatic tests have given similar values.[13]

Fructose

The occurrence of fructosuria is estimated to be approximately 1:130,000.[14] This asymptomatic abnormality of decreased utilization of dietary fructose is uncommon, as is another inherited condition, fructose intolerance, which is associated with symptoms of vomiting and liver disturbances. The quantitative methods for determination of fructose are similar to those for inulin, a polysaccharide of fructose. A method recommended by Pileggi and Szustkiewicz[6] is that of Heyrovsky,[15] in which the fructose is determined spectrophotometrically by the violet color produced when it is reacted with indole-3-acetic acid in HCl.

Galactose

Galactosuria occurs in some normal newborn infants usually from two to six days after birth[16] and in the inherited diseases of galactose intolerance and galactosemia. Quantitative tests on urine are rarely performed, but an enzymatic method utilizing galactose dehydrogenase in a redox reaction monitored by the increase in absorbance at 340 nm has been described.[17] Normal infants less than two weeks old excrete up to 1.39 mmole/L (25 mg/dl). Older individuals normally excrete less than 0.56 mmole/L (10 mg/dl).

Pentoses

Pentosuria has been categorized according to its etiology. Three categories described are[6]:

1. Alimentary: This results from the ingestion of fruits that contain large quantities of pentoses, e.g., prunes, grapes, and cherries. This is a temporary cause of pentosuria.
2. Reactive: This category includes those stimuli that result in pentosuria, e.g., such drugs as morphine, cortisone, and antipyretics, and fever and allergy.
3. Essential: This is a recessively inherited abnormality in the enzyme, xylotol dehydrogenase, which has a decreased affinity for nicotine adenine dinucleotide phosphate. It is harmless, and the pentose excreted is L-xyloketose (L-xylulose).

The qualitative tests rely upon the reducing characteristics of pentose and on their reaction with acid to produce furfural, which gives color reactions with phloroglucinol (Tollens' test),[18] orcinol (Bial's test),[19] or benzidine (Tauber's test).[20] The furfural reaction has been used in the quantitative determination of pentoses using a p-bromoaniline acetate reagent to give a pink color with the furfural.[21] Specific enzymatic assays for the measurement of D-xyloketose and L-xyloketose use the D-xyloketose and L-xyloketose dehydrogenases.[22]

Quantitation of xylose is occasionally requested. Xylose is absorbed principally in the jejunum and is not metabolized. Its absorption has been used in the differential diagnosis of intestinal malabsorption. A 25 g dose of xylose is administered, and urine and blood specimens are analyzed to determine the absorption. Normally, adults will excrete at least 26.6 mmoles (4 g) xylose in a 5-hour period.[23] In order to ascertain that renal disease is not interfering with the test, the blood level determined should be 2.4 ± 1.07 mmole/L (36 ± 16 mg/dl).

Lactose

The disaccharide lactose is excreted in the urine in several conditions:

1. In pregnancy and during lactation,
2. In intestinal disease, e.g., celiac disease, sprue, Giardia lamblia infestation,
3. While taking medication, e.g., neomycin, kanamycin,
4. In lactose intolerance due to lactase deficiency in the mucosa of the small bowel, and
5. In an exclusive milk diet.

Persons with lactose intolerance exhibit intestinal cramping and fullness after ingesting food that contains lactose. This is usually followed by diarrhea. The watery stool has a pH of less than 6 due to the bacterial formation of acids from the unabsorbed sugar.

Screening tests for lactose use lead acetate and ammonium hydroxide (Rubner's test)[24] or a furfural test (Tollens' test). A specific quantitative method for determination of lactose in urine utilizes galactosidase to hydrolyze the lactose to glucose and galactose and the quantitation of these products by the o-toluidine method.[25]

Analysis of Sugars by Gas Chromatography

Carbohydrates in urine may be measured by gas liquid chromatography.[26] This analytic technique overcomes the disadvantages of (1) the nonspecificity of tests based on reducing characteristics, (2) reactions given by other substances, and (3) interfering substances present in urine that affect the enzymatic assays. In preparation for gas chromatographic analysis, the sugars are derivatized to o-trimethylsilyl (TMS) ethers. These derivatives may be separated in a variety of polar and nonpolar phases. For a detailed discussion, the reader is referred to a review of the subject.[27]

Mucopolysaccharides (Glycosaminoglycans)

The detection of mucopolysacchariduria and the identification of the specific mucopolysaccharides excreted have been important in the delineation of the inherited diseases grouped as mucopolysaccharidoses.

The mucopolysaccharidoses are disorders of connective tissue concerned with enzyme deficiencies (Table 6.3). These are rare diseases ranging from an incidence of 1:150,000 to 1:1,000,000, and they are characterized by skeletal and facial abnormalities. The sub-stances excreted in the urine, acid mucopolysaccharides, are high molecular weight molecules composed of carbohydrate chains with repeating units of uronic acids and sulfated hexosamines.[28] An example of such a repeating unit is shown in Figure 7.2.

Screening tests for urinary acid mucopolysaccharides are based upon (1) the metachromasia or color changes produced as the acidic group reacts with the basic groups of a dye, e.g., Alcian blue and toluidine blue dyes,[29] and (2) the precipitation with acidified albumin[30] or quaternary ammonium salts, e.g., cetyltrimethyl ammonium bromide[31] or cetylpyridinium chloride.[32] Normally chondroitin 4-sulfate and 6-sulfate and hyaluronic acid appear in the urine. The first two are excreted in excessive amounts in some mucopolysaccharidoses. A quantitative microprocedure for the determination of total urinary acid mucopolysaccharides that requires only 50 μl of urine is based upon complex formation with the cationic dye Alcian blue.[33,34]

The distinction of the type of mucopolysaccharide present is made by several methods. Ion exchange chromatography is used, followed by colorimetric reactions performed on the eluate fractions to determine the various hexosamines and uronic acids.[35] Gas liquid chromatography is also used to separate and quantitate the glucosamines and galactosamines present.[36] Other methods

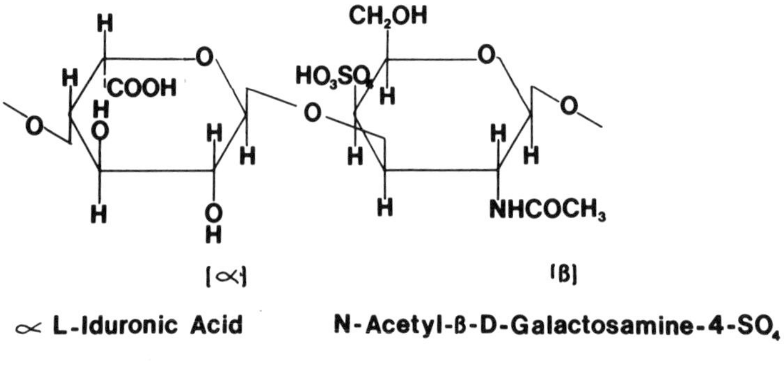

α L-Iduronic Acid   N-Acetyl-β-D-Galactosamine-4-SO$_4$

Figure 7.2. One of the repeating units of dermatan sulfate. Others are α-L-iduronic acid-2-SO$_4$ and β-D-glucuronic acid, each attached to N-acetyl-β-D-galactosamine-4-SO$_4$.

used to classify the type of mucopolysaccharides present in urine are electrophoresis on cellulose acetate[37,38] (Fig. 6.7) and thin-layer chromatography.[39,40] In addition, enzymes are used to determine specific components of the glycosaminoglycans, including the isomers.[35] For an evaluation of laboratory methods and a flow chart for the use of these tests in the analysis of urinary mucopolysaccharides, the reader is referred to a report by Pennock.[35] Extensive discussions of mucopolysaccharidoses by Sly[41] and Dorfman and Matalow[42] are available.

Mucolipidoses

The mucolipidoses are characterized by some clinical similarities to the mucopolysaccharidoses. However, this group of abnormalities is biochemically distinguishable by the absence of mucopolysacchariduria in all but one type. The mucolipidoses exhibit either deficient enzyme activity or increased activity of lysosomal enzymes in tissues and body fluids. The types of mucolipidoses, their defects, and the fluid or body tissue used for the detection of the defect are shown in Table 7.2.

Methods for the detection and separation of oligosaccharides are thin-layer chromatography[43] and high pressure liquid chromatography.[44] Analysis of the excess or deficient activity of the enzymes that are related to the type of mucolipidosis can be performed.[45] Those that are performed on urine are indicated in Table 7.2.

AMINOACIDURIAS

Aminoaciduria can result from several causes, e.g., metabolic lesions of liver disease or enzyme deficiencies of inherited disease. One type of aminoaciduria exhibits an increased blood concentration of amino acids that eventually are filtered through the glomerulus, exceed the absorptive capacity of the tubules, and are excreted in the urine. This is known as the "overflow" type of aminoaciduria. The second type of aminoaciduria results from a defect in the reabsorptive capability of the renal tubules. It can be distinguished from the first type because the blood concentration of amino acids is normal. Conditions that fall in this second type are Fanconi's syndrome, cystinosis, Wilson's disease, and toxic damage to the kidney.

Total Amino Acids

The most commonly performed screening test for aminoaciduria is thin-layer chromatography in one dimension with color development with ninhydrin.[46,47] This method is discussed in Chapter 6. Total amino acid urinary excretion is measured quantitatively after removal of interfering materials, e.g., uric acid, by treatment with cation exchange resins. The isolated amino acids are treated with sodium β-napthoquinone-4-sulfonate, and a brownish orange color develops with the addition of acid formaldehyde. This is measured at 470 nm in a spectrophotometer.[48] A simpler method that gives com-

TABLE 7.2. MUCOLIPIDOSES AND THEIR CHARACTERISTICS

Type	Defect	Laboratory Investigation
Fucosidosis	Deficient fucosidase	Serum fucosidase
G_M-gangliosidosis	Deficient β-galactosidase	Urine, leukocytes
Mucolipidosis I	Increased β-galactosidase and other hydrolases	Urine
Mucolipidosis II	Increased β-galactosidase and other hydrolases	Serum
Mannosidosis	Acid α-mannosidase deficiency	Metachromatic granules in urine
Mucosulfatidosis	Arylsulfatase-A deficiency	Mucopolysaccharides in urine, arylsulfatase in urine

From Sly WS.[41]

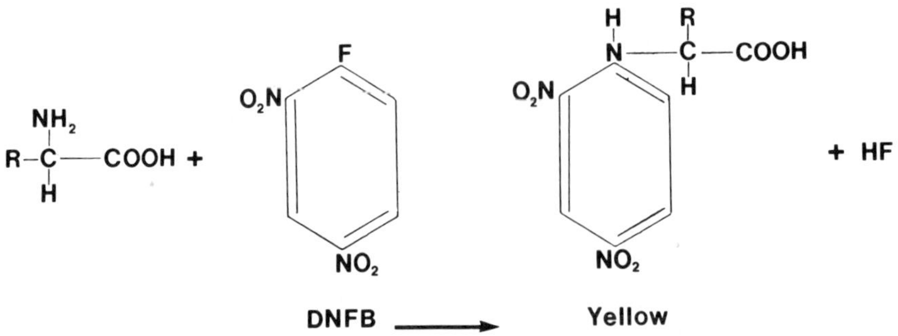

Figure 7.3. Reaction of amino acid with 1-fluoro-2,4-dinitrobenzene.

parable results utilizes the reaction of amino acids with 1-fluoro-2,4-dinitrobenzene (DNFB) to develop a yellow color measured at 420 nm[49] (Fig. 7.3).

The normal adult range for total amino acids in urine is 50 to 200 mg/24 hours,[50] that for children of 2.5 to 12 years of age is 3.3 to 6.2 mg/kg/24 hours,[51] and that for infants is 3.8 to 6.5 mg/kg/24 hours.[49]

Quantitation of Individual Amino Acids

Analysis of the individual amino acids is done either by a reaction that is specific for the amino acid or by a separation of the amino acids and reaction with ninhydrin or DNFB. Some chemical tests that do not require prior separation follow:

1. Urinary cystine is reduced to cysteine, the sulfhydryl groups of which reduce phosphotungstic acid to give tungsten blue which is measured at 600 nm.[52]
2. Urinary histidine is measured by its interference in the formation of a blue complex of copper with biscyclohexanone oxaldihydrazone (cuprisone).[53]
3. Urinary tyrosine, tyramine, and other p-alkalated phenol derivatives give red complexes when reacted with nitrosonaphthol in nitric acid.[54]
4. Glycine is determined by a micromethod based on the formation of formaldehyde in the reaction of glycine with ninhydrin.[55]

5. Hydroxyproline is in high concentration in collagen. It is important in the diagnosis of bone disease or collagen disease. Colorimetric tests usually employ oxidation to a pyrrole type compound and condensation with Ehrlich's reagent (p-dimethylaminobenzaldehyde).[56]

Quantitative analysis of each of the amino acids present in a urine specimen is commonly done by column chromatography. The analysis of each amino acid requires a 24-hour collection of urine under refrigeration or preserved with thymol, toluene, or chloroform. The pH is adjusted to 2.0 with concentrated HCl and applied to a two-column system, one of which separates the neutral and acidic amino acids and the other for the separation of the basic amino acids. The use of high pressure pumps, small resin beads, automatic color development with ninhydrin, and the computerized calculation of the concentration of each fraction (amino acid) allows the determination of the array of amino acids in urine in about six hours. Details of column chromatographic methods may be found in several reviews.[57,58,59]

URINARY PROTEINS

Proteins found in urine enter from (1) the blood, (2) the kidney and urinary tract, and (3) extraneous sources, such as the vagina and prostate. The proteins entering via the blood plasma must be able to pass through the filtration barriers in the glomerulus. They must also travel the entire tubule and urinary tract without being completely reabsorbed or disintegrated in order to appear in the urine. Proteins arising from the blood are found in the urine because:

1. The glomerulus has allowed either a larger amount of proteins or a larger size of proteins to pass, and
2. The tubules cannot or have not reabsorbed these proteins at their usual capacity.

The majority of the proteins found in the urine arise from the blood plasma. Only a few originate in the urinary tract. Table 7.3 lists some of the urinary proteins and their expected concentration in the urine of healthy adults.

Techniques for the Quantitation of Total Protein in Urine

Originally, the distinction of proteins in the urine was between albumin and globulin or others. As more sensitive techniques were developed for detecting proteins and quantitating them in biologic fluids, the list of proteins that have been found in the urine has grown.

One of the screening tests discussed in Chapter 4, the organic acid precipitation test, is widely used for the quantitation of total urinary protein. A 24-hour urine is collected, and the turbidity that is created with an anionic organic acid, e.g., sulfosalicylic acid, is measured either by visual comparison with standard protein solutions for semiquantitative estimation or in a spectrophotometer for quantitation.[71] In most laboratories, the comparison of the turbidity of the urine precipitate is made with that of several protein solutions of known concentration by measuring their absorbances in a spectrophotometer at 400 to 500 nm. This method of determining the total protein concentration has several problems[72]:

1. The organic acids generally do not precipitate albumin and each of the globu-

lins and other proteins (e.g., mucoproteins) to the same extent.
2. The composition of the standard solutions is not identical to the composition of the types of proteins in the urine.
3. The absorbance readings are based upon the amount of light scattered by the precipitate and thus depend to a large extent on the size of the aggregate. The size of the aggregate is concentration, time, and temperature dependent.
4. Other nonprotein substances react, e.g., x-ray contrast media.

In spite of these drawbacks the turbidimetric methods remain in wide use. A modified Shevy-Stafford method[73] has been reported to be very sensitive to a wide spectrum of proteins, including albumin, globulin, free kappa and lambda light chains, and hemoglobin even when the amount is less than that detectable by a reagent strip test.[74] This method uses Tsuchiya's reagent, a solution of phosphotungstic acid in acid alcohol, to precipitate the protein. The precipitate is measured by volume in a tube following centrifugation. This is similar to Esbach's method,[75] which uses picric acid as the precipitating agent, and the volume of precipitate is read in a calibrated tube after allowing the precipitate to settle for 30 minutes.

Methods that are considered to give more accurate results employ precipitation of the proteins, dissolution of the protein precipitate, and then color formation with Lowry's copper-phenol reagent[76] or a biuret reagent.[77] Lowry's reagent reacts with phenolic groups of amino acids in proteins, whereas the biuret reagent reacts with molecules with two peptide bonds $HNC=0$ or two of the following adjacent groups: $CONH_2$, CH_2NH_2, $CSNH_2$, $C(NH)(NH_2)$. Dye-binding methods utilizing Coomassie blue[78,79] and Ponceau S[80] are more recent colorimetric methods for quantitating the total protein content of urine. These tests are based upon the change in the wavelength of maximal absorbance of the dye when it is complexed with protein. They are less subject

TABLE 7.3. PROTEINS OF NORMAL HUMAN URINE

	Concentration (mg/day)				Range (5-95%)				Molecular Mass	Isoelectric Point
	A*	B	C	D	A mg/day	B mg/day	C mg/day	D		
Prealbumin		0.04		0.025[63]		0.01-0.13			61,000	4.7
Albumin	7.8	5.0	6.1		3.6-14.1	2.5-28.8	1.64-34.2		67,000	4.9
α₁-Antitrypsin		0.15		0.3[64]		0.04-0.63			45,000	4.0
α₁-Acid glycoprotein (orosomucoid)	0.37	0.45			0.18-0.67	0.021-2.33			44,100	2.7
α₂-Macroglobulin									820,000	5.4
α₂-HS glycoprotein	0.34	0.23			0.13-0.69	0.07-1.12			49,000	4.3
Lysozyme			0.15				0.02-0.45			10.5-11.0
Fc fragment of IgG	0.2			0.133[65]	0.1-0.4					
Lambda free light chains	3.4		1.3		1.2-7.2		0-7.6		23,000-46,000	4.6-6.7
Kappa free light chains			2.2				0-9.0		23,000-46,000	
β₂-Microglobulin	0.12		0.04	0.014[66]	0.06-0.21		0-0.14	.03-0.37[66]	11,000	5.4-5.7
Transferrin	0.38	0.17	0.69		0.32-0.47	0.04-0.45	0-3.5		90,000	5.9
Haptoglobin			0.09				0-0.95		100,000	4.1
IgA 11S (secretory)†				1.1[67]						
IgA-75	1.4	0.25	0.54		0.7-2.7	0.08-0.42	0-2.25			
IgM			0.3				0-1.34			
IgG	3.2	3.06	1.98	2.9[68]	1.2-6.5	0.90-6.28	0.2-6.5	1.1-4.8[68]	150,000	5.8-7.3
Retinol binding protein				1.35[69]						4.4-4.8
Zn α₂-globulin									41,000	3.8
Tamm-Horsfall†				40.0[67]						3.2
Urokinase										
β₂-Glycoprotein				0.32[69]						
Fibrin split products				<2.0[70]						
Ceruloplasmin				0.5[69]					160,000	4.4
Hemopexin				0.2[69]					80,000	
Gc globulin				0.025[69]					50,000	

*A, radial immunodiffusion, Bergaard[60]; B, rocket electrophoresis, Weeke[61]; C, automated nephelometry, Hemmingsen and Skaarup[62]; D, other references noted.
†Originate in the kidney or urinary tract.

to variation in dye binding from one protein to another and thus less dependent upon the relative amounts of the various types of proteins present in the specimen.

Since most proteins have a strong absorbance in the ultraviolet at 279 nm and also at 210 nm, the absorbance of protein solutions at one or the other of these wavelengths has been used to calculate the protein concentration. The absorbance at 280 nm is due principally to the absorbance of tyrosine and tryptophan, whereas that at 210 nm is due to the peptide bond.[81] Thus the absorbance of a solution of urinary proteins at 280 nm is an indication of the number of tyrosine and tryptophan residues, and this varies from one protein to another. Since the composition of the proteins in a given urine specimen is unknown, some error occurs when the absorbance of a solution of urinary proteins is compared with a standard solution of known concentration of a defined protein mixture or a solution of pure albumin. The turbidity of the urine and the presence of other compounds that absorb light at these wavelengths make a separation and purification step necessary prior to absorbance measurements.

Methods of Concentrating Urinary Proteins

Normally urine has such a low concentration of protein (approximately 0.1 g/L) that some method of concentration is required in order to analyze the types of protein that are present. Methods that are employed in the medical laboratory are:

1. Collodion bags with negative pressure,[82]
2. Cellulose acetate membranes with capillary or centrifugal[83] force,
3. Hollow fibers,[84] and
4. Cellulosic tubes and dialysis against polymers such as polyethylene glycol.[85,86]

The proteins that remain to be analyzed after concentration depend to some extent upon the method employed for concentration. Each of the methods listed employs a filter that has a certain pore size which will allow molecules of some lower molecular weight (or size) to be removed while retaining those proteins with molecular weights or sizes larger than the pore size.

A very convenient apparatus for use in the clinical laboratory is the Amicon Minicon Concentrator,* a disposable microconcentrator that will accept 0.75 to 5.0 ml of specimen and is capable of a maximum concentration ratio of 100-fold. The urine sample is inserted in a plastic tube, one side of which is separated from a spongelike material by a porous membrane. The concentration occurs by gravity and is also influenced by the hydrophilicity of the sponge across a membrane that has a molecular weight cutoff value of either 15,000, 25,000, 75,000, or 125,000. The membrane with a 15,000 cutoff, for example, would be used to retain the low molecular mass proteins. There is no necessity for pressure, vacuum, centrifugation, or technician attention in this method. However, a loss of low molecular weight proteins in tubular proteinuria following the concentration of urine in the Minicon B-15 Concentrator has been reported.[87]

The other methods listed also use membranes of various materials with pore sizes that can be selected. However, they require negative pressure or centrifugal force for filtration to occur.

Bergaard[60] quantitated urinary proteins immunochemically after using a method of concentration described by Everall and Wright[88] that utilizes negative pressure and Visking dialysis tubing. The Visking tubing designated 8/32 retains proteins down to 30,000 to 40,000 daltons whereas the 12/32 tubing retains proteins down to 10,000 to 15,000 daltons.

A concentration of urinary protein to give approximately 20 to 30 g/L is sufficient for their separation and detection by electrophoretic methods that employ a conventional cellulose acetate and a pH 8.6 barbiturate buffer system.[86] Immunochemical reac-

---

*Amicon Corporation, Lexington, Massachusetts.

tions usually require 0.1 to 0.5 mg/ml for observation to be made.

Methods of Separation and Quantitation of Urinary Proteins

The development of separation techniques, immunologic methods for identification, and sensitive optical methods has enabled investigators to study the individual proteins that are excreted normally and in unusual or disease states.[60–70,89–92]

Several methods that are used to separate, identify, or quantitate urinary proteins as fractions or individual entities are:

1. Electrophoresis on cellulose acetate, agar, or polyacrylamide gel,
2. Two-dimensional electrophoresis,
3. Isoelectric focusing,
4. Immunoelectrophoresis/rocket electrophoresis,
5. Nephelometry of antigen-antibody complexes,
6. Radial immunodiffusion, and
7. Radioimmunoassay.

Electrophoresis, Isoelectric Focusing, and Immunoelectrophoresis/Rocket Electrophoresis. Electrophoresis separates the proteins on the basis of their net charge in a buffer at a specified pH, usually 8.6, in an electric field. Albumin has one of the lower isoelectric points, approximately 4.6, which results in its mobility toward the anode. Serum proteins are routinely fractionated by electrophoresis at pH 8.6 on cellulose acetate into five fractions (bands). These are, from anode to cathode:

1. Albumin,
2. α_1-Globulin,
3. α_2-Globulin,
4. β-Globulin, and
5. γ-Globulin.

Frequently, a normal serum protein electrophoresis is made simultaneously with that of urine for a reference. The proteins in urine concentrates are electrophoresed in the same manner as serum on cellulose acetate.

The pattern obtained on normal urine shows a small band corresponding to human serum albumin and broad, ill-defined protein bands in the α, β, and γ areas.[91] This method, which separates proteins into groups and is thus a rather crude separation method, has its greatest use in detecting narrow bands of homogeneous protein (spikes) of an immunoglobulin and/or free light chains in cases of multiple myeloma. Electrophoretic patterns of serum are useful in the investigation of renal loss of protein to determine if the loss represents a selective or sieving loss or a nonselective loss associated with renal tubular disease.

The proteins that have been separated can be quantitated by staining the protein with a dye, commonly Ponceau S, followed by a destaining reagent to give an unstained background with the five stained bands. Amido black, bromphenol blue, and Coomassie blue have been used as protein stains on electrophoretic patterns. The selection of a stain or dye is based upon the type of support medium that has been used in the electrophoresis and upon the affinity of the protein to be studied for the dye. For example, Ponceau S is a very good stain for proteins that have been separated on cellulose acetate because each of the protein fractions has about the same affinity for the stain and also because Ponceau S does not stain the cellulose acetate itself. This contrasts with polyacrylamide gel, which retains the Ponceau S and which cannot be destained to give a colorless background.

The fractions on the stained pattern are then quantitated by scanning the pattern in a densitometer and obtaining an integration of the absorbance of the protein in the individual bands or by removing the bands, eluting the dye from them, and measuring the absorbance in a spectrophotometer. The method of scanning densitometry is used in many clinical laboratories at this time.

Electrophoresis on agar or acrylamide gel in place of the cellulose acetate for the support has an added separation quality, that is, the separation according to molecular size.[92] The concentration of agar in the agar gel and the amount of polymerization within the polyacrylamide gel determines the restriction of mobility of the larger molecules. Patterns of urinary proteins obtained by electropho- resis and immunoelectrophoresis on agar gel are shown in Figures 7.4 A,B. The addition of sodium dodecyl sulfate (SDS) to the protein and the polyacrylamide gel negates the effect of charge differential, and, therefore, the molecular mass controls the flow of proteins through the gel. SDS-polyacrylamide gel has been reported to give more clinically useful information about urinary protein content than chromatography on Sephadex G 100, electrophoresis on cellulose acetate, im- munoelectrophoresis, and polyacrylamide gel without SDS.[93] Two-dimensional elec- trophoresis, i.e., electrophoresis sequentially at right angles, in a variety of buffers with different pH has been used to increase the resolution of urinary proteins.[94]

Isoelectric focusing is electrophoresis in a gradient of pH so that the resolution of pro- tein separation is improved by a focusing of the proteins into narrow bands according to their isoelectric points. Quantitation of the fractions or individual proteins that appear as bands upon separation by isoelectric focusing is made in the same manner as that described for separation made by electrophoresis on cellulose acetate. Over 250 urinary proteins have been resolved by a method employing isoelectric focusing in one dimension and by SDS polyacrylamide gel in the other.[95] Dia- grams of the pattern achieved by this method are shown in Figure 7.5.

Immunoelectrophoresis employs antisera to proteins to create precipitin lines by which the various proteins of the urine are iden- tified or quantitated (Fig. 7.4 B). The Laurell or rocket electrophoresis method is a quan- titative immunoelectrophoretic technique.[96] It is based on the relationship of mobility to concentration and upon the precipitation of antigens and antibodies at optimal propor- tions. Electrophoresis of the urinary protein takes place in a gel that contains antibodies specifically directed to one protein. Whenever the protein moving through the gel reaches a concentration that represents

optimal proportion to the antibody concen- tration in the gel, a precipitin line forms. The distance of migration measured from the point of application of the specimen to the precipitin line is proportional to the con- centration, and thus a comparison of the dis- tance of migration of unknown to standard solutions allows the unknown concentra- tion to be calculated. Rocket electrophore- sis requires the antigen to be known and the antibody to be specific. Only one kind of protein can be quantitated in one assay system. Nine serum proteins that are nor- mally found in urine have been quantitated by rocket electrophoresis on concentrated urine specimens.[61]

Nephelometry, Radial Immunodiffusion, and Radioimmunoassay. The scattering of light by antigen-antibody complexes forms the basis for the nephelometric immunoassay of pro- teins.[97] This method is used in many labora- tories to quantitate individual serum pro- teins. An automated nephelometric im- munoassay has been compared with the rock- et electrophoretic immunoassay for the quantitation of urinary proteins.[98] The au- tomated nephelometric immunoassay was found to be more sensitive and more precise than the rocket method on unconcentrated urine.

Radical immunodiffusion was among the first immunologic methods used to quantitate proteins normally found in urine.[99,100] The antibody specific for the protein to be quanti- tated is embedded in the agar. The urine protein concentrate is placed in a well in the agar, and the distance (radius) of the precipi- tin line that forms a circle around the well is related to the concentration of the protein. This method is subject to variation due to temperature, prozone reactions in antigen excess, and the difficulty in measuring the distance of diffusion when the precipitin line is diffuse. Some of these problems are over- come by assaying standard solutions of known concentration simultaneously.

Radioimmunoassay has also been used to determine the concentration of individual proteins in urine. It is a method utilizing

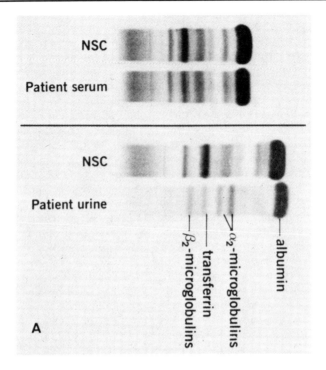

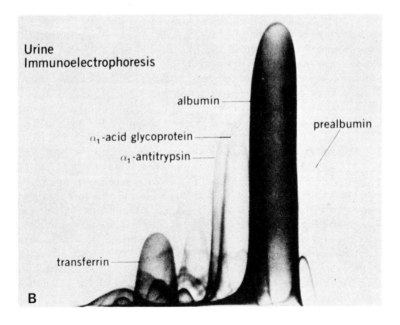

Figure 7.4. Electrophoretic patterns of urinary proteins. **A.** Agarose gel pattern (urine protein = 550 mg/24 hours). **B.** Immunoelectrophoresis, agar gel, showing individual protein precipitin lines. (From Killingsworth LM, Cooney SK, Tyllia MM: Diagnostic Med 3:71, 1980.)

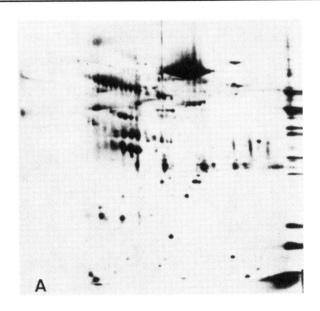

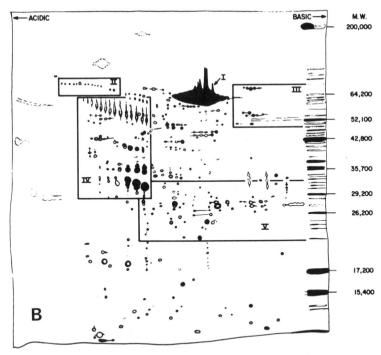

Figure 7.5. Urinary proteins demonstrated by electrophoresis and isoelectric focusing (ISODALT technique). **A.** Pattern of urinary proteins from a 59-year-old normal male. **B.** Diagram of the pattern shown in **A.** I, includes serum albumin; II, unknown proteins; III, amylase, IgG heavy chains; IV, probably contains α_1-antitrypsin, actin, haptoglobin β chains; V, rows of IgG light chains. (From Anderson NG, Anderson NL, Tollaksen SL: Proteins of human urine. 1. Concentration and analysis by two-dimensional electrophoresis. Clin Chem 25:1199, 1979.)

TABLE 7.4. TOTAL PROTEINURIA AND RENAL DISEASE

Proteinuria gm/day	Category	Implication for Renal Disease
0–0.2	Undetectable, intermittent	Pyelonephritis, nephrolithiasis, renal tumor
<0.5	Minimal/intermittent	Chronic glomerulonephritis, tubular disorders
0.5–4.0	Moderate/continuous	Many types of renal disease, pyelonephritis with hypertension
>4.0	Heavy	Marked glomerular permeability, chronic and acute glomerulonephritis, pericarditis, congestive heart failure

From Relman A and Levinsky NG.[104]

radioactively labeled antigen to compete with the unlabeled antigen located in the specimen for participation in complex formation with the antibody in the reaction. The amount of radioactivity in the immunoprecipitate is thus inversely related to the concentration of antigen in the specimen. The sensitivity of this method is superior to that of the other methods discussed here.[101] It is, therefore, a very useful method for the quantitation of individual urinary proteins. It has been used for determining IgG,[68] albumin,[102] and β_2-microglobulin[103] in the study of renal function and for the early detection of renal allograft rejection.

Significance of Proteinuria

Protein excretion is generally greater during the day than at night. This has been attributed to increased activity during the day. Five types of proteinuria have been categorized on the basis of the total protein excretion in a 24-hour period.[104] These types and their correlation with disease are given in Table 7.4.

Exercise Proteinuria

It has been found that the excretion of protein increases during exercise from 0.04 g/L to as much as 5 g/L.[105] Data on 15 plasma proteins acquired on urine specimens before and after exercise showed increases of up to

50-fold in some proteins.[106] The proteins that were found to increase significantly with exercise are listed in Table 7.5.

Exercise proteinuria does not appear to be simply an increased normal proteinuria found at rest. The glomerular origin of exercise proteinuria is demonstrated by the small effect that exercise has on the excretion of the low molecular weight proteins.[107] However, there is some increase of the lower molecular weight proteins in exercise urine. These are carbonic anhydrase and lysozyme (muramidase). Most of the proteins excreted after exercise have a molecular weight range of 45,000 to 160,000. Studies using lysozyme indicate that not only is the glomerular per-

TABLE 7.5. SEVERAL URINARY PROTEINS MARKEDLY INCREASED FOLLOWING EXERCISE

Prealbumin (tryptophan-rich)
Albumin
α_1-Acid glycoprotein (orosomucoid)
Zn-α_2-glycoprotein
Transferrin
3 S γ_1-globulin
γ-G-globulin
Carbonic anhydrase
Lysozyme

From Poortmans JR.[106,107]

meability increased with exercise but also the tubular binding mechanism for lysozyme appears to be saturated.[107] The explanation for this is not certain.

Postural or Orthostatic Proteinuria

For many years, it has been known that certain individuals exhibit proteinuria upon standing after having been in a recumbent position. This has been regarded as a benign condition, although several investigators perceive it as an indication of underlying renal disease.[108,109] The total protein excretion is generally below 1.5 g per day, and electrophoresis on SDS-acrylamide shows approximately 40 percent low molecular weight proteins, 40 percent medium molecular weight proteins, and 20 percent high molecular weight proteins.[91] Electrophoretic and immunoelectrophoretic analyses of proteins in transient postural proteinuria give patterns similar to those of normal urine, i.e., principally albumin.[110]

The Proteinuria of Pregnancy

Many women demonstrate proteinuria during pregnancy. This is generally a transient proteinuria that disappears after delivery. This kind of proteinuria has been categorized into four groups, shown in Table 7.6 along with the type of pattern that is associated with each group.[111] The proteinuria of pregnancy is generally not associated with renal disease unless the complications listed in Table 7.4 create an insult to the kidney which leads to renal disease.

Glomerular Proteinuria

Proteins appearing in the urine that originate in the blood get there by passing the glomerular filtration barriers. Alterations in glomerular permeability may result in increased permeability of a selective character, in which case the glomerulus continues to control to some extent which proteins from the blood appear in the urine. Three terms have been used to describe the alteration of glomerular permeability: selective, moderately selective, and nonselective. In selective permeability, molecules larger than usual may appear in the urine, although such proteins as IgM, α_2-macroglobulin, and low density β-lipoprotein do not pass the glomerulus to any degree, and albumin is clearly the predominant protein present.[86]

Glomerular permeability may be altered to the extent that there is none or only moderate selectivity occurring. In moderately selective permeability, proteins such as α_2-macroglobulin pass into the urine. The nonselective type results in a protein excretion pattern that is representative of a dilute serum—in other words, all serum proteins are represented. Selective proteinuria is indicative of a better prognosis than the finding of a nonselective type regardless of the etiology of glomerular disease.[112]

Overflow Proteinuria

An increased concentration of a low molecular weight protein in the urine can result from an increase in its concentration in the circulating blood plasma. Examples of this

TABLE 7.6. PROTEINURIA OF PREGNANCY

Condition	Selective	Poorly or Nonselective	Tubular or Mixed Tubular
Toxemia of pregnancy			
Fetal death or involvement	×		
No fetal involvement		×	
During delivery		×	
During urinary tract infections		×	×
No other clinical symptoms		×	

Adapted from Charret F, Manuel Y, Pelissier B: In Manuel Y, Revillard JP, Betuel H (eds): Proteins in Normal and Pathological Urine, 1970, pp. 220–223. Courtesy of University Park Press.

type of proteinuria are the increased excretions of immunoglobulin light chains (Bence-Jones proteins) in some patients who have multiple myeloma, hemoglobin in the case of intravascular hemolysis, and myoglobin in instances of muscle trauma. The interaction of myoglobin, hemoglobin, and Bence-Jones proteins that are positively charged in the luminal fluid with the negatively charged Tamm-Horsfall or uromucoid protein in the lining of the distal nephron has been suggested as one cause of acute renal failure.[113] The clinical association of acute renal failure with increased concentrations of myoglobin, hemoglobin, and Bence-Jones proteins is well known.[114-116]

Tubular Proteinuria

Tubular proteinuria is the term used whenever the low molecular weight proteins (less than 40,000) appear in the urine. These low molecular weight (LMW) proteins normally pass the glomerulus but are reabsorbed by the tubular cells and catabolized there. In disease or malfunction of the renal tubules, these proteins are not disposed in the tubules and appear in the urine.[117] Tubular damage and the increased excretion of low molecular weight proteins in the urine were found in workers who were exposed to cadmium dust.[118] This correlation led to the investigation of the urinary excretion of low molecular weight proteins in an attempt to define renal tubular damage or malfunction in various diseases. The assay of β_2-microglobulin, a molecule that shows similar structural characteristics to immunoglobulin light and heavy chains, is a popular procedure for assessing tubular ability to reabsorb or catabolize low molecular weight proteins.[103]

Protein Hormones—Human Chorionic Gonadotropin (HCG) and Pregnancy Tests

One protein hormone commonly measured in the urine is HCG, which is secreted by the placenta. It is measured most frequently to determine the presence of active placental tissue in pregnancy. Thus, pregnancy tests are generally tests that determine HCG. Other tissues that secrete HCG are those of trophoblastic tumors and a few nontrophoblastic tumors. Measurement of this hormone is helpful in the diagnosis of these tumors and the evaluation of the efficacy of treatment.

HCG is a glycoprotein consisting of two noncovalently linked subunits, α and β. The α peptide is essentially identical to the subunits of luteinizing hormone (LH) and follicle-stimulating hormone (FSH). The β peptide units appear to be unique to each of these hormones. The only known function of HCG is the support of corpus luteum that occurs in the eighth day after ovulation in maternal blood. This function is essential to the survival of the corpus luteum and, therefore, to the pregnancy itself. After the seventh week, the placenta gradually replaces the corpus luteum, and at the tenth week of gestation, HCG secretion reaches a maximum level of 500,000 to 1,000,000 IU per day.

Bioassay methods were previously used to determine urinary HCG. These were the Ascheim and Zondek (A-Z) test which utilized corpus luteum formation in mice, the rabbit test based on ovulation (Freidman test), the *Xenopus laevis* (clawed toad) test based on egg extrusion, and the male *Rana pipiens* (frog) test based on sperm release. These bioassay tests have been replaced with immunoassay tests, e.g., radioimmunoassay, radioreceptor, hemagglutination inhibition, latex agglutination inhibition, and latex agglutination.

In the hemagglutination inhibition test, antiserum to HCG and the patient's urine are mixed, and red blood cells coated with HCG are added. When HGC is present in the urine, it complexes with the antiserum, and no reaction occurs when HCG-coated red cells are added. However, if HCG is not present, the antiserum to HCG is available to complex with the HCG-coated red cells, which causes agglutination to occur. The agglutination of the cells causes them to settle in the bottom of the tube in a homogeneous diffuse pattern. When no agglutination of red cells takes place (HCG is present in the urine), the cells settle to the bottom of the tube in a doughnut pattern. These patterns are shown in Figure 7.6.

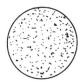

+ AGGLUTINATION
HCG absent

– AGGLUTINATION
HCG present

Figure 7.6. Patterns in the hemagglutination inhibition test for urinary HCG.

Latex particle agglutination is similar to the hemagglutination inhibition test except that latex particles are used in place of the red cells. The agglutination that occurs in the case of a urine that has no HCG is observed visually as the presences of clumping of the particles. This test takes only a few minutes and is commonly made on glass slides. The direct particle agglutination test is performed with latex particles that are coated with antiserum to HCG. When this is mixed with urine, if HCG is present, agglutination occurs.

Radioimmunoassays for HCG, in order to avoid cross-reactivity to FSH and LH, must utilize antisera specific for the HCG β chain. These procedures can be done in about five hours. Radioreceptor assays utilize receptors obtained from bovine ovaries. These assays are faster but tend to have a greater cross-reactivity with LH.[119] The radioimmunoassays will generally detect as little as 0.005 IU/ml, and the hemagglutination inhibition tests detect approximately 0.5 IU/ml, whereas the latex agglutination tests will detect about 1.0 IU/ml. The results of the tests are generally reported as positive or negative, although the author much prefers the report to read, for example, "1.0 IU/ml or greater HCG detected" in the case of a positive latex agglutination inhibition test. This use of the lower limit of detection of HCG for the report does not confuse the issue of whether the test is positive for pregnancy or not. Attention must be given to situations and substances that cause false negative and false positive reactions to occur (Table 7.7).

Serum HCG reaches detectable concentrations (5 mIU/ml) within 24 hours after implantation and reaches peak levels at about 70 days after the last menstrual period. Radioimmunoassay tests become positive in 90 percent of women at the time of the first missed menses.[120] Hemagglutination inhibition tests are positive in 80 to 90 percent of individuals 14 days after the first missed menses, and latex agglutination inhibition tests are positive in 21 days.

Whenever trophoblastic tumors are present, i.e., hydatiform mole or choriocarcinoma including testicular choriocarcinoma, the levels of HCG are very high. Frequently they are over 5,000,000 mIU/ml (480,000 ng/ml). Some patients, however, do not exceed a level of 5,000 mIU/ml. In all these patients, dilution and quantitative determination of HCG are useful in confirming evidence of trophoblastic tumors and in following therapy or surgical removal.

Proteins Originating in the Kidney

One well-known protein that originates in the kidney is the Tamm-Horsfall or uromucoid protein that is produced in the tubules.[121] This mucoprotein is capable of inhibiting several viruses. It is the major protein of casts found in urinary sediment and of renal stones.[122,123] Immunoelectron and immunofluorescent studies have shown that this protein is located almost exclusively along the surface membranes of the distal tubules and collecting tubules.[124,125]

Secretory IgA is found in the urine. The 7S portion of the IgA is synthesized in the plasma cells beneath the epithelial surface of the mucous membrane, and the secretory piece is added by the epithelial cells during

TABLE 7.7. CAUSES OF INACCURATE IMMUNOASSAY TESTS FOR HUMAN CHORIONIC GONADOTROPIN IN URINE

Type of Test	Causes of Results that Are	
	False Positive	False Negative
Hemagglutination inhibition and latex agglutination inhibition	Increased LH midcycle and at menopause	Early pregnancy, ectopic pregnancy, threatened abortion, second and third trimester when HCG decreases
	Drugs, e.g., phenothiazines, promethazine, methadone	
	Proteinuria 1 g/day	
Radioimmunoassay chain specific	None reported	None reported
Radioreceptor assay	Cross reaction with LH	None reported

From Krieg AF: Pregnancy tests and evaluations of placental function. In Henry JB (ed): Clinical Diagnosis and Management by Laboratory Methods, 1979, pp. 680–90. (Courtesy of W. B. Saunders Co.)

IgA transit across the epithelial surface to the lumen.[126] Antibody activity of urinary IgA to *Escherichia coli* has been reported,[127] and patients with rheumatoid arthritis who have high serum titers of rheumatoid factor have been shown to excrete secretory IgA rheumatoid factor in their urine.[128]

Six other proteins of renal origin have been noted.[129] The characteristics, site of synthesis in the kidney, and function have not been well defined. However, one of these is thought to be secreted from the urogenital tract. Substances that cross-react with antibodies to renal tissue are also found in the urine. The excretion of these tissue breakdown products in the urine has been termed "histuria."[130] Antigens of basememt membrane tissue have been demonstrated in urine,[131] and the excretion of kidney brush border antigens has been shown to be a quantitative indicator of tubular damage.[132]

Urinary Enzymes

Proteins of a special nature that occur in urine are the enzymes. Some investigators recommend that, in addition to other urinary studies, three enzyme determinations should be done[133]: (1) typical brush border enzyme, e.g., alanine aminopeptidase, (2) a lysosomal enzyme, e.g., β-glucuronidase, and (3) a low molecular weight enzyme that passes the glomerular membrane and is usually reabsorbed by the tubules, e.g., lysozyme. The urinary excretions of three enzymes in three types of renal disease are shown in Figure 7.7. Urokinase is an enzyme of renal origin that plays a role in intravascular hemostasis and the prevention of obstruction of urinary tract by clot formation.[134] Urinary lactate dehydrogenase is known to increase significantly in nephrotoxicity, whereas γ-glutamyltransferase is increased in renal malignancy but decreased in all other renal disorders.[135,136] Not all of the enzymes that are present in urine are of renal origin, but the excretion of those that are and those that originate in other tissues is a useful indicator of renal disease[137] and renal allograft rejection.[138,139]

Protein Summary

Knowledge of the proteins present in the urine under various circumstances has advanced considerably in the past decade. This has been due in part to the improvement of analytic techniques and the introduction of renal transplantation. Table 7.8 lists several typical proteins that are excreted in renal disease. For a comprehensive text on proteinuria, the reader is referred to the book by Pesce and First.[67]

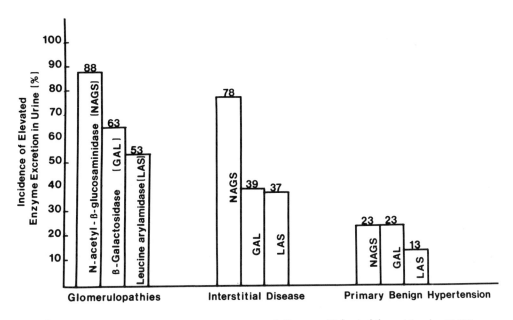

Figure 7.7. Urinary enzyme excretion in renal disease. (Adapted from Maruhn D.[137])

TABLE 7.8. INDIVIDUAL PROTEINS TYPICALLY EXCRETED IN SEVERAL TYPES OF PROTEINURIA

Glomerular		Tubular	Overflow
Selective *(40,000–70,000 daltons)*	*Nonselective* *(40,000–>300,000 daltons)*	**Tubular** *(<40,000 daltons)*	**Overflow** *(Variable)*
Albumin	Albumin	β_2-Microglobulin	Myoglobin
Transferrin	Transferrin	Kappa free light chains	Hemoglobin
Albumin dimers	IgG	Lambda free light chains	Lambda free light chains
Fc fragments	α_2-Macroglobulin	Lysozyme	Kappa free light chains
IgG light chains		Retinol-binding protein,	IgG
α_1-Antitrypsin		α_1-Microglobulin,	IgA
		fibrin split products	IgM

SUMMARY

The special tests discussed in this chapter that are performed to evaluate renal function or diseases are the urinary protein assays.

Those that are performed to evaluate pregnancy, toxic conditions, metabolic disturbances or defects in the body are:

1. Tests for urinary carbohydrates and mucopolysaccharides,
2. Tests for urinary proteins, and
3. Tests for human chorionic gonadotropin.

These special tests are occasionally performed in the same laboratory as the routine urinalysis. However, in many laboratories, these tests are done in clinical chemistry or special laboratories.

The inclusion of this material in a book on urinalysis is made to furnish a more complete understanding of the importance of the kidney and the urine in the evaluation of health or disease. In the future, it is expected that the determination of urinary proteins and the use of special microscopic techniques will be more common and play a greater role in the investigation of renal disease.

Review Questions

More than one multiple choice response may be correct. Select all correct ones.

1. Justification of quantitative results for assays on urine in units of mass of analyte per unit mass of creatinine is based upon:
   A. The metabolic feedback relationship between the analyte and creatinine
   B. The excretion of the analyte in terms of renal function
   C. The identical units of analytes and creatinine
   D. The constancy of the excretion rate of creatinine
   E. The difficulty in obtaining a precise 24-hour urine volume
2. Which of the following quantitative tests for glucose is more specific for the β form of glucose?
   A. Glucose oxidase test
   B. o-Toluidine test
   C. Benedict's test
   D. Folin-Wu test
   E. Rubner's test
3. The normal 24-hour urinary excretion of glucose is:
   A. 0-0.25 g
   B. 0.25-5.0 g
   C. 5.0-5.5 g
   D. 5.5-6.5 g
   E. 6.5-12.5 g

4. Match one item from Group A with the correct item in Group B.

Group A
__ A. Fructosuria
__ B. Pentosuria
__ C. Galactosuria
__ D. Lactosuria

Group B
1. Milk diet solely
2. Vomiting and liver disturbance
3. Over 25 mg/dl for infants less than two weeks old
4. Ingestion of fruits
5. Mucopolysaccharides are characterized chemically by their content of:
   A. Uronic acid
   B. Sulfated hexosamines
   C. Glucose
   D. Mucus
   E. Mucoprotein
6. Methods for the quantitative determination of mucopolysaccharides are:
   A. Complex formation with Alcian blue
   B. Ion exchange chromatography and color reactions
   C. Gas liquid chromatography
   D. Electrophoresis in barium acetate on cellulose acetate
   E. Enzymatic analysis of sugar constituents
7. Match the substance sought in the examination of urine with the mucolipidosis listed.

   A. G_M-gangliosidosis
   B. Mannosidosis
   C. Mucosulfatidosis
   D. Fucosidosis

   1. Leukocytes
   2. Metachromatic granules
   3. Arylsulfatase
   4. None
8. Diseases or condition associated with overflow aminoaciduria are:
   A. An increased serum amino acid concentration

SPECIAL TESTS

171

B. Liver disease
C. Renal tubular disease
D. Inherited enzyme deficiency
E. Cystinosis

9. Reagents that react with most isolated amino acids in their quantitative measurement are:
   A. Para-dimethylaminobenzaldehyde
   B. 1-Fluoro-2,4-dinitrobenzene
   C. Ninhydrin
   D. 2,4-Dinitrophenylhydrazine
   E. β-Napthoquinone-4-sulfonate

10. The quantitative analysis of all amino acids present in a urine specimen customarily is performed:
    A. On a 24-hour urine specimen
    B. By anonic ion exchange chromatography
    C. By cationic ion exchange chromatography
    D. By color development with ninhydrin
    E. In an automated analyzer

11. Sources of protein in the urine are:
    A. The hair
    B. The spleen
    C. The blood
    D. The kidney
    E. The urinary tract

12. Turbidimetric methods for the quantitation of urinary proteins that employ organic acids have the following problems:
    A. Technically difficult, require ultraviolet light
    B. Do not precipitate all urinary proteins to same extent
    C. Standards are not identical to specimens
    D. Size of aggregate is critical
    E. Are not specific for proteins

13. Match the following methods or reagents for quantitative determination of proteins with the principle of the method (principle may be used more than once).

Methods
A. Coomassie blue
B. Absorbance at 210 nm
C. Absorbance at 280 nm
D. Lowry's
E. Biuret
F. Ponceau S

Principles or Reactions
1. Molecules with two adjacent HNC=O
2. Shift of absorbance maxima upon complex formation
3. Tyrosine and other phenols
4. Tyrosine, tryptophane, phenylalanine
5. The number of peptide bonds

14. Methods that are used to quantitate specific individual proteins are:
    A. Electrophoresis
    B. Isoelectric focusing
    C. Rocket electrophoresis
    D. Nephelometry of antigen-antibody complexes
    E. Radial immunodiffusion

15. The urinary protein electrophoretic pattern obtained in glomerulonephritis differs from that of renal tubular disease because in the latter:
    A. α_2 and β_2 bands are increased
    B. All protein fractions are increased
    C. The α_1 and γ-globulins are increased
    D. No increase in protein occurs

16. The method for quantitation of urinary proteins that employs electrophoresis in agar-containing specific antiserum is:
    A. Radial immunodiffusion
    B. Rocket electrophoresis
    C. Isoelectric focusing
    D. Immunoelectrophoresis
    E. Agar gel electrophoresis

17. The most sensitive method for the quantitation of a specific protein is:
    A. Radial immunodiffusion
    B. Radioimmunoassay
    C. Isoelectric focusing
    D. Nephelometry of antigen-antibody complexes
    E. Rocket electrophoresis

18. Proteinuria can result from which of the following?
    A. Pregnancy

    B. Exercise

    C. Cadmium poisoning

    D. Multiple sclerosis

    E. Gastroenteropathy

19. A condition associated with overflow proteinuria is:

    A. Cadmium poisoning

    B. Methanol poisoning

    C. Postural change to vertical position

    D. Immunoglobulin light chain proteinuria

    E. Glomerulonephritis

20. Proteins that originate in the kidney are:

    A. Albumin

    B. Secretory IgA

    C. β_2-Microglobulin

    D. Tamm-Horsfall protein

    E. α_2-Macroglobulin

21. The upper limit of the normal excretion of proteins in the urine is:

    A. 10 mg/L

    B. 50 mg/L

    C. 100 mg/L

    D. 1,000 mg/L

    E. 2 g/L

22. Match the urinary enzymes with the condition or function for which they are useful indicators.

    A. Alanine aminopeptidase

    B. β-Glucuronidase

    C. Lysozyme

    D. Lactate dehydrogenase

    E. Glutamyltransferase

    1. Nephrotoxicity

    2. Brush border integrity

    3. Tubular reabsorption

    4. Lysosomal activity

    5. Renal malignancy

    6. Intravascular renal blood flow

23. Human chorionic gonadotropin (HCG) has the following characteris-

    A. Composed of four subunits

    B. Unique β-peptide units

    C. Glycoprotein

    D. β-Peptide unit in common with FSH and LH

    E. Unique α-peptide unit

24. In the hemagglutination test for HCG, an increase in the concentration of HCG in urine is indicated when:

    A. No agglutination occurs

    B. Cells settle to bottom of tube in a doughnut pattern

    C. Agglutination occurs

    D. Cells settle to bottom in a diffuse, homogeneous pattern

    E. Cells are lysed

25. The most sensitive and specific test for HCG is:

    A. Latex agglutination

    B. Radioreceptor assay

    C. Hemagglutination inhibition

    D. Radioimmunoassay (β-HCG)

    E. Spectrophotometric assay

26. Increased concentrations of HCG in the urine are found in which of the following conditions?

    A. Pregnancy

    B. Hydatidiform mole

    C. Choriocarcinoma

    D. Pituitary adenoma

    E. Multiple myeloma

27. False positive tests for HCG may be caused by:

    A. Phenothiazine administration

    B. Proteinuria

    C. Menopause

    D. Early pregnancy

    E. Glycosuria

(See Appendix for answers.)

Case Studies

Case Study 1

A 79-year-old retired college professor who had been active and in good health gradually experienced general weakness, difficulty in breathing upon exertion, and cold intolerance. The laboratory results showed:

    Hemoglobin: 1.24 mmole/, (8 g/dl), low

    Hematocrit: 0.23 (23%), low

    Blood urea nitrogen: 57.4 mmole/L (161 mg/dl), high

Creatinine: 848 μmole/L (9.6 mg/dl), high

Creatinine clearance: 7.5 ml/min, low

The physician requests a urine protein electrophoresis and suspects chronic renal failure to be the diagnosis.

Questions

1. Why is chronic renal failure a likely diagnosis?
2. What kind of urine protein electrophoretic pattern do you expect to find in chronic renal failure?
3. What kinds of proteins will be present?

Answers

1. Chronic renal failure occurs in later life, and it is accompanied by marked anemia, uremia, low renal clearance tests, and tubular reabsorption insufficiency.
2. In chronic renal failure, one expects to find a combined glomerular-tubular pattern.
3. The specific kinds of proteins present will be representative of middle and low molecular weight proteins, e.g., albumin, transferrin and β_2-microglobulins.

Case Study 2

A 55-year-old woman was admitted to the hospital for evaluation of general malaise. For the past two months the patient had been aware of fatigue and low back pain. Her weight loss was 9 kg. She had arthalgia. Physical examination revealed mild hypertension and hepatosplenomegaly.

Laboratory results were:

Characteristic	Finding
Hemoglobin:	1.21 mmole/L (8.5 gm/dl), low
Hematocrit:	0.29 (29%), low
Erythrocyte sedimentation rate:	38 mm/hour, high
WBC:	5×10^9/L ($5 \times 10^3/\mu$l), low normal
Differential:	0.40 segmented neutrophils

0.55 lymphocytes
0.20 immature lymphocytes
0.30 plasmacytes
The red cells were normocytic, normochromic, and, on occasion, were seen in rouleaux formation

Serum creatinine:	212 mmole/L (2.2 mg/dl), high
Blood urea nitrogen:	12.3 mmole/L (34.5 mg/dl)
Serum albumin:	48 g/L (4.8 gm/dl), normal
Total protein:	70 g/L (7.0 gm/dl), normal
Urinalysis:	Protein 3+ Sediment showed numerous RBC, 4 to 7 WBC, 3 to 5 hyaline casts/high power field, no red cell casts

The serum congealed after being placed in the refrigerator overnight. Serum cryoglobulins were present.

Quantitation of the immunoglobulins in serum revealed:

IgM: 20 g/L (2 g/dl), approximately 10 times normal
IgA: 0.3 g/L (0.3 g/dl), low
IgG: 5.5 g/L (0.55 g/dl), low

Serum protein electrophoresis and immunoelectrophoresis on warmed serum showed an IgM-kappa monoclonal spike. Urine protein electrophoresis and immunoelectrophoresis showed the presence of free kappa light chains (Bence-Jones protein). No rheumatoid factor was demonstrable in the cryoprecipitate. The bone marrow revealed infiltration by plasma cells (myeloma cells). The diagnosis of multiple myeloma (myelomatosis) was made.

Questions

1. What evidence does this patient have of renal disease?
2. What are the most likely explanations (two) for the renal disease in this patient?
3. What type(s) of proteinuria does this patient have? (Exercise, overflow, glomerular, postural or orthostatic, pregnancy)

Answers

1. Renal disease is exhibited by the elevated serum creatinine and blood urea nitrogen and the proteinuria. The finding of red cells and casts in the urine microscopic examination is significant. The number of white cells is also increased.
2. The most likely explanations for the renal disease in this patient are:
   (a) Persons with multiple myeloma are occasionally subject to infection. In this particular case the presence of white cells may reflect a urinary tract infection.
   (b) More likely, however, is the known association between proteinuria of myeloma and subsequent renal disease thought to be caused by the lodging of excess and abnormal protein in the glomeruli and the swamping of tubular reabsorptive sites in the tubules by the low molecular weight immunoglobulin light chains (Bence-Jones protein).
3. This patient has overflow proteinuria and probably also has some glomerular proteinuria.

REFERENCES

Introduction

1. Banda PW, Tuttle MS, Sherry AS, Blois MS: Total creatinine content of the first morning urine is independent of dietary change. Clin Chem 26:535, 1980.
2. Greenblatt DJ, Ransel BJ, Harmatz JS: Variability of 24-hour urinary creatinine excretion by normal subjects. J Clin Pharmacol 16:321, 1976.
3. Walker MS: Urinary free 11-hydroxycorticosteroid/creatinine ratios in early morning urine samples as an index of adrenal function. Anal Clin Biochem 14:203, 1977.
4. Rao LGS: Predicting fetal death by measuring estrogen and creatinine ratios on early morning samples in urine. Br Med J 2:874, 1977.
5. Gurson CT, Sauer G: Urinary chromium excretion, diurnal changes and relationship to creatinine excretion in healthy and sick individuals of different ages. Am J Clin Nutr 31:1162, 1978.

Definitive Tests for Carbohydrates and Mucopolysaccharides in Urine

6. Pileggi VJ, Szustkiewicz CP: Carbohydrates. In Henry RJ, Cannon DC, Winkelman JW (eds): Clinical Chemistry, 2nd ed. New York, Harper & Row, 1974, p 1268.
7. Benedict SR: A reagent for the detection of reducing sugar. J Biol Chem 5:485, 1909.
8. Harding VJ, Downs CE: Notes on a Shaffer-Somogyi copper reagent. J Biol Chem 101:487, 1933.
9. Pileggi VJ, Szustkiewicz CP: Carbohydrates. In Henry RJ, Cannon DC, Winkelman JW (eds): Clinical Chemistry, 2nd ed. New York, Harper & Row, 1974, pp 1300–1302.
10. Kingsley GR, Getchell G: Direct ultramicro glucose oxidase method for determination of glucose biological fluids. Clin Chem 6:466, 1960.
11. Weatherburn MW, Logan JE: A simplified quantitative enzymatic procedure for glucose in urine. Diabetes 15:127, 1966.
12. Kadish AH, Hall DA: A new method for the continuous monitoring of blood glucose by measurement of dissolved oxygen. Clin Chem 11:869, 1965.
13. Caraway WT: Carbohydrates. In Tietz N (ed): Fundamentals of Clinical Chemistry, 2nd ed. Philadelphia, Saunders, 1976, p 259.
14. Lasker M: Essential fructosuria. Human Biol 13:51, 1941.
15. Heyrovsky A: A new method for the determination of inulin in plasma and urine. Clin Chim Acta 1:470, 1956.
16. Dahlqvist A, Svenningsen NW: Galactose in the urine of newborn infants. J Pediatr 75:454, 1969.
17. Kelly S: Biochemical Methods in Medical Genetics. Springfield, Ill., Thomas, 1977, pp 106–108.
18. Hawk PB, Oser BL, Summerson WH: Practical Physiological Chemistry, 13th ed. New York, McGraw-Hill, 1947, p 845.
19. Militzer WE: Note on the orcinol reagent. Arch Biochem 9:85, 1946.
20. Tauber H: A color test for pentoses. Proc Soc Exp Biol Med 37:600, 1937.

21. Roe JH, Rice EW: A photometric method for the determination of free pentoses in animal tissues. J Biol Chem 173:507, 1948.

22. Hickman J, Ashwell G: A sensitive and stereospecific enzymatic assay for xylulose. J Biol Chem 234:758, 1959.

23. Reiner M, Cheung HL: Xylose. In Meites S (ed): Standard Methods of Clinical Chemistry. New York, Academic, 1965, vol 5, p 257.

24. Pileggi VJ, Szustkiewicz CP: Carbohydrates. In Henry RJ, Cannon DC, Winkelman JW (eds): Clinical Chemistry, 2nd ed. New York, Harper & Row, 1974, p 1311.

25. Toseland PA: Specific determination of plasma and urinary lactose. J Clin Pathol 21:112, 1968.

26. Horning EC, Horning MG: Human metabolic profiles obtained by GC and GC/MS. J Chromatogr Sci 9:129, 1971.

27. Wells WW: Gas liquid chromatography of carbohydrates. In Curtis, HCh, Roth M (eds): Clinical Biochemistry Principles and Methods. New York, Walter deGruyter, 1974, vol II, pp 931–943.

28. DiFerrante N: The measurement of urinary mucopolysaccharides. Anal Biochem 98, 1967.

29. Berry HK, Spinanger J: A paper spot test useful in the study of Hurler's syndrome. J Lab Clin Med 55:136, 1960.

30. Carter CH, Wan AT, Carpenter DG: Commonly used tests in Hurler's syndrome. J Pediatr 73:217, 1968.

31. Renaurt AW: Screening for inborn errors of metabolism associated with mental deficiency or neurologic disorders or both. N Engl J Med 274:384, 1966.

32. Pennock CA: A modified test for glycosaminoglycan excretion. J Clin Pathol 22:379, 1969.

33. Whiteman P: The quantitative measurement of Alcian blue-glycosaminoglycan complexes. Biochem J 131:343, 1973.

34. Whiteman P: The quantitative determination of glycosaminoglycans in urine with Alcian blue 8GX. Biochem J 131:351, 1973.

35. Pennock CA: An evaluation of methods suitable for a clinical laboratory study of abnormal glycosaminoglycan excretion. In Holton JB, Ireland JT (eds): Inborn Errors of Skin, Hair, and Connective Tissue. Baltimore, University Park Press, 1975, pp 267–282.

36. Greiling H: Glycosaminoglycans. In Curtius HCh, Roth M (eds): Clinical Biochemistry Principles and Methods. New York, Walter de Gruyter, 1974, vol II, pp 958 960.

37. Whiteman P: Acid mucopolysaccharide excretion in the mucopolysaccharidoses. Determination of glycosaminoglycans in urine and amniotic fluid using new microanalytical technique. In Holton JB, Ireland JT (eds): Inborn Errors of Skin, Hair, and Connective Tissue. Baltimore, University Park Press, 1975, pp 257–261.

38. Wessler E: Analytical and preparative separation of acidic glycosaminoglycans by electrophoresis in barium acetate. Anal Biochem 26:439, 1968.

39. Humbel R, Chamolls NA: Sequential thin-layer chromatography of urinary acidic glycosaminoglycans. Clin Chim Acta 40:290, 1972.

40. Lippiello L, Mankin HJ: Thin-layer chromatographic separation of the isomeric chondroitin sulfate, dermatan sulfate and keratan sulfate. Anal Biochem 39:54, 1971.

41. Sly WS: The mucopolysaccharides. In Bondy PK, Rosenberg, LE (eds): Metabolic Control and Disease, 8th ed. Philadelphia, Saunders, 1980, pp 545–581.

42. Dorfman A, Matalow R: The mucopolysaccharidoses. In Stanbury JB, Wyngaarden JB, Frederickson DS (eds): The Metabolic Basis of Inherited Disease, 3rd ed. New York, McGraw-Hill, 1972, pp 1218–1272.

43. Humbel R, Collart M: Oligosaccharide in urine of patients with glycoprotein storage disease. I. Rapid detection by thin-layer chromatography. Clin Chim Acta 60:143, 1975.

44. Knudsen PJ, Eriksen PB, Fenger M, Florentz K: High performance liquid chromatography of hyaluronic acid and oligosaccharides produced by bovine testes hyaluronidase. J Chromatogr 187:373, 1980.

45. Von Figura K, Lögering M, Mersmann G, Kresse H: San Filippo B disease: Serum assays for detection of homozygous and heterozygous individuals in three families. J Pediatr 83:607, 1973.

Aminoacidurias

46. Kelly S: Biochemical Methods in Medical Genetics. Springfield, Ill., Thomas, 1974, pp 17–25.

47. Saifer A: Rapid screening methods for the detection of inherited and acquired aminoacidopathies. In Bodansky O, Latner AL (eds): Advances in Clinical Chemistry. New York, Academic, 1971, vol 14, pp 145–218.

48. Sobel C, Henry RJ, Chiamori N, Segalove M: Proc Soc Exp Biol Med, 95:808, 1957.

49. Goodwin JF: The colorimetric estimation of plasma amino nitrogen with DNFB. Clin Chem 14:1080, 1968.

50. Henry RJ: Clinical Chemistry, Principles and Technics. New York, Harper & Row, 1964, p 575.

51. Ibbott F: Amino acids and related substances. In Henry RJ, Cannon DC, Winkelman JW (eds): Clinical Chemistry, Principles and Technics, 2nd ed. New York, Harper & Row, 1974, p 575.

52. Ibbott F: Amino acids and related substances. In Henry RJ, Cannon DC, Winkelman JW (eds): Clinical Chemistry, Principles and Technics, 2nd ed. New York, Harper & Row, 1974, pp 592–595.

53. Gerber MG, Gerber DA: A simple screening test for histidinuria. Pediatrics 43:40, 1969.

54. Udenfriend S, Cooper JR: The chemical estimation of tyrosine and tyramine. J Biol Chem 196:227, 1952.

55. Alexander B, Landwehr G, Seligmann AM: A specific method for the colorimetric determination of glycine in blood and urine. J Biol Chem 160:51, 1945.

56. Schulman JD, Lustberg TJ, Kennedy JL, Museles M, Seegmiller JE: A new variant of maple syrup urine disease (branched chain ketoaciduria). Am J Med 49:118, 1970.

57. Van Steirteghem AC, Young DS: Amino acids. In Blackburn S (ed): Physiological Fluids in Amino Acid Determination, 2nd ed. New York, Dekker, 1978, pp 263–309.

58. King JS: Observations on the ninhydrin-positive substances in human urine. Clin Chim Acta 9:441, 1964.

59. Gerritson T, Niederwieser A: Amino acids. In Curtius HCh, Roth M (eds): Clinical Biochemistry Principles and Methods. New York, Walter deGruyter, 1974, pp 1062–1121.

Urinary Proteins

60. Berggard I: Plasma proteins in normal human urine. In Manuel Y, Revillard J, Betuel H (eds): Proteins in Normal and Pathological Urine. Baltimore, University Park Press, 1970, pp 7–19.

61. Weeke EOB: Urinary serum proteins. Peeters H (ed): Protides of Biological Fluids. New York, Pergamon, 1974, vol 21, pp 363–379.

62. Hemmingsen L, Skaarup P: The 24-hour excretion of plasma proteins in the urine of apparently healthy subjects. Scand J Clin Lab Invest 35:347, 1975.

63. Poortmans JR, Jeanloz RW: Quantitative immunochemical determination of 12 plasma proteins excreted in human urine collected before and after exercise. J Clin Invest 47:386, 1968.

64. Takayanagi N: Study of the variation of urinary protein pattern referring to histopathological changes in renal diseases. Acta Pathol Jpn 25:75, 1975.

65. Vaughn JH, Jacox RF, Gray BA: Light and heavy chain components of γ-globulins in urines of normal persons and patients with agammaglobulinemia. J Clin Invest 46:266, 1967.

66. Pharmacia Diagnostics: Phadebas β_2-Micro Test Radioimmunoassay. Grafiska, Sweden, Upplands, 1976.

67. Pesce AJ, First MR: Proteinuria, An Integrated Review. In Cameron JS, Glassock RJ, de Strihou CY (eds): Kidney Disease. New York, Dekker, 1979, vol 1, p 74.

68. Woo J, Floyd M, Longley MA, Cannon DC: Radioimmunoassay for immunoglobulin G in serum and urine. Clin Chem 25:2015, 1979.

69. Poortmans JR: The level of plasma protein in normal human urine. In Peters H (ed): Protides of Biological Fluids, 16th Colloquim. Oxford, Pergamon, 1969, pp 603–609.

70. Gonick HC, Stiehm ER, Saldana LF: Comparison of serum and urine fibrin split products and urinary beta-glucuronidase in the diagnosis of renal transplantation. Curr Probl Clin Biochem 9:259, 1978.

71. Bradley M, Schumann GB, Ward PCJ: Examination of urine. In Henry JB (ed): Todd, Sanford, Davidsohn Clinical Diagnosis and Management by Laboratory Methods, 17th ed (vol II). Philadelphia, Saunders, 1979, p 604.

72. Cannon DC, Olitzky I, Inkpin JA: Proteins. In Henry RJ, Cannon DC, Winkelman JW (eds): Clinical Chemistry, 2nd ed. New York, Harper & Row, 1974, pp 428–429.

73. Shevky MC, Stafford DD: A clinical method for the estimation of protein in urine and body fluids. Arch Intern Med 32:222, 1923.

74. Freeman JA, Beeler F: Laboratory Medicine—Clinical Microscopy. Philadelphia, Lea & Febiger, 1974, pp 287–288.

75. Esbach G: Dosage clinique de l'albumine (modification du procede de 1974). Bull Therap (Fr) 98:497, 1880.

76. Lowry OH, Roseborough NJ, Farr AL, Randall RJ: Protein measurement with the Folin phenol reagent. J Biol Chem 193:265, 1951.

77. Frier E: Determination of urine protein with biuret reaction. In Grant GH, Kachmar JF: The proteins of body fluids. In Tietz N (ed): Fundamentals of Clinical Chemistry. Philadelphia, Saunders, 1976, pp 363–364.

78. Miller N, Mezel LM, Grindler EM, Staley J: Evaluation of a new Coomassie blue G 250 (CBB) method for CSF and urine protein. Clin Chem 25:1071, 1979.

79. Heick HMC, Bégin-Heick N, Acharya C, Mohammed A: Automated determination of urine and cerebrospinal fluid proteins with Coomassie brilliant blue and the Abbott ABA-100. Clin Biochem 13:81, 1980.

80. Pesce MA, Straude CS: A new micromethod for determination of protein in cerebrospinal fluid and urine. Clin Chem 19:1265, 1973.

81. Schultze HE, Heremans JF: Molecular Biology of Human Proteins. New York, Elsevier, 1966, vol 1, pp 101–104.

82. Grant GH: The proteins of normal urine. J Clin Pathol 10:360, 1957.

83. Windisch RM, Bracken MM: Cerebrospinal

fluid proteins: Concentrations by membrane ultrafiltration and fractionation by electrophoresis on cellulose acetate. Clin Chem 16:416, 1970.

84. Mondorf AW, Scherberich JE, Reitinger W: Quantitative immunological determination of brush-border protein in urine. Contrib Nephrol 1:119, 1975.

85. Colover J: A microtechnique by protein concentration suitable for quantitative electrophoresis of cerebrospinal fluid. J Clin Pathol 14:559, 1961.

86. Manuel Y, Revillard JP: Study of urinary proteins by zone electrophoresis, methods and principles of interpretations. In Manuel Y, Revillard JP, Betuel H (eds): Proteins in Normal and Pathological Urine. Baltimore, University Park Press, 1970, pp 153–171.

87. Lindstedt G, Lundberg P: Loss of tubular proteinuria pattern during urine concentration with a commercial membrane filter cell (Minicon B-15 system). Clin Chim Acta 56:125, 1974.

88. Everall PH, Wright GH: Low pressure ultrafiltration of protein-containing fluids. J Med Lab Technol 15:209, 1958.

89. Berggärd I: Studies on the plasma proteins in normal human urine. Clin Chim Acta 6:413, 1961.

90. Berggärd I, Risinger C: Quantitative immunological determination of albumin in normal human urine. Acta Soc Med Upsal 66:217, 1961.

91. Balant L, Fabre J: Clinical relevance of different electrophoretic methods for the analysis of urinary proteins. Curr Probl Clin Biochem 9:216, 1978.

92. Grubb A: Combined use of electroendosmosis—free agarose gel and polyacrylamide gel in some electrophoretic procedures. In Peeters H (ed): Protides of the Biological Fluids. New York, Pergamon, 1974, vol 21, pp 649–652.

93. Balant L, Mulli JC, Fabre J: Urinary protein analysis with sodium dodecyl sulfate polyacrylamide gel electrophoresis, a comparison with other techniques. Clin Chim Acta 54:27, 1974.

94. Felgenhauer K, Hagedorn D: Two-dimensional separation of human body fluid proteins. Clin Chim Acta 100:121, 1980.

95. Anderson NG, Anderson NL, Tollaksen SL: Proteins of human urine. 1. Concentration and analysis by two-dimensional electrophoresis. Clin Chem 25:1199, 1979.

96. Laurell CB: Electroimmunoassay. Scand J Clin Lab Invest 29[Suppl 124]:21, 1972.

97. Ritchie RF: Theory and practice of automated nephelometry. In Peeters H (ed): Protides of Biological Fluids. New York, Pergamon, 1974, vol 21, pp 569–578.

98. Borg N, Hemmingson L, Skaarup P: Evaluation of quantitative methods for determination of protein in urine. Clin Chim Acta 64:247, 1975.

99. Schultze HE, Heremans JF: Molecular Biology of Human Proteins. New York, Elsevier, 1966, vol 1, p 670.

100. Mancini G, Carbonara AO, Hereman JF: Immunochemical quantitation of antigens by single radial immunodiffusion. Immunochemistry 2:235, 1965.

101. Skelly DS, Brown LP, Besch PK: Radioimmunoassay. Clin Chem 19:146, 1973.

102. Woo J, Floyd M, Cannon DC: Radioimmunoassay for urinary albumin. Clin Chem 24:1464, 1978.

103. Evrin PE, Peterson PA, Wide L, Berggärd I: Radioimmunoassay of β_2-microglobulin in human biological fluids. Scand J Clin Lab Invest 28:439, 1971.

104. Relman A, Levinsky NG: Clinical examination of renal function. In Strauss MB, Welt LG (eds): Diseases of the Kidney. Boston, Little, Brown, 1963, pp 85–86.

105. Poortmans JR, Kerchore E van: La proteinurie d'effort. Clin Chim Acta 7:229, 1962.

106. Poortmans JR: Proteinuria after muscular work. In Manuel Y, Revillard JP, Betuel H (eds): Proteins in Normal and Pathological Urine. Baltimore, University Park Press, 1970, pp 229–234.

107. Poortmans JR: High and low-molecular weight protein excretion in exercise proteinuria. In Peeters H (ed): Protides of Biological Fluids. New York, Pergamon, 1974, vol 21, pp 375–378.

108. King SE: Albuminuria (proteinuria) in renal disease. II. Preliminary observations on the clinical course of patients with orthostatic albuminuria. NY State J Med 59:825, 1959.

109. Lecocq FR, McPhaul JJ, Robinson RR: Fixed and reproducible orthostatic proteinuria. V. Results of a five-year follow-up evaluation. Ann Intern Med 64:557, 1966.

110. Robinson RR: Postural proteinuria. In Manuel Y, Revillard JP, Betuel H (eds): Proteins in Normal and Pathological Urine. Baltimore, University Park Press, 1970, pp 224–228.

111. Charvet F, Manuel Y, Pellisier B: Proteinuria of pregnancy. In Manuel Y, Revillard JP, Betuel H (eds): Proteins in Normal and Pathological Urine. Baltimore, University Park Press, 1970, pp 220–223.

112. Revillard JP, Fries D, Salle B, Blanc N, Traeger J: Proteinuria in glomerular disease. In Manuel Y, Revillard JP, Betuel H (eds): Proteins in Normal and Pathological Urine. Baltimore, University Park Press, 1970, pp 188–197.

113. Clyne DH, Kant KS, Pesce AJ, Pollak VE: Nephrotoxicity of low molecular weight serum proteins: Physiochemical interactions between myoglobin, hemoglobin, Bence-Jones proteins and Tamm-Horsfall mucoprotein. Curr Probl Clin Biochem 9:299, 1978.

114. Baker SL, Dodds EC: Obstruction of the renal tubules during the excretion of hemoglobins. Br J Exp Pathol 6:247, 1925.

115. Blackburn CRB, Hensley WJ, Grant DK, Wright FB: Studies on intravascular hemolysis in man. The pathogenesis of the initial stages of acute renal failure. J Clin Invest 33:825, 1954.

116. DeFronzo RA, Humphrey RL, Wright JR, Cooke CR: Acute renal failure in multiple myeloma. Medicine 54:209, 1975.

117. Strober W, Waldman TA: The role of the kidney in the metabolism of plasma proteins. Nephron 13:35, 1974.

118. Friberg L: Health hazards in the manufacture of alkaline accumulators with special reference to cadmium poisoning. Acta Med Scand 138[Suppl 124]:1, 1950.

119. Saxena BB, Hasan SH, Haour F, Schmidt-Gullwitzer M: Radioreceptor assay of human chorionic gonadotropin: detection of early pregnancy. Science 184:793, 1974.

120. Krieg AF: Pregnancy tests and evaluations of placental function. In Henry JB (ed): Clinical Diagnosis and Management by Laboratory Methods. Philadelphia, Saunders, 1979, pp 680–690.

121. Hoyer JR, Seiler MW: Pathophysiology of Tamm-Horsfall protein, Kidney Int 16:279, 1979.

122. McQueen EG: The nature of urinary casts. J Clin Pathol 15:367, 1962.

123. Boyce WH, King JS, Fielden ML: Total non-dialyzable solids in human urine. XIII. Immunological detection of a component peculiar to renal calculous matrix and to urine of calculous patients. J Clin Invest 41:1180, 1962.

124. Bichler KH, Ideler V, Harzmann R: Uromucoid excretion in normal individuals and stone formers. Curr Probl Clin Biochem 9:309, 1978.

125. McKenzie JK, McQueen EG: Immunofluorescent localization of Tamm-Horsfall mucoprotein in human kidney. J Clin Pathol 22:334, 1969.

126. Tomasi TB, Tan EM, Solomon A, Prendergast RA: Characteristics of an immune system common to certain external secretions. J Exp Med 121:101, 1965.

127. Tourville DR, Bienstock J, Tomasi TB: Natural antibodies of human serum, saliva, and urine reactive with Escherichia coli. Proc Soc Exp Biol Med 128:722, 1968.

128. Bienstock J, Tomasi TB: The nature of γA in normal urine. In Manuel Y, Revillard JP, Betuel H (eds): Proteins in Normal and Pathological Urine. Baltimore, University Park Press, 1970, pp 59–62.

129. Hermann G, Vaux St Cyr Ch de: Les proteines urinaires provenant du tissu renal. In Peeter H (ed): Protides of the Biological Fluids. Amsterdam, Elsevier, 1964, vol 12, pp 494–498.

130. Antoine B, Neveu T: Tissue-like macromolecules in pathological urine (histuria). In Manuel Y, Revillard JP, Betuel H (eds): Proteins in Normal and Pathological Urine. Baltimore, University Park Press, 1970, pp 244–259.

131. Mahieu P, Maqhuin-Rogister G: Purification of basement membrane antigens from normal human urine by affinity chromatography. In Peeters H (ed): Protides of Biological Fluids. New York, Pergamon, 1974, vol 21, pp 467–471.

132. Scherberich JE, Mondorf WA: Excretion of kidney brush border antigens as a quantitative indicator of tubular damage. Curr Probl Clin Biochem 9:281, 1978.

133. Burchardt U, Haschen RJ, Krosch H: Clinical usefulness of enzyme determinations in urine. Curr Probl Clin Biochem 9:106, 1978.

134. Andrassy K, Ritz E: Isolation and renal localization of urokinase. Curr Probl Clin Biochem 9:330, 1978.

135. Plummer DT, NGAHA ED, Wright PJ, Leathwood PD, Blake ME: The sensitivity of urinary enzyme measurements for detecting renal injury. Curr Probl Clin Biochem 9:71, 1978.

136. Hautmann R: Diagnosis of renal disorders: Comparison of urinary enzyme patterns with corresponding tissue patterns. Curr Probl Clin Biochem 9:58, 1978.

137. Maruhn D: Evaluation of urinary enzyme pattern in patients with kidney diseases and primary benign hypertension. Curr Probl Clin Biochem 9:135, 1978.

138. Price RG: Urinary n-acetyl-β-D-glucosaminidase (NAG) as an indicator of renal disease. Curr Probl Clin Biochem 9:180, 1978.

139. Gonick HC, Stiehm ER, Saldanhia LF: Comparison of serum and urine fibrin split products and urinary beta-glucuronidase in the diagnosis of renal transplant rejection. Curr Probl Clin Biochem 9:257, 1978.

Karen Lorimor and Darlean Brown

	CHAPTER 8

Quality Control and Management in Urinalysis

Objectives

It is expected that the information presented in this chapter will enable the student to:

1. List six activities in the laboratory that comprise a quality control program.
2. List ten major errors in urine testing.
3. List six criteria for evaluating urine controls that are prepared in the laboratory.
4. Identify three factors that are important in the use and storage of lypophilized urine controls.
5. Identify four situations at which time a control solution should be analyzed.
6. Identify three errors in the use of the Clinitest.
7. Identify two frequent misuses of the glucose oxidase strip test.
8. Identify the three errors that affect most of the chemical tablet and strip test results.
9. Identify three steps in the procedure for the microscopic examination of urinary sediment where variation is likely to occur.
10. Identify two major reasons for participation in a proficiency survey program.
11. List three general steps in the quality control preventive maintenance program.
12. State the three parts of a safety program.
13. List the four areas of biohazard safety control.
14. Identify compatible and incompatible chemicals.
15. Identify safety items that should be present in the laboratory for individual, personal protection from chemical hazards.
16. Identify the most important precaution in electrical safety and personnel fire safety.

17. List four important factors to be considered in planning a urinalysis laboratory.
18. Describe the typical workflow sequence in a urinalysis laboratory.
19. List the steps in sequence for planning a laboratory.
20. List four factors to be considered in staffing a urinalysis laboratory.
21. Identify seven items that are considered in establishing the cost of the urinalysis.
22. Identify four items that are considered in the estimation of the effectiveness of a laboratory procedure.
23. Relate the direct, indirect, and net induced costs, and the quality and years of life to the cost effectiveness of a urinalysis test.
24. Analyze laboratory situations and identify the quality control area that is involved and the effect the quality control process had on each situation.

The management of a urinalysis laboratory requires a knowledgeable and skilled individual, the supervisor or manager, who can effectively perform all the usual management functions of planning, organizing, monitoring, and evaluating. These functions occur in a setting that requires adeptness in interpersonal communications, technical know-how, and an awareness of the ethical and moral responsibilities of reporting accurate data and cost containment.

In the preceding chapters about the various aspects of urinalysis, a broad view of the testing of urine has been presented. In this chapter, the discussion of the management and quality control of a urinalysis laboratory will be restricted to the laboratory that performs the typical routine chemical and microscopic analyses of urine. The special tests on urine are performed in the clinical chemistry and immunology divisions of many laboratories because the techniques and equipment used for serum analyses can be used for many urine tests as well. If these tests were to be performed together with the routine tests in a urinalysis laboratory, larger space and additional and more sophisticated equipment would be required. The management functions and processes discussed in this chapter will be those of quality assurance, safety assurance, planning and staffing, and cost

awareness. More comprehensive discussions of laboratory management functions can be found in the literature specifically directed to management and quality control[1-7] and safety.[8,9]

The routine urinalysis is an important part of every series of observations on an individual. If the individual is healthy, is an outpatient, or is a hospital patient, the result of the routine urinalysis can assist the physician with a diagnostic problem or provide clues that aid in recognizing some other unsuspected disorder. With this in mind, care should be taken with the normal as well as abnormal urine.

Quality control in the urinalysis laboratory includes monitoring of patient preparation, specimen collection, transportation and handling of specimen, performance of the test, instrument performance, and reporting of results. Any time there is a breakdown at any point in this process, the quality of both the specimen and the result reported to the physician is sacrificed. The major intent of quality control in the urinalysis laboratory is to eliminate errors through a comprehensive and standardized internal and external quality control program. Quality control in urinalysis is sometimes considered very lightly because of the difficulties that can arise in the implementation of the quality control program due to variability and subjectivity in the testing procedures. The detrimental effects of substandard quality control, however, can be very significant to the patient suffering from renal distress. All care should be given by the technologist in urinalysis to achieve the highest quality of work possible.

Free and Free[10] summarize the difficulty of achieving this goal by listing ten major errors in urine testing (Table 8.1). All personnel working in the urinalysis laboratory should be familiar with these errors. In addition, knowing the correct approach to urine testing should be appreciated and steps taken to prevent errors. The information in Table 8.2[10] suggests that for each correct technique there are many improper techniques.

The initial step in achieving quality in the urinalysis laboratory is preparation of technical procedures for the laboratory personnel

TABLE 8.1. TEN MAJOR ERRORS IN URINE TESTING

1. Failure to test fresh specimen
2. Use of unclean collection containers
3. Inadequate care of reagents
4. Poor technique in testing
5. Failure to mix urine specimen (blood, casts, bacteria)
6. Improper recording of results
7. Failure to recognize implications of a result
8. Disregard for a result (believing some other answer is more important)
9. Inadequate understanding of interfering substances (too little emphasis or too much)
10. Failure to recognize that any result is only part of the picture

From Free AH, Free HM: Rapid Convenience Urine Tests: Their Uses and Misuses. Lab Med 9:12, 1978.

TABLE 8.2. PROBLEMS WITH INDIVIDUAL CHEMICAL TESTS ON URINE

Correct Approach	Incorrect Approach
Use fresh urine	Delay in testing of urine without refrigeration
Quality control acceptable for reagent strips	Use expired reagent strips or ignore incorrect chemical reactions
Store reagents properly and tightly	Leave caps loose on bottles and allow moisture to collect inside, fail to refrigerate unstable reagents and overheat room temperature reagents
Be aware that normal as well as abnormal results are significant	Believe urine results have little significance in the overall diagnostic picture of the patient
Follow directions and carefully time chemical tests	Dip in, out, and read, time span of 10 seconds to 5 minutes is not important—depends on how fast the technologist is
Accept only clean, proper collection bottles	The salad dressing jars, perfume bottles, and Coke bottles are really unique
Be familiar with interfering substances	Cross-reactions and interfering substances considered unimportant in urine results
Proper mixing of urine	Mixing not done because it is not always necessary with clear urines and urine may leak if inverted
Accurate recording of results	Interpretation of chemical tests are sometimes unclear, recording of result not checked by supervisor during training of new personnel
Personnel qualified and properly trained	New personnel always start out in urinalysis because it is easiest to do and least significant

Adapted from Free AH, Free HM: Rapid Convenience Urine Tests: Their Uses and Misuses. Lab Med 9:12, 1978.

to follow when doing urine testing. Instructional procedures prepared by the laboratory should be available for the hospital (nursing units) or clinics to follow during collection of urine specimens. These procedures should include instructions for proper collection, information about preservatives, and the techniques to follow during handling. In addition to the technical procedures, a comprehensive quality control program must be established and well defined.

Once technical and quality control procedures have been defined, training and education of all laboratory personnel working in the urinalysis laboratory are necessary to guarantee that the procedures will be followed identically by all personnel. If individual techniques are allowed, quality will be lost.

The final step in maintaining good quality control is frequent monitoring by the supervisor.

QUALITY OF THE SPECIMEN

The quality of the specimen will be determined by the techniques used for patient preparation and collection. This is usually the responsibility of the nursing staff, except that for outpatients the laboratory usually carries out the procedure of preparation and collection. In these instances, careful instruction must be given to the patient on proper techniques for collection of a midstream urine sample or, if the sample is for culture, proper methods and materials for cleansing prior to collection of the sample. Following collection, specimen must be sent to the laboratory immediately or within a short period of time. Time lapse from collection to analysis should not be more than three hours, preferably no longer than one hour. If the specimen cannot be assayed immediately, care must be taken to refrigerate the specimen or keep it on ice. Collection of a 24-hour urine or other timed specimen must be properly carried out in order to achieve the most accurate excretion of hormones and urinary constituents. The procedures for collection and the need for a creatinine assay to determine the adequacy of

the 24-hour urine collection are discussed in Chapters 2 and 7.

For urine cultures, the quality of the specimen received will reflect the bacterial number in the urinary tract. Consequently, the urine must be placed on ice immediately after collection and remain on ice during transportation to the laboratory. Once in the laboratory, the specimen is given priority and processed at once. Any time a specimen that has not been properly collected and held on ice is received in the laboratory for culture, the collector (nursing staff) should be notified of its unacceptability and requested to collect a new specimen.

Enforcement of the guidelines must be uniform on all shifts and among all areas of the institution and laboratory. In certain instances, independent judgment is required by the supervisor or the director.

REAGENTS, METHODS, AND QUALITY ASSURANCE

Quality Control Material

Negative and positive control materials must be assayed each day, by each working shift, and whenever reagents are changed, e.g., whenever a new bottle of dipsticks is opened. Control materials may be prepared in-house or purchased commercially.

If the urine control is to be prepared in-house, certain criteria must be met:

1. Ease of preparation. Time is important, and the control material should be made easily in a short period of time.
2. Ease of use. It should be no more difficult to test than a routine urine specimen.
3. Control values. Normal and abnormal levels of the urinalysis need to be controlled.
4. Appearance. It should resemble normal urine.
5. Stability. The stability period should be sufficient to eliminate the need for frequent preparation.
6. Availability of material. Constituents to

be used in preparation of the control material should be available in the laboratory.

Many techniques and procedures are available for the preparation of quality control material. All use approximately the same format for preparation, including the constituents added (Table 8.3).[11] The reagents used are pulverized, dissolved, brought to volume, and stored at room temperature. These controls are stable for six to nine months.

The acceptable range of readings for the urine control solution is established by assaying the control solution at least 30 times and calculating the mean and the standard deviation for each test to be performed. The mean plus or minus 2 standard deviation becomes the 95 percent range, i.e., the acceptable limits in most laboratories.

Commercial controls are available for assessing the quality of the specific gravity and chemical analysis portion of the urinalysis (Table 8.4). These controls come as lyophilized tablet or liquid samples and in varying concentrations. Among these are Kova-trol,* QC-U,† Tek-Chek,‡ and Urintrol.§ The importance of proper reconstitu-

tion and the use of correct diluents in each of these controls cannot be overemphasized. Storage time should be noted by recording the date when it is received in the laboratory and also when it is opened. Limits for temperature of storage as well as the expiration date must be observed.

Whether control material is purchased commercially or prepared in-house, a negative check should be performed, and the positive check should fall in the area where the level of activity or response is borderline positive/negative. This area is where discriminatory judgment is critical and where proper performance is crucial. A positive control level 10 to 100 times the critical value is of little value in monitoring the sensitivity of a reagent and/or technique.

The value of using these control solutions is highest where they are used:

1. Daily for reagent strips or tablets that are in opened bottles,
2. Whenever a new bottle of reagent

*ICL Scientific, Fountain Valley, California.
†General Diagnostics, Morris Plains, New Jersey
‡Ames Division, Elkhart, Indiana
§Harleco, Gibbstown, New Jersey

TABLE 8.3. REAGENTS FOR PREPARATION OF QUALITY CONTROL SOLUTIONS AND THEIR EXPECTED VALUES

Reagent	Low Control		High Control	
	1 L	Concentration	1 L	Concentration
Sodium chloride AR*	5.0 g	500 mg/dl	10.0 g	1,000 mg/dl
Urea AR	5.0 g	500 mg/dl	10.0 g	1,000 mg/dl
Creatinine AR	0.5 g	50 mg/dl	0.5 g	50 mg/dl
Glucose AR	3.0 g	300 mg/dl	15.0 g	1,500 mg/dl
30% Bovine albumin	5.0 ml	150 mg/dl	35 ml	1,050 mg/dl
Whole normal blood (with Hct 40-45) (Hb 13-15 g/dl)	100 L	1.3-1.5 mg/dl	—	—
Acetone AR	—	—	2 ml	160 mg/dl
Chloroform AR	5 ml	0.5 ml/dl	5 ml	0.5 mg/dl
Distilled water	To 1 L		To 1 L	

Adapted from Bradley GM, Schumann GB, Ward PCJ: In Henry JB (ed): Clinical Diagnosis and Management by Laboratory Procedures, 16th ed, 1979, Vol 1, p 565. Courtesy of W. B. Saunders Co.
*AR = Analytical Reagent

TABLE 8.4. COMMERCIAL QUALITY CONTROL MATERIALS

Analyte	Method	Expected Test Result	
		Low Control	High Control
pH	Reagent strip (Ames)	6	6
Protein	Reagent strip (Ames)	2+	4+
Glucose	Reagent strip (Ames)	+	3+
Ketone	Reagent strip (Ames)	Negative	Small
Blood	Reagent strip (Ames)	Small to moderate	Negative
Protein	Precipitation	2+	3-4+
Glucose	Benedict's	1+	3+
	Testape (Lilly)	2+	3+
	Clinitest (Ames)	Trace	3+
Ketone	Acetest	Negative	Small
Specific gravity	Refractometer	1.006	1.020
Osmolality (mOsm/kg)	Freezing point depression	305	660

Adapted from Bradley GM, Schumann GB, Ward PCJ: In Henry JB (ed): Clinical Diagnosis and Management by Laboratory Procedures, 16th ed, 1979, Vol 1, p 565. Courtesy of W. B. Saunders Co.

strips or reagent solution is opened or a new reagent is prepared,

3. Whenever a personnel shift changes or there is a new employee, and
4. Whenever a new control solution is made. This should be checked against the current solution using tablets or strips from the same bottle.

Specific Gravity

The measurement of the specific gravity with a hydrometer (urinometer) is easy to do but is subject to inaccuracy. Because of the inaccuracy of these instruments, they must be checked against solutions of known specific gravity. A deviation of ± 0.003 or greater is unsatisfactory.

The quality control should be done at least daily and preferably by each shift measuring the specific gravity of distilled water at room temperature. This specific gravity must be 1.000. If the urinometer does not give a reading of 1.000, appropriate corrections must be applied to all readings taken with the urinometer. When specific gravity is measured using the urinometer, care must be taken to use an appropriate volume of urine and the proper sized vessel. The urinometer must be allowed to float freely, or the reading will be

inaccurate. If the volume is not sufficient to float the urinometer, the specific gravity cannot be taken.

The refractometer is a much more precise instrument than is the urinometer. This instrument rarely needs recalibration, and performing the zero check is usually all that is needed. It is an accurate instrument for determining the amount of dissolved material. For urine it is calibrated on an empirical scale in terms of specific gravity. In addition, it is temperature compensated between 60F (15.6C) and 100F (37.8C). The refractometer is calibrated by the manufacturer, but the zero check can be recalibrated following the manufacturer's directions if necessary. Use a 5 percent (weight/volume) solution of sodium chloride to check the accuracy of the reading. This solution should read 1.022 ± 0.001.

Because only one drop of urine is needed in order to determine the specific gravity with the refractometer, QNS (quantity not sufficient) specimens are less likely to occur and better quality results are obtained than with the urinometer.

Besides the daily zero and function checks, quality control material is used to assess precision. When using the urinometer or the refractometer, two controls should be used, one with a low specific gravity and the other with a high specific gravity.

Critical Steps and Monitoring of the Individual Physical/Chemical Tests on Urine

Dipstick testing has become quite popular in the last two decades because of ease of use and reliability. This form of rapid, convenient testing may be significant not only in renal disease but also in relation to other diseases of the body. Information can be provided in acute diagnostic situations and in monitoring treatment of disease.

As mentioned earlier, errors may occur while using the dipstick simply because it is so easy to use. The common uses and misuses associated with each test on reagent strips are discussed below. Detailed descriptions and information on each of these tests may be found in Chapter 5. The critical steps in each of the chemical tests and common sources of error should be described and discussed as a part of the technical procedures in the laboratory notebook in the urinalysis laboratory.

Sugar Tests.

*Clinitest Tablets.** The Clinitest tablet is used to test for the presence of urine-reducing sugar. Although the procedure consists simply of mixing a specific amount of water and urine plus the Clinitest tablet, attention must be paid to the mixture during the boiling phase. High sugar concentrations (3 percent or greater) produce a passthrough phenomenon. Color change involves a rapid change to bright orange and on to a brown which may match the 1 percent color interpretation block. If the mixture is not observed during boiling, the orange color may be missed, and the resultant brown misinterpreted as a low result. Large amounts of protein may cause increased foaming and slow the boiling action. One drop of octyl (or caprylic) alcohol may be added to the test tube before adding the Clinitest tablet.

Clinitest tablets are quite stable unless exposed to moisture. A second misuse is failure to close the container tightly between tablet removal, thus allowing moisture to enter the bottle. No reaction occurs when this happens.

Two-drop Clinitest Tablets. This is a modified procedure of the Clinitest tablet test in which two drops of urine are used instead of the five drops in the traditional Clinitest procedure. Misuse may result if the number of drops of urine used is incorrect or if color charts are mixed. The five-drop procedure shows colors for 0.25, 0.5, 0.75, 1, and 2 percent glucose, whereas in the two-drop procedure color chart, increments are trace, 0.5, 1, 2, 3, and 5 percent.

*Clinistick** and *Chemstrip.†* The glucose oxidase enzyme test strip has two frequent misuses: failure to recognize both the high sensitivity and specificity of the enzyme test, and the effect of ascorbic acid by causing inhibition of a reaction. The sensitivity of the enzyme test is 0.1 percent, whereas that of the reducing tablet test is 0.2 percent. Thus, instances may occur where the enzyme test is positive and the reducing test is negative. Large amounts of ascorbic acid (50 mg/L or greater) in the urine may cause a delay or blockage of the second part of the reaction involving peroxidase and, consequently, cause a false negative in the enzyme test.

Tes-Tape.‡ This product employs the glucose oxidase enzyme and peroxidase methodology. One common misuse relates to using the tape after the two months allowed after opening. In addition, the reaction must proceed for two minutes with all urine specimens containing over 0.25 percent glucose.

*Diastix.** The Diastix enzyme test for glucose is also affected in high humidity, and the container must be tightly capped between uses. Matching of the colors is sometimes difficult because the shades of brown at the upper levels of the color chart are not easily distinguished. One advantage of the Diastix is that it is less affected by ascorbic acid inhibition than are the other glucose oxidase enzyme tests.

*Ames Division, Elkhart, Indiana

†BMC, Houston, Texas
‡Lilly, Indianapolis, Indiana

Protein Tests. The Albustix* and also the protein portion of the multidipsticks react by the protein error of indicators. The strip reagent is buffered at a pH of 3, and any changes in protein will cause a yellow to blue color change. Stale urine (highly alkaline) may cause false positives if the buffer is overcome. Excessive contact with the urine may wash the buffer out of the test strip.

Some technologists fail to use the color chart when reading protein. Close comparison of the dipstick to the color chart will lessen the chance of missing the trace urines whose reaction is only a slight tinge of green.

Ketone Tests. Whether the technologist uses the dipstick or tablet ketone test, there are two major aspects of misuse. One relates to protection of the product from moisture and the other to the incidence of urinary excretion of ketones. If exposed to room humidity for only a few hours, the reagent will become nonreactive. It is one of the most moisture-sensitive dip and read reagents. Urine collected during a BSP excretion test may give a false positive ketone test.

Occult Blood Tests. The Hemastix* and/or the multidipstick procedure employs a reaction with hemoglobin in the urine. Some technologists have learned to relate the positive blood occult blood test with red blood cells found in the microscopic examination of the urine. It should be remembered that red cells may not always be present if the urine has become alkaline due to age. Red cells and casts deteriorate in alkaline urine. A fresh, acid urine must be used if this comparison is to be of any value. In addition, red blood cells may hemolyze in a hypotonic urine specimen, resulting in a positive chemical test even when cells are not visible under the microscope.

Bilirubin Tests. Bililabstix or Ictotest Tablets and Chemstrips.†* One error while testing for bilirubin is using urine that has been allowed to stand before testing. Bilirubin

glucuronide is rapidly hydrolyzed to free bilirubin and oxidized to biliverdin, which has less or no reactivity with the dipstick test. The Ictotest is not affected to the same degree, but comparison between the methods is difficult.

A second error with the dipstick test for bilirubin is not using the color comparison chart. Color reaction for this test is not as marked and vivid as the other reagent areas, and consequently positive reactions can be missed.

Urobilinogen. Fresh urine must be used when testing for urobilinogen or false negative results will occur. Urobilinogen is rapidly oxidized to urobilin, which is not reactive with the reagent employed in the method. False positive reactions due to interfering substances can usually be ruled out because of their immediate reactivity with the color reagent, since elevated amounts of urobilinogen develop the red-orange color gradually over the 60-second reaction time.

pH Measurement. A problem in measurement of pH relates to the runover phenomenon seen while using the multiple reagent strip. If care is not taken to remove the last drop of urine from the strip by touching it to the side of the urine container, it will run down over the strip and carry the acid buffer from the protein area to the pH area. This is most noticeable with a urine of pH 7 or higher when the pH area would normally be green or blue. With runover there will be an orange color beginning at the edge of the pH area caused by the acid carried over from the protein area.

Nitrite Test. The test for nitrite in urine is primarily for the detection of bacteriuria. There are no false positive reactions since metabolism of nitrate to nitrite by bacteria is the only way nitrite can appear in the urine. Stale urine for nitrite testing is unacceptable because of the possible production of nitrite by the bacteria present as a result of contamination rather than clinical infection. Again, the importance of a fresh urine is emphasized.

*Ames Division, Elkhart, Indiana
†BMC, Houston, Texas

Runover resulting from excess urine present on the dipstick has been discussed, but, at the same time, properly moistened dipsticks are crucial to the quality of the result. Care should be taken to avoid incomplete dipping and to assure that the reagent strip is thoroughly and evenly moistened.

The timing should be observed and followed when using reagent strips. Allow the proper reaction time to elapse without an excessive amount of time, as directed.

Semi-automated Instruments for Chemical Analysis

Semi-automated instruments are available for performing the hand-dipped portion of the urinalysis. These systems maintain consistency and reproducibility among technologists. The errors during analysis that have been mentioned earlier are somewhat controlled by eliminating subjective visual interpretation of color changes. False positive results may occur with intensely colored urine, in which case such specimens should be read by eye. Glucose, ketone, urobilinogen, and nitrite tests show high reproducibility (greater than 90 percent), with the deviations being no more than one color increment away. A low proportion of false positive results occurs in the protein determination. Significant interference from bilirubin does result, however, in the urobilinogen section in concentrations above 32 mg/L. In the bilirubin section about 16 percent false negative results occur.

Table 8.5 summarizes the false positive and false negative results for the N-Multistix* read with the Clini-tek, observed by Peele, Gadsden, and Crews.[12]

Quality control advantages to using semiautomated systems include:

1. Elimination of subjective visual interpretation,
2. Self-calibration before the reading of each stick, and
3. Reflectance limits set to avoid excess error toward either false negative or false positive results

*Ames Division, Elkhart, Indiana

TABLE 8.5. RESULTS FOR DETERMINATION OF VARIOUS ANALYTES BY CLINI-TEK*

	Negative	Trace	+1	+2	+3
Glucose (g/L)					
0	90	10	—	—	—
1	1	97	2	—	—
2.5	—	5	95	—	—
5	1	—	8	91	—
10	—	—	—	13	87
Ketone† (mg/L)					
0	100		—	—	—
150	5		94	1	—
400	1		5	94	—
800	—		—	14	86
Albumin (g/L)					
0 (n=200)	195		5	—	—
0.30	—		77	23	—
1.00	—		—	82	18
3.00	—		—	—	100
Occult blood‡ (g/L)					
0	92		8	—	—
0.616	—		69	31	—
3.08	—		1	68	31
30.8	—		1	99	

	Negative	Positive
Nitrite (g/L)		
0 (n=300)	296	4
2	5	95
5	1	99

From Peele JD, Gadsden RH, Crews R: Evaluation of Ames' "Clini-Tek." Clin Chem 23:2238. © Clinical Chemistry, 1977.

*100 determinations at each concentration, unless otherwise specified.

†Ketone concentration expressed as milligrams of acetoacetic acid/L.

‡Occult blood concentration expressed as grams of hemoglobin/L.

QUALITY CONTROL OF MICROSCOPIC EXAMINATION

To a certain extent, the chemical analysis of urine can be controlled by good quality reagents and techniques, but the microscopic examination is entirely dependent on the technologist's judgment, which derives from education, experience, and careful study of the urine sediment. All personnel must follow the procedure exactly and interpret the results carefully. Some possible errors in analysis of the sediment are:

1. No standardized procedure for centrifugation (speed and time of centrifugation),
2. The quantity of urine left in the tube after pour-off for resuspension of the sediment,
3. The amount of sediment added to the slide (1 drop, 2 drops, 0.1 ml) for examination, and
4. No standardization for examining the sediment (e.g., with or without a coverslip).

The average amount of urine centrifuged is approximately 10 ml. The time and speed of centrifugation may vary from technologist to technologist and must be noted in the written procedure for microscopic examination. It may be advantageous to attach a note to the centrifuge indicating the proper length of time for centrifuging and the speed desired. The speed should be known after QCPM (quality control preventive maintenance) of the centrifuge is completed.

When the supernatant is decanted, an unknown volume of urine remains, varying from one to two drops to 1 ml. Uniformity is difficult to maintain, but this step is critical to precise microscopic assays. As the volume of remaining urine increases, the sediment becomes more dilute, resulting in decreased cell counts per field. A technique must be established for pouring off supernatant, and all technologists must be familiar with it.

The amount of sediment added to the glass slide may vary simply because the sediment is usually poured onto the slide or transferred by pasteur pipette. Uniformity of depth is lost. Some sediments will run on the slide and be shallow whereas others may remain in drop form and be deeper. The depth of the sediment will cause variations in the microscopic count. Use of a coverslip, always of a uniform size, may help control depth, but the concentration of the urine will still cause some variation. Tapping the coverslip will cause the cellular elements (epithelial cells,

casts) to move to the edge of the coverslip, and touching the coverslip, once mounted, should not be allowed.

A standardized procedure (Kova System*) has been developed to eliminate some of the imprecision associated with the microscopic examination. This system not only offers accuracy and reproducibility but also is rapid and easy to do. The Kova System uses a 12 ml graduated Kova-tube, a Kova-petter (used during decanting of the supernatant), stain, and a Kova-slide. The centrifuge tube is designed to measure exactly 12 ml of urine. The specimen is then centrifuged at 1,500 rpm (400 G) for 5 minutes, and the Kova-petter is inserted after centrifugation. The construction of this transfer pipette is such that it fits into the Kova-tube and allows exactly 1 ml of supernatant to remain after decanting. One drop of stain (optional) is added to the remaining urine. The sediment is resuspended, and the Kova-petter is reinserted to transfer the sediment to the slide. The plastic slide is designed with semicircular covered examination chambers of a specific standard depth and volume. The sediment is drawn into the chamber by capillary action.

By using the Kova System, the errors inherent in the traditional method are controlled. In addition, the crossover of urine specimens when more than one specimen is put on a slide is prevented, since each specimen section is contained.

The reproducibility of the results obtained with the traditional method and the Kova system of examination of urinary sediment was checked by Braden[13] and by Kurtzman and Boyd.[14] The results of 30 examinations of the same urine by both methods are shown in Table 8.6.

A quality control material is available with the Kova System that consists of a freeze-dried preparation of human serum and a diluent containing an aqueous suspension of stabilized human red blood cells and organic particles that simulate leukocytes.

The method involves preparation of the control, chemical testing, and performing the

---

*ICL Scientific, Fountain Valley, California.

TABLE 8.6. REPRODUCIBILITY OF KOVA SYSTEM AND STANDARD METHOD RESULTS FOR URINARY SEDIMENT EXAMINATION

Cells	Mean	SD	CV
KOVA SYSTEM			
WBCs	11.4	1.55	13%
RBCs	2.0	0.35	18%
Epithelial cells	2.7	0.47	17%
STANDARD METHOD			
WBCs	18.0	8.28	46%
RBCs	2.2	0.98	46%
Epithelial cells	3.2	1.31	40%

From Braden M: Evaluation of Kova® System. Courtesy of ICL Scientific.

microscopic examination. Mixing of the diluent prior to pouring into the freeze-dried urine is critical. Vortexing may be necessary to resuspend the sediment thoroughly. Lower counts will result if this resuspension is not complete.

MONITORING QUALITY CONTROL

Monitoring quality control in the urinalysis laboratory is essential for assuring good results. A means of monitoring must be established which includes a report sheet for recording the quality control results in an organized format (Fig. 8.1).[15]

The College of American Pathologists (CAP) Inspection and Accreditation Program[16] requires that acceptable limits be indicated on the quality control report sheet and that all personnel be familiar with the range. If an unacceptable result is received, indicating a bad bottle of dipsticks, expired reagents, or other source of error, this must be recorded or documented, and the test must be repeated. The out-of-limits response should indicate the problem and whatever corrective action was taken. A specific form for this documentation is necessary (Fig. 8.2).[15] It is the responsibility of the supervisor to monitor the thoroughness of the quality control recording.

Proficiency testing materials provide an excellent means for monitoring and assessing the accuracy of the patient results. There are several programs available from both professional and governmental agencies. In order to be accredited by CAP, a laboratory must also participate in the CAP proficiency testing program.[17] CAP offers mandatory as well as optional survey programs. The Comprehensive Hematology/Clinical Microscopy Series (H) is mandatory for accreditation, and lyophilized specimens are provided quarterly for bilirubin, hemoglobin, osmolality, pH, protein, reducing substances (glucose), specific gravity testing, and the identification of an object in a 2 by 2 inch transparent photograph of urine sediment. Other CAP survey programs, Basic Urine Chemistry Series (U) and Advanced Urine Chemistry Series (N) are available for those laboratories that do routine quantitative urine testing. The Basic Survey set (U) provides urine for sodium, potassium, calcium, phosphorus, urea, osmolality, protein, creatinine, glucose, and amylase. In addition to the analytes indicated, two urine protein standards are supplied during the year for the calibration of instruments used in quantitative protein procedures. The Advanced Survey set (N) includes analytes, such as 17-ketosteroids, 17 ketogenic steroids, vanillylmandelic acid (VMA), estriol, total catecholamines, urinary free cortisol, aldosterone, total metanephrines, and 5-hydroxyindole acetic acid. The Basic Urine Chemistry Series (U) and the Advanced Urine Chemistry Series (N) are optimal survey programs and are not necessary for CAP accreditation.

Normally, if a laboratory is CAP accredited and subscribes to the necessary survey programs, this fulfills the requirements for Clinical Laboratory Improvements Act (CLIA, 1967) licensure, Joint Commission on Accreditation of Hospitals (JCAH), and Medicare approval.

The proficiency testing survey program also provides a means for appraising the laboratory performance relative to that of its peer laboratories. Specimens that are sent to each individual laboratory are compared to

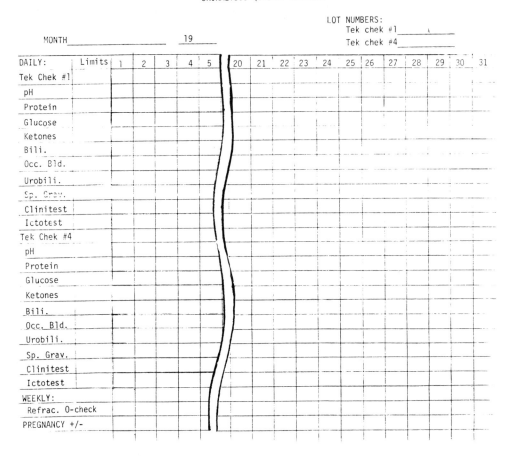

Figure 8.1. Form for recording urinalysis quality control data. (Figures 8.1–8.6, 8.8, courtesy of Hermann Hospital.)

other laboratories using the same methodology and instrumentation. A participant summary is included with the evaluation report, as is a referee summary. The referee summary lists the actual result obtained for each constituent (mean and standard deviation if applicable). All participants are then compared to the referee result. The participant summary lists all laboratories categorized by methods and/or instruments. These data can be very valuable during eval-

uation of a new method or instrument and can also be used for troubleshooting a constituent or assay that has exceeded acceptable limits.

The importance of monitoring the evaluation report returned from the proficiency testing agency is twofold. First, it is imperative that all results exceeding 2 standard deviations be corrected immediately in order to maintain the quality of the patient results. Second, CAP inspection and accreditation

OUT OF LIMITS REPORT
DEPARTMENT OF PATHOLOGY
HERMANN HOSPITAL/THE UNIVERSITY HOSPITAL

PROCEDURE _____

DATE   OUT OF LIMITS REPORT

Figure 8.2. Out-of-limits report for urinalysis.

guidelines state that: "There must be evidence of active review of survey or proficiency testing results."[16]

A laboratory procedure outlining the steps to be taken for review is necessary for clarification (Fig. 8.3). The supervisor of the urinalysis section and the laboratory director are responsible for reviewing the survey evaluation report. Such review may be documented in a manner similar to the procedural example given in Figure 8.4 or more simply on the bottom of the evaluation report in the area indicated.[11]

QUALITY CONTROL AND PREVENTIVE MAINTENANCE OF INSTRUMENTS AND EQUIPMENT

Quality control and preventive maintenance (QCPM) may be divided into separate functions in the urinalysis laboratory. Quality con-

trol of instruments and equipment may be defined as "those periodic actions required by the operator to assure that the instrument is operating at optimal conditions." Preventive maintenance of an instrument may be defined as "those periodic actions by the operator such as cleaning, replacement of parts, and recalibration. These actions assure that the instrument or equipment is maintained at optimal conditions for the maximum length of time."

The QCPM program established for the urinalysis laboratory should include a written laboratory procedure (Fig. 8.5), daily maintenance checks, periodic maintenance checks, and troubleshooting and/or correcting instruments problems.

Laboratory equipment most often found in the urinalysis laboratory includes refrigerator/freezer, water and dry baths, centrifuges, refractometers, and microscopes.

Refrigerator/Freezer Units

The primary quality control required for this equipment is daily monitoring and recording of temperatures. This must be done for accreditation purposes. Reagents and controls must be maintained at around 4 to 6C in order to assure stability. If freezer storage is required, routine laboratory reagents and controls should be stored around $-20C$. Regardless of temperature used, the acceptable limits must be clearly stated.

The type of thermometer used may vary depending on the materials stored. In the routine urinalysis laboratory, a regular glass thermometer may be acceptable but the best thermometer to use is the maximum/minimum (MM) thermometer. This type of thermometer is excellent for assessing the temperature variability in a given period of time (between readings). The MM thermometer will give three readings: (1) the temperature at time of reading, (2) the warmest temperature obtained since the last reading, and (3) the coldest temperature obtained since the last reading. Using these three temperatures, one can know im-

PROFICIENCY TESTING SURVEYS

This procedure outlines the responsibilities and record keeping for proficiency
testing surveys. The intent of a proficiency testing survey, regardless of its
source, is to assess the accuracy of laboratory performance relative to that of
its peer laboratories. To achieve this end, proficiency testing materials will
be treated in a manner identical to that given to routine clinical samples.

Handling of Materials for Proficiency Testing:

All materials for proficiency testing will be delivered to the Quality Control
section. The Quality Control Coordinator will distribute these materials to
the appropriate laboratories with instructions on the tests to be performed and
the dates by which these tests must be completed. These test materials shall
be processed in a manner identical to that for routine clinical samples, i.e.,
without special precaution, and they shall be assayed in the next run without undue
delay. The results on these test materials will be submitted to the Quality Control
Coordinator for the purpose forwarding to the appropriate proficiency testing
agency. The Quality Control Coordinator may submit materials to the sections as
blind clinical samples.

Supervisors are encouraged to make maximum use of these testing materials by: (a)
submitting them for testing using the routine method, by more than 1 laboratory
or medical technologist, and (b) assaying these materials using "nonroutine" or
"backup" methods.

Permanent survey materials such as 35 mm slides and stained smears or slides will
be kept by the Quality Control section for review purpose.

Review of Results:

Results from the Proficiency Testing Agency will be mailed to Quality Control
section, and copies will be sent to the appropriate sections by the Quality Control
Coordinator. These results shll be reviewed by the supervisor; results exceeding limits
of 2 S.D. should be handled according to Quality Control procedure "Monitoring of
Proficiency Surveys". The Quality Control Coordinator and the supervisor should
discuss these survey results with their laboratory techonologists. Original copies
of survey results shall be kept in the Quality Control section, and may be examined
by the laboratory director.

_____   _____
Quality Control Coordinator   Laboratory Director

Figure 8.3. Quality control procedure for proficiency testing surveys.

mediately what the temperature is, how cold
it has been, and how warm it has been. As the
supervisor monitors this, he can quickly tell if
the door has been open for an excessive
amount of time, allowing the temperature to
rise, or if the refrigerator/freezer was mal-
functioning without anyone's knowledge.

This maximum/minimum thermometer
can be purchased from a laboratory supply
house and is inexpensive.

Calibration of the thermometers is necessary regardless of the type used. Calibration
may be achieved by testing the thermometer
against a National Bureau of Standards
(NBS) certified thermometer. Calibration
should be done within or near the temperature range in which it is to be used. Refrigerator thermometers should be calibrated
near 0 to 4C, freezers near -10 to -20C, and
so on. Both the NBS thermometer and the

MONITORING OF PROFICENCY TESTING SURVEYS

Upon receipt of each survey report from the Proficiency Testing Agency, copies
will be distributed by the Quality Control Coordinator to the following members
for review: The supervisor and the laboratory director will initial the original survey copy which will be filed in the Quality Control Section.

PROFICIENCY TESTING SURVEY
REVIEWED BY

QC COORDINATOR_____ DATE_____

SUPERVISOR_____ DATE_____

LABORATORY DIRECTOR_____ DATE_____

Any result exceeding the limits of 2 standard deviations or otherwise judged unsatisfactory must be given immediate attention by the supervisor, by repeating the
sample or reviewing the slides, results, etc. No later than 1 week after receipt
of the survey report the supervisor will submit to the Quality Control Coordinator
a written report stating the cause(s) of the deviations and the corrective actions
to be taken. This report will be studied and initialed by the Quality Control Coordinator and laboratory director. This report ultimately will be filed with the
corresponding survey in the Quality Control Section.

_____   _____
Quality Control Coordinator   Laboratory Director

Figure 8.4. Monitoring of proficiency testing surveys.

thermometer being calibrated should be held
in water, mineral oil, or other suitable fluid to
avoid a rapid change in temperature while
reading. Recalibration is required when a
thermometer calibrated in one temperature
range is to be used in another temperature
range, when a thermometer is suspected of
being damaged due to dropping or other accidents, or on an annual basis to assure continued accuracy.

Preventive maintenance on the refrig-
erator/freezer units is minimal. Defrosting
should be done monthly or when necessary.
Cleaning and decontamination are very important. If cultures and/or blood and urine
specimens are stored, decontaminate with a
1:100 dilution of sodium hypochlorite every
three to five months. The compressor and
motor check should be done once each year.

This is usually accomplished by the maintenance department.

All preventive maintenance should be
documented along with daily temperatures.
If any fluctuation occurs in temperature, corrective action must be taken immediately.
This should also be documented. Small booklets may be used for recording temperature
and preventive maintenance.

Waterbaths and Dry Heat Blocks

Quality control of waterbaths and dry heat
blocks simply entails daily recording of the
temperature. Acceptable temperature ranges
should be clearly stated, and the thermometers used should be calibrated near this temperature. Complete documentation of the
temperature and initialed entries by the urinalysis technologist are necessary. The dry

QUALITY CONTROL AND PREVENTIVE MAINTENANCE
OF REFRIGERATOR/FREEZERS

Standards to be Achieved and Maintained:

1.   Temperature of the refrigerator compartment must be _____ $\pm$ 2°C.

2.   Temperature of the freezer compartment must be _____ $\pm$ 2°C.

Quality Control Prodcedure:

1.   Record the highest (H) and lowest (L) temperature from the Maximum –
      Minimum thermometer maintained in the refrigerator and the freezer
      compartments in the QCPM Book each morning. The procedure for using the
      Taylor Maximum-Minimum thermometer is as follows:

      a.   To record the minimum index (L), refer to the left hand side of the
            thermometer. Read the bottom edge of the index.
      b.   To record the maximum index (H), refer to the right hand side of the
            the thermometer. Read the bottom edge of the index.
      c.   Record the minimum index in the QCPM Book under "Low", and the
            maximum index under "High". Initial all entries.

      The upper left-hand side of the thermometer is in minus degrees. The
      upper right-hand side of the thermometer is in positive degrees.

2.   Reset each index after taking the two readings by placing the ceramic
      magnet across the U-tube in a horizontal position and draw downward
      slowly until the indices come to rest on the tops of the mercury columns.

3.   If mercury becomes separated, grasp the thermometer firmly at the upper
      end giving a number forceful downward swings, until the columns are reunited.

Person(s) Responsible:

Laboratory or medical technologist to be designated by the Supervisor.

Out-of-Limits Instructions:

1.   Check thermostat setting and readjust if necessary.

2.   Inform the Supervisor if unable to achieve or to maintain within temperature
      range.

Figure 8.5. Example of a preventive maintenance procedure.

heat block temperature may be monitored by placing a test tube filled with water in one of the wells and inserting the thermometer. The water level must approximate that of the test volumes used and be deep enough to cover the thermometer bulb.

Preventive maintenance involves cleaning the baths and changing the water at least monthly. Distilled water should be used to prevent rusting of the interior of the water-bath. A bacterial inhibitor may be added to control bacterial growth. In the dry baths, daily cleaning is necessary. Spilled material must not be allowed to dry on the block. Tube holes should be cleaned monthly.

Documentation of the preventive mainte-nance as described in the quality control pro-cedure (Fig. 8.5) is required.[16] A booklet is

QCPM of Refrigerator/Freezers

Preventive Maintenance Procedure:

1. Defrost monthly or when necessary. Defrost deep chest type freezer 2 times
    a year.

2. Cleaning and decontamination - Remove expired materials and clean every 3
    months. If cultures or specimens are stored, decontaminate once every 6
    months with 1:100 Clorox^R.

3. Compressor, motor check - Call Hospital Maintenance for system check once per
    year unless there have been service or repairs during that year.

4. Document all actions in the OCPM Book. Initial all entries.

| Quality Control Coordinator | Director, Quality Control | Chairman, Department of Pathology and Laboratory Medicine |

Figure 8.5. (Cont.)

provided for the technologist to record the required data (Fig. 8.6).[15] The same form used for refrigerator/freezer units may be used for the water baths and dry heat blocks.

Refractometers

The TS (total solids) meter is the refractometer most commonly used in the clinical laboratory. Quality control includes weekly zero checks and function checks. Sodium chloride (5 percent w/v) is used for monitoring the function check. This solution must read 1.022 ± 0.001 on the specific gravity scale. The sodium chloride solution must be sealed tightly to assure that the concentration does not change. The solution in a sealed bottle is stable indefinitely.

The zero check is performed with deionized water at ambient temperatures (20 to 30C). The value for specific gravity should be 1.000 ± 0.05 percent (one-half division). The zero setting should rarely need adjusting, but if it is necessary, instructions are provided with the instrument. Results that are not within acceptable limits must be documented and corrected before patient

testing can proceed. Readjustment of zero can be done in accordance with the manufacturer's instructions. If the function check is unacceptable, it should be reported to the supervisor. A fresh solution of sodium chloride may be tried to correct the problem prior to any other corrective action.

Preventive maintenance on the refractometer includes cleaning of the prism and plastic cover with a soft dry cloth after each use. Weekly, the instrument, tubing, waste container, and stand should be cleaned with a mild detergent or disinfectant. The light source should be checked and replaced if necessary. Again, documentation of adjustments to zero, repairs, and cleaning are necessary.

Microscopes

Quality control and preventive maintenance on microscopes is primarily preventive maintenance. All microscopes should be covered when not in use. Objectives should be kept clean by frequent use of a lens cleaner. Harsh solvents should not be used for cleaning the objectives. Eyepieces and objectives

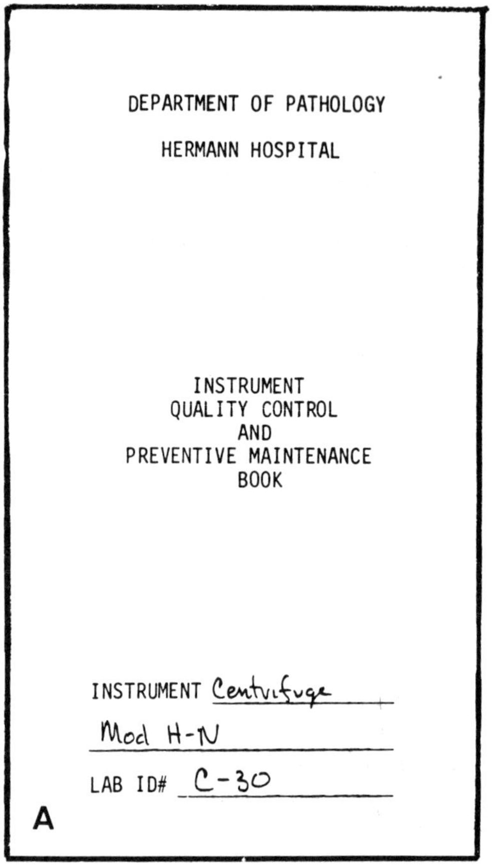

DEPARTMENT OF PATHOLOGY

HERMANN HOSPITAL

INSTRUMENT
QUALITY CONTROL
AND
PREVENTIVE MAINTENANCE
BOOK

INSTRUMENT _Centvifuge_

Mod H-N

LAB ID# _C-30_

A

| PREVENTIVE MAINTENANCE & REPAIRS | |
Date	Action Taken
19 Nov 78	Angle head
	Brushes completely worn-down
	commutator groved
	needs replacement — for last
	service
	Centrifuge cleaned
	Expect brushes to wear quickly
	Setting RPM
	1/2 1350 725OKG
	3/4 2200 65OXG
	full 2750 1OOOXG
	Timer OK — 5min ≅ 5min

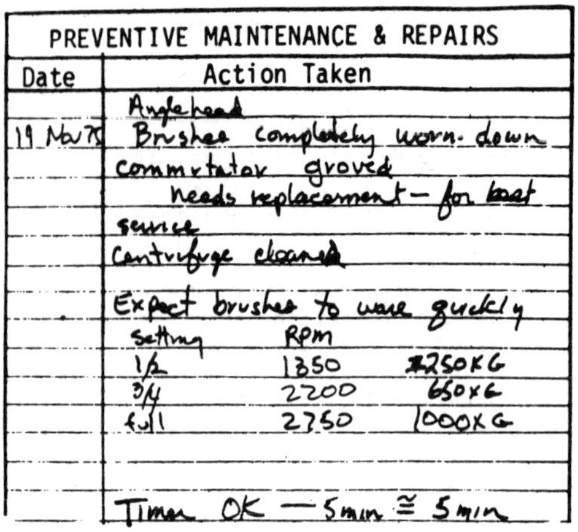

B

Figure 8.6. Booklet for recording quality control and preventive maintenance on equipment. **A.** Cover. **B.** Record page.

should not be disassembled for cleaning because of the risk of dust entering into the microscope or objectives.

Centrifuges

Tachometers are used as a means of calibrating the speed of the centrifuge in revolutions per minute. The rpm determined for each centrifuge setting should be recorded and attached to the centrifuge for easy reference. It should be remembered that this value of rpm is only a factor involved in determining centrifugal force. The efficiency of a centrifuge must be calculated in relative centrifugal force, a number times gravity. The relative centrifugal force is calculated from the calibrated rpm and the radius of the head plus the carrier. The reason for calculating the relative centrifugal force is that rpm when applied to a centrifuge does not give any indication of the force applied to samples in the centrifuge.

More specifically, instructions for the use of the machine should always be stated in terms of relative centrifugal force, or G values. These terms give a true measurement of the force exerted by the machine, since both the speed of the centrifuge and the radius of the centrifuge head will cause some variance. Once the radius of the centrifuge head is known and the speed is found, the G value can be determined from a nomograph (Fig. 8.7).[17] A photoelectric tachometer works well in determining rpm. The machine operates by shining a beam of light onto a small piece of reflecting tape on the centrifuge head. The light beam reflecting from this tape is received by the photoelectric cell, which inte-

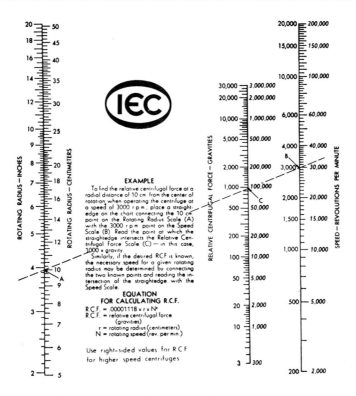

Figure 8.7. Nomogram for calculating relative centrifugal force. (From International Equipment Co, Division of Damon, Needham Heights, Massachusetts.)

grates these flashes and gives a direct reading in rpm. The tachometer is standardized by pointing it at a fluorescent light. The instrument is simple to operate, and instructions are provided on the unit itself. The cost of a photoelectric tachometer is reasonable.

Calibration should be done on each centrifuge every three to four months. Variations in the G value will occur between centrifuges because of differences in head radius (if they are made by different manufacturers). The timer of the centrifuge can be checked for accuracy rather simply. Check the timer with a stopwatch, and if the timer is inaccurate, replace it or indicate the deviation (if greater than one minute) on the timer. Timer checks should be done every three to six months.

The preventive maintenance schedule includes periodic lubrication of the shaft and inspection as well as replacement of the graphite brushes if necessary. These graphite brushes gradually wear down as the centrifuge is operated at high speed, and if the graphite is allowed to wear away completely, the retainer spring of the brush will make contact with the smooth surface of the internal parts of the centrifuge and cut grooves or scratches in its surface. Should this occur, new brushes wear excessively quickly, and deposits of graphite may cause arcing and burning that decrease the efficiency of the motor and may damage the motor. It cannot be overemphasized that proper maintenance is vital to the efficiency and longevity of the centrifuge. Although lubricating and checking the brushes can be done by the manufacturer or the maintenance department, it is simple enough to assign to the technologist, and this assures continued awareness of centrifuge care by the personnel. This preventive maintenance should be done every three months. Daily cleaning of the centrifuge is necessary for control of biohazard conditions. This can be accomplished by wiping with a 3 percent phenolic solution.

The centrifuge should be checked for unusual vibrations to assure proper balancing. All shields, cups, or carriers should contain a cushion and be of the same weight. Urine specimens should always be balanced with a tube of the same size and amount of liquid. Usually, visual observation is acceptable. The tubes of equal size and volume should be placed in opposite positions in the centrifuge head.

Familiarity with the components of a centrifuge and a preventive maintenance schedule will assure maximum performance of the machine. In addition, the preventive maintenance program will prevent or reduce breakdown periods that impair efficiency of patient care service.

DOCUMENTATION AND MONITORING OF QUALITY CONTROL AND PREVENTIVE MAINTENANCE

Once the maintenance program for each piece of equipment or instrument has been established in the urinalysis laboratory, procedures must be written describing the action to be taken while performing quality control preventive maintenance on the equipment. A standardized format should be used in writing these procedures. It should include:

1. Standards to be achieved and maintained:
   Indicate the temperature, calibration, and checks to be done on each piece of equipment and the specific temperature, calibration, and other measurements with acceptable deviation ranges.
2. Quality control procedure:
   A step-by-step procedure should be given for the quality control of the equipment or instrument.

3. Persons responsible:
   It should be emphasized that assigning responsibility for each task eliminates the uncertainty as to who was supposed to do the QCPM and monitoring by the supervisor is made easier. This controls the chances of an unauthorized person performing functions outside his job description.
4. Out-of-limits report:
   Complete instructions should be given on what to do if the instrument or equipment does not meet the standards indicated above. At this point, the supervisor should be notified if troubleshooting cannot correct the unacceptable result.
5. Preventive maintenance procedure:
   Detailed instructions for doing the preventive maintenance should be given and explained. This information is generally obtained from the manufacturer's instruction manual.

An example procedure using this format is provided in Figure 8.5.[15] Separate procedures should be written for each piece of equipment. Small booklets may be used for recording the QCPM on the equipment. The pages may be reduced to 5 by 7 inches and folded in the center. An example is provided in Figure 8.6. By printing on both sides of the paper, then folding, a cover can be placed on the outside and the booklet bound or stapled. Each piece of equipment should have its own booklet for individual QCPM documentation. The right side of the sheet is used for daily recording of temperatures. The spaces at the top of this side are left open to allow flexibility between equipment. The example is for a combination refrigerator/freezer using a maximum/minimum thermometer. The four empty columns could just as well be used for recording tachometer readings on a centrifuge.

The left side of the sheet is for recording out-of-limits action or routine preventive maintenance, such as defrosting, cleaning, decontamination. The review by the supervisor can be noted for accreditation purposes.

These booklets may be attached to the equipment or kept close to the instrument at all times. This will speed the time used for QCPM considerably. The personnel will include it as part of their initial start-up if it is well organized and accessible.

In summary the quality control maintenance program is composed of three steps:

1. Regular evaluation of instrument performance by established criteria,
2. Documentation of the evaluation results, and
3. Correction or adjustment of malfunction to result in compliance of the instrument's function with the established criteria.

SAFETY IN THE URINALYSIS LABORATORY

The primary purpose of a safety program is to maintain an environment within which one can function with a minimum of risk. The safety program, if well planned, will state the hazards, give the procedure to follow to prevent an accident, and the action to follow should an accident occur. Procedures must be written, organized into a safety manual, and available for review by all employees. The responsibility for safety can be broken into three divisions: (1) individual, (2) supervisory, and (3) educational or instructional programs.

Each individual in the laboratory whether student or employee has the responsibility to learn the safety and health hazards associated with his work. In addition, the employee should be familiar with the safety procedures established by the laboratory. Any accident that occurs must be reported immediately to the supervisor, whether it be a biologic accident, chemical spill, fire, or electrical problem. Familiarity and use of safety equipment are mandatory.

The supervisor has the responsibility of giving the necessary direction, including complete safety procedures to be followed and seeing that all procedures are followed.

He must be familiar with proper safety techniques and the use of safety equipment. By being alert to possible safety hazards, laboratory workers can prevent most accidents.

Education of the employees may be carried out by the supervisor or a designated safety officer whose sole duty is educating and monitoring. The initial establishment of procedures and protocol begins with the safety officer who, after reviewing federal, state, and local regulations, determines policies to be followed.

Safety can be categorized as follows: (1) biohazard safety, (2) chemical safety, (3) fire safety, and (4) electrical safety.

Biohazard Safety

Biohazard safety involves primarily the control of the spread of hepatitis and, to a lesser extent, bacterial infections. All specimens should be considered highly infectious, since there is no way of knowing which are positive specimens at the time of analysis. With this in mind, specific areas of control may be established:

1. Disinfection of work areas and equipment,
2. Storage and disposal of biologic specimens and waste,
3. Precautions in the laboratory, and
4. Identification of hepatitis patients and proper labeling of specimens.

Disinfection of Work Areas and Equipment

Processing the urine specimens involves a high degree of risk to the technologist, and decontamination procedures reduce the chance of infection. Bench tops should be cleaned at the end of each shift or more often if required. The most effective and economical disinfectant is a 1:100 solution of sodium hypochlorite. All bench top surfaces should be cleaned thoroughly and the solution allowed to stand approximately 10 minutes to allow maximum effectiveness. Small quantities of the sodium hypochlorite solution should be made daily or every other day so that it is always fresh. It becomes less active as it loses its strength. Recording the date on the bottle will aid in avoiding the inadvertent use of weak solution.

A stronger solution of sodium hypochlorite, 1:10, should be used to decontaminate the skin or articles that have come in contact with known sources of hepatitis. A 3 percent phenolic solution can be used when the use of sodium hypochlorite is inadvisable, such as on equipment made of stainless steel. In addition, the use of 10 percent sodium hypochlorite on human hands may cause reddening or soreness. If an employee appears to have a sensitivity to either of these two chemicals, any soap that produces a good lather can be used for handwashing. The intent is to dilute the organisms.

All glassware that has come in contact with biologic materials should be totally immersed in a 1:10 solution of sodium hypochlorite or a comparable disinfectant and allowed to soak at least 15 minutes before being washed. Fresh sodium hypochlorite must be used to maintain effectiveness.

Telephones, sample holders, handles (refrigerator doors, drawers) must be disinfected frequently or after a spill occurs with a 1:100 solution of sodium hypochlorite. Microscopes, refractometers, and centrifuges should be wiped down with a mild solution of 3 percent phenol. The reservoir for collecting the fluid as it is dispensed from the refractometer should contain sodium hypochlorite or 3 percent phenol.

Storage and Disposal of Biologic Specimens and Waste

Specimens that are kept for a period of time must be covered to prevent the potential hazard of spillage and aerosol production.[18] All specimens and such contaminated items as gauze, pipettes, and urine containers must be disposed of in appropriate waste containers lined with autoclave bags. Each work area should be equipped with an autoclave waste bag, and all items that come in contact with the biologic material must be put into this bag.

Regular housekeeping trash containers should be available for material not consi-

dered contaminated. All biologic material is then autoclaved before disposal. It is imperative that the housekeeping staff be able to recognize the difference between the two types of waste. Under no circumstances should the housekeeping staff be allowed to come in contact with the autoclave trash. Most autoclave bags are orange or have specific warnings to differentiate them from nonhazardous trash. The autoclave bags should be tightly closed during transport to the autoclaving area. While handling the autoclave bags, the staff must wear gloves to eliminate contact with the skin.

Precautions for Personnel

One important precaution directed toward reducing the risk of infection involves frequent and proper handwashing while working with specimens and before leaving the urinalysis laboratory. The proper handwashing technique involves using hot water at a temperature comfortable to the hands and a suitable hand soap, preferably containing phenol. Lather should be induced by using the friction of one hand upon the other, with special attention given to the area around the fingernails. The hands should be lathered for one minute, followed by thorough rinsing and drying.

Laboratory coats or uniforms should be worn to provide a protective barrier against contamination of skin and clothing. The laboratory coat should be buttoned at all times and removed before leaving the laboratory for meals or at the end of the work day.

It is important that laboratory requisitions (i.e., physicians' results) be kept separate from specimens insofar as possible and kept free of biologic fluid, since such forms may serve as carriers of the hepatitis virus if they are contaminated with body fluids. Any laboratory form or request slip contaminated with biologic fluid must be rewritten, and the contaminated slip must be placed in an autoclave bag.

Mouth pipetting presents one of the more serious sources of potential infection. Pipetting by mouth of any biologic sample should be prohibited. Safety bulbs should be used and decontaminated by soaking in 3 percent phenolic solution for a minimum of 30 minutes at least monthly. Mechanical pipettes, if used, must be decontaminated following the procedure indicated above, and the pipette tips must be disposed of in an appropriate reservoir for autoclaving.

Other oral routes of transmission besides mouth pipetting include smoking, eating, drinking, and the application of cosmetics and contact lenses. These activities increase the chance of infection within the laboratory. Tight regulations must be applied not only for control of hepatitis but also to satisfy accreditation guidelines. No eating, drinking, smoking, or application of cosmetics and contact lenses should be allowed in any area of the laboratory or clerical area that handles the processing of patient specimens or request and report forms. Food, beverages, and coffee cups should not be stored in the analytic area or in the refrigerators containing biologic materials or reagents. A specified refrigerator in an area not contiguous with the analytic area should be assigned for this purpose. Fingers, pencils, and other fomites also serve as an oral route of transmission.

During the initial processing of large volumes of specimens when the potential for infection increases, gloves should be worn. If there is a break in the skin because of a cut or scratch, finger cots will protect the open wound area. The importance of using gloves and finger cots because of the direct transmission into the bloodstream cannot be overemphasized.

Prevention of biohazardous aerosols can be accomplished by decontaminating centrifuges regularly, allowing centrifuges to come to a complete stop before opening the lid, and capping specimens prior to centrifugation. In addition, care in preventing splashes during disposal of urine is necessary.

Identification of Hepatitis Patients and Proper Labeling of Specimens

The laboratory safety procedures should include a method for the identification of hepatitis patients (Fig. 8.8).[15] A list of known or highly suspect hepatitis patients may be posted in the laboratory to alert personnel to the potential hazards. By doing this, special precautions and labeling of specimens can be done to assure control of the hazards during analysis.

Biohazard labels must be affixed to all specimens before they are brought to the laboratory, and the request slip must be kept separate to avoid contamination. If it is necessary to aliquot the specimen, biohazard labels must be attached to all secondary containers. CAP inspection and accreditation guidelines indicate that the biohazard label must be retained throughout the transmission of the specimen in the laboratory.

Chemical Safety

The practice of chemical safety involves proper use, storage, and waste disposal of chemicals. By implementing established safety rules, the technologist will develop a habit of good chemical safety.

Storage of Chemicals

Chemical storage in stockrooms should be kept to a minimum in order to have an annual turnover of all chemicals. Small containers are more advantageous unless the quantity used dictates the need for larger volumes. The purchase of small volumes maintains a fresher inventory of chemicals and eliminates the hazard of chemical changes due to aging. All chemicals should be dated when they are received and when they are opened. Old, undated chemicals should be disposed of if there is any indication of a possible explosion or fire hazard.

Incompatible chemicals should be stored separately,[8] and separate areas should be allocated for acids and alkalies. Ideally, chemicals are stored separately in four grous: (1) flammable, (2) toxic, (3) corrosive, and (4) reactive.[19] Caps must be tight to control the escape of fumes. Preferably, acids and alkalis should be stored in cabinets painted with anticorrosive paint and in which there are no plumbing fixtures. Fumes can quickly corrode and damage a metal cabinet without proper protective paint. A list of incompatible chemicals is given in Table 8.7.[8]

IDENTIFICATION OF HEPATITIS PATIENTS

References:

1. Duckworth, J. K., Col. Amer Path. 30: 412-419, 1976.

2. Viral Hepatitis, W. H. O. Technical Report No. 512, 1973.

Principle:

Laboratory personnel should consider all biological materials as possible sources of hepatitis virus. However, in cases of known or highly suspected hepatitis, the utilization of an Hepatitis Patients List and biohazard labels provides additional awareness of the risk surrounding these patients and their specimens, as well as providing helpful information in the event of an accident involving laboratory personnel.

Procedure:

A. Hepatitis Patients List:

1. A list of all known or highly suspect hepatitis patients will be prepared by the office of Laboratory Administration.

2. The following types of patient's will be included on the list:

   a. Patients who have been tested for the presence of the HB_s Ag and found to be positive by the RIA laboratory.

   b. Patients who are admitted with a diagnosis of hepatitis and placed in "Enteric Isolation".

   c. Patients who are admitted and known to be carriers of HB_s Ag and are placed on "Needle Precaution".

3. The RIA laboratory will be responsible for calling the Laboratory Administration office on a daily basis to inform them of whether or not they have new HB_s Ag (+) patients for the list.

4. The Infection Control office will be responsible for informing the Laboratiory Administration office of newly admitted Hepatitis patients or patients which are suspected of Hepatitis.

5. Designated personnel in the charting and records area will be responsible for deleting names from the Hepatitis List resulting from discharge or expiration.

6. The cutoff time for receiving additional names for the list will be 3:30 p.m.

Figure 8.8. Safety procedure for the identification of hepatitis patients.

Use of Chemicals. Personnel using toxic and/or corrosive chemicals must be properly attired and use techniques to prevent a chemical accident. The proper attire includes a long laboratory coat, safety glasses, gloves, and use of acid carriers for transporting. At no time should a laboratory employee use corrosive chemicals without proper eye protection. Safety goggles may be used, but a full-face safety mask provides greater protection. Laboratory coats and gloves may prevent damage to clothing and skin, and pipetting by mouth is prohibited. The acid carrier is rubberized with a handle and a lid so that if

Identification of Hepatitis Patients

7. The list will be updated, xeroxed, and distributed only to the Clinical and Anatomical laboratories.

8. The office Laboratory Administration will be responsible for retaining the master copies of the Hepatitis Patients List.

9. The Hepatitis Patients List will be amended only when new patients are to be added to the list. Therefore, a Hepatitis list will remain in effect until superseded by a new list.

B. Biohazard Labels:

1. Before entering the Clinical or Anatomical laboratories all biological materials from the hemodialysis unit, hepatitis patients (enteric isolation), and chronic carriers (needle precaution) will be identified by a fluorescent red biohazard label and the specimen placed in a plastic zip-lock bag, a styrofoam container or lilly bucket. The laboratory request slip will be attached to the outside of the plastic bag.

2. To facilitate this procedure, the hemodialysis unit and all isolation carts will be supplied with biohazard labels and plastic bags. All collectors will equip their blood collection trays with biohazard labels and several plastic bags.

3. Laboratory personnel will handle biohazardous specimen according to the procedure on "Collection and Transportation of Biohazardous Specimens".

4. If it is necessary to aliquot the specimen into a secondary container in the laboratory area, biohazard labels must be attached to all secondary containers.

5. The biohazard labeling system shall prevail throughout all steps of specimen handling and through all steps of specimen analysis.

6. All in-house pools of biological materials used or control material will require a biohazard label until proven negative by RIA for HB_s Ag.

_____   _____
Safety Coordinator   Laboratory Director

Figure 8.8. (Cont.)

the glass bottle is accidentally dropped and broken, the acid will be contained and the employee will be protected. The acid carriers, which are available in various sizes, may also be used for storage of chemicals. Only one bottle of corrosive material should be carried at a time.

Spill kits and a respirator mask are helpful if an accident should occur. Spill kits are available from several chemical companies and provide a means for easy clean-up at minimal risk. The material available in the spill kits consists of two different compounds which are to be used either for an acid spill or an alkali spill. They are simple to use and have indicators present to alert the user when the spilled solution has been neutralized. Once neutralized, the chemical can be effectively cleaned up and disposed of. Respirator masks provide a source of clean air during a chemical spill when fumes are overpowering. These masks should be placed in a location easily available to employees for use in an accident involving another person who is overcome by fumes. Several types of masks are available, and small facial masks with

TABLE 8.7. INCOMPATIBLE CHEMICALS

Chemical	Keep Out of Contact with
Acetic acid	Chromic acid, nitric acid, perchloric acid, peroxides, permanganates, glycol
Acetylene	Chlorine, bromine, copper, fluorine, silver, mercury
Ammonia, anhydrous	Mercury, chlorine, iodine, bromine, calcium, hypochlorite, hydrofluoric acid (anhydrous)
Ammonium nitrate	Flammable liquids, chlorates, nitrates, sulfur, finely divided organic and combustible materials
Aniline	Nitric acid, hydrogen peroxide
Bromine, chlorine, fluorine	Ammonia, acetylene, butadiene, methane, propane, hydrogen, benzene, turpentine
Carbon, activated	Calcium hypochlorate, all oxidizing agents
Chlorates	Ammonium salts, metal powders, sulfur, finely divided organic or combustible materials
Chromic acid	Acetic acid, naphthalene, camphor, glycerin, alcohol, flammable liquids, turpentine
Copper	Acetylene, hydrogen peroxide, sodium azide
Flammable liquids	Ammonium nitrate, chromic acid, hydrogen peroxide, nitric acid, sodium peroxide, halogens
Oxalic acid	Silver, mercury
Perchloric acid	Acetic acid, alcohol, paper, wood, flammable liquids
Potassium, sodium, lithium	Carbon tetrachloride, water, carbon dioxide
Potassium permanganate	Glycerin, ethylene glycol, benzaldehyde, sulfuric acid
Silver	Acetylene, oxalic acid, tartaric acid, ammonium compounds

canisters containing chemicals that remove or neutralize contaminants are sufficient for protection. However, these are not to be used for smoke protection during a fire. When selecting the respirator, this should be taken into consideration.

Ethers tend to absorb and react with oxygen from the air to form unstable peroxides. The peroxides can detonate with extreme violence when they become concentrated by evaporation or distillation, when combined with other compounds to create explosive mixtures, or when disturbed by unusual heat, shock, or friction.

Peroxides may form in freshly distilled and unstabilized ethers within two weeks. Exposure to the air, as in opened and partially emptied containers, accelerates the formation of peroxides, and exposure to light will also increase the formation of peroxides, although this is not fully understood. Refrigeration does not prevent the formation of peroxides.

The following properties of ether make it potentially dangerous:

1. It is highly flammable because of a low flash point (−45C for ethyl ether). The flash point is the temperature at which a chemical gives off a vapor sufficient to ignite.
2. When in contact with air, peroxide formation takes place. Peroxides are highly explosive.
3. Specific gravity is less than 1, and the vapor density is greater than 1. (Ether vapor is heavier than air and will, therefore, dissipate in a room without any warning.)

Because of the potential explosive and flammability hazards associated with ether, the quantity of ether on hand should be kept to a minimum. Small containers will be used up faster and eliminate storage of open containers. Ether should never be stored in a refrigerator unless it is explosion-proof. Flammable safety cabinets may be used for storage.

All ethers should be dated when they are received and when they are opened. Outdated ether may be disposed of after a method involving the removal of peroxides has been utilized. Ether should be stored at temperatures not to exceed 30C (86F). It should never be allowed to evaporate to dryness without taking the necessary precautions to neutralize any possible peroxides.

A ventilation hood should always be used when working with ether to control the escaping fumes. A velocity check on the hood should be performed regularly to assure that the necessary velocity rate is maintained. The vent of the hood, kept in a partially closed position, will form a protective barrier and prevent an accident to the employee.

Eyewash stations and safety showers may save an employee the loss of an eye and/or permanent disfigurement. All employees must know how the equipment operates. In case of an accident in which a chemical has splashed in the eye, immediately hold the eye open and rinse with water for a minimum of 15 minutes.[19] It is of the utmost importance to remove contact lenses, since these will hold the chemical and prevent thorough cleansing.

If a spill occurs in the clothing or skin, immediate rinsing under the safety shower could prevent permanent damage. All contaminated clothing should be removed, and the employee should wash for a minimum of 15 minutes.

Disposal of Waste Chemicals. Waste disposal is a problem to which no simple solution exists. No matter what means is used for disposing—down the drain, burning, or burying—pollution results. Until recommendations can be provided, the laboratory must resort to the most efficient, yet safe, process.

If the chemicals are miscible with water, the most efficient means of disposal is down the laboratory drain. Large amounts of water should accompany the chemical to create an effective dilution.

Electrical Safety

Electrical malfunction of the instruments and equipment used in the urinalysis laboratory may cause fires and/or an electrical shock which could result in death to an employee. Since electrical accidents usually are preventable, certain guidelines must be established to maintain a safe environment.

All electrical equipment should have a periodic inspection (every six months to one year), at which time proper grounding and leakage of current are checked. All electrical cords are checked for frayed ends, broken plugs, exposed wires, and for the presence of a safety ground wire. The safety ground wire serves the purpose of allowing excess current to be channeled properly to the ground instead of through the human operator. It must be present on all equipment with metal cases, frames, or covers. It is perhaps the most important of all preventive procedures in electrical safety.

Employees should know where the circuit breaker boxes are in order to assure a fast response during an electrical fire or electrical shock. Equipment should always be unplugged before maintenance is performed. Equipment that has had liquid spilled on it and has come in contact with the electrical wiring should be immediately unplugged and allowed to dry. Safety procedures should be written indicating what should not be done, such as not handling electrical connections with damp hands or when standing in or near water. The importance of electrical safety should be emphasized, and all personnel must be responsible for daily electrical monitoring and reporting of unsafe situations and equipment.

Specific guidelines must be written and available for the personnel to follow should an accident involving electrical shock occur. The sequence to follow after electrical shock may be stated as follows:

1. Shut off the power or carefully remove the power contact from the victim using an insulator (a nonconductor of electricity). Use a glass pipette, heavy rubber or asbestos gloves, or simply a hand in a glass beaker to push the vic-

tim or power supply to the side. Do not attempt to touch the victim while he is still in contact with the electrical current. If this should happen, the rescuer will also become part of the circuit and will also be electrocuted.

2. Once the power source has been controlled, medical help should be summoned and cardiopulmonary resuscitation applied.

3. No attempt should be made to move the victim while waiting for medical assistance. Keep the victim warm—a fire blanket could serve this purpose.

Fire Safety

Fire in the laboratory calls for prompt action to extinguish the fire or evacuate occupants. The laboratory personnel have the sole responsibility for emergency procedures, which consist of the following steps to prevent injury and limit the spread of the fire:

1. Alert personnel in the immediate area of the fire and evacuate the area.
2. Confine the fire by closing doors and windows tightly.
3. Notify the proper authorities immediately of the fire and location so that the internal fire brigade and fire department can reach the scene of the fire.

In minor situations where the fire may be easily extinguished without calling the fire department, the first two steps of alerting and confining the fire should still be taken. If a small benchtop fire cannot be controlled, all personnel must be familiar with the procedure for reporting the fire. Promptness is of uppermost importance as every second lost increases the risk of equipment and possibly lives being lost.

In the urinalysis laboratory, a fire extinguisher and fire blanket must be available. The type of fire extinguisher is dependent upon what fire risks are present. Usually a dry chemical or CO_2 type is sufficient for all types of fires that could occur. Demonstrations on the use of fire extinguishers and fire

blankets should be conducted by the supervisor or safety officer. Evacuation routes must be posted, and all personnel must be familiar with the closest exits. Conducting fire drills that encompass the use of extinguishers, fire blankets, notification procedures, and evacuation is the most important precaution in preventing loss of human life.

Storage and use of flammable materials must be kept to a minimum. These materials should be stored in a safety cabinet, preferably vented to the outside of the building. Safety cans are used to store small volumes of flammable materials and to control the disposal of flammable wastes. Care should be taken to use flammable chemicals under a ventilation hood.

Monitoring Accidents

Once these safety procedures and policies have been established, the majority of situations that can result in accidents hopefully will be prevented or controlled. Accidents that do occur, whether biologic, chemical, fire, or electrical, must be reported, and an accident report must be prepared. The purpose of the accident report is to provide a record and a detailed description of the circumstances surrounding the accident. This report provides a means of thorough investigation and correction of the causative situation. Such records can serve as an indicator of the types of accidents, frequency, weaknesses in the safety program, frequency of accidents by the same individual, and the effectiveness of the safety program.

PLANNING A URINALYSIS LABORATORY

Initial Planning

There are several important factors to consider in planning a well-organized, efficient urinalysis laboratory. These include[20]:

1. The approximate number of tests to be performed,
2. The types of tests to be performed, e.g., routine, special, and so on,

3. The number of personnel required to operate the laboratory at its fullest capacity, and
4. Educational activities (numbers of students, teaching equipment, and space).

Once these factors have been reviewed, one is ready to undertake the task of actually drawing the plans for the laboratory. The following set of questions was designed to cover all aspects of designing and planning:

1. How much space will be needed to provide the services desired?
2. How much of this space should be designated to stand-up work benches and how much to sit-down bench space?
3. How much storage space will be needed?
4. How much countertop space will be needed for equipment? How much floor space will be needed for equipment?
5. How much countertop space will be needed for books, files, and so on?
6. How much extra space will be needed for teaching purposes?
7. How many sinks will be needed, and where should they be located?
8. Will there be need for a hood?

Physical Layout

The next phase of planning involves working with scale models until the desired arrangement is achieved. A pattern of the flow of work should be kept in mind (Fig. 8.9).

There should be a designated area to receive all incoming specimens. From this point, specimens can be easily moved to the processing area and then to the centrifuge. The original container is stored for a specified time period and then discarded. Each laboratory should determine its own time limit, but an eight-hour shift is usually sufficient. After centrifugation, the samples that require confirmation tests are tested, and all samples are then taken to the microscope for sediment examination.

If the laboratory can be arranged to keep the work flow moving smoothly, efficiency is greatly improved. With this in mind, draw a floor plan using one-quarter-inch scale. Put in standing and sit-down work benches. After the positions for the work benches have been determined, put in overhead cabinets, then drawers, and undercounter cabinets. Place the sinks in a convenient location. It would be ideal to have a sink for discarding specimens and one strictly for handwashing. Show this and alternate plans to the staff who will be working in the area, get feedback from them, and move things around until the most practical working arrangement is obtained. This is the time to arrange everything for the convenience of the staff.

Utilities and Services

Once these permanent fixtures have been placed, lighting, flooring, wall color, heating and air-conditioning, ventilation, electrical outlets, and telephones should be considered.

Good lighting is essential for the laboratory to function properly. Fluorescent lights generally work extremely well and will allow for the reading of fine details. A good choice of lighting, along with pastel or white walls, creates an air of space and cleanliness.

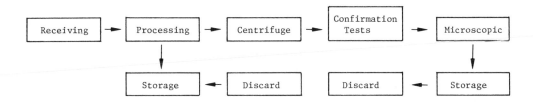

Figure 8.9. A typical work flow pattern.

A cushioned floor would be the most comfortable, but unless it is resistant to stains and chemicals, it may not be the wisest choice. A durable flooring is most desirable.

Heating and air-conditioning are generally preplanned in the original scheme of the building. However, it may be necessary to have individual control units available in the laboratory for needed adjustments. Ventilation, too, is usually preplanned. The laboratory performing only routine urinalysis examinations may not need to install a hood, but if there is a chance of expansion, this is the time to consider the possibility of a hood and where it may be installed.

Electrical outlets will not be a problem if electrical strips are installed along each work bench. This allows for the addition of new equipment, which can be placed conveniently without interrupting the work flow. Ill-placed electrical outlets have made many laboratories look completely disorganized.

The telephone should be centrally located between work benches. Files and log books should be in close proximity to minimize the time used in search of reports and specimens.

Equipment

Equipment for the urinalysis laboratory is minimal. Most laboratories can operate with a microscope, a centrifuge, an instrument to read specific gravity, a refrigerator, and a waterbath. The refrigerator and the waterbath are optional pieces of equipment. Some of the more modern laboratories have a great deal of sophisticated automation, but the same results and the same degree of quality can be obtained in a laboratory with no automation.

The size of the centrifuge will depend, of course, on the number of specimens to be processed. Generally, a 24-hour-specimen size with speed controls and a timer is sufficient. The centrifuge should be placed on the stand-up workbench away from the microscope to reduce the chance of vibration interfering with microscopic examinations.

A good quality microscope is essential, and all efforts should be made to keep it clean and in good working condition.

The size of the refrigerator (optional) will depend on the workload and whether specimens will be refrigerated to be tested in batches or if they will be tested as they arrive in the laboratory. If storage will not be a major problem, a small tabletop model would work quite well. It will be just large enough for reagents, controls, and any samples that may need to be saved for whatever reason. Whichever model is chosen, tabletop or floor model, it should be placed where it will not obstruct the work flow.

There are several mechanisms available for reading the specific gravity of urines. The most widely used is the simple hand-held refractometer. It has proven to be very accurate and requires only a few drops of urine. A more advanced model with a pump unit is also available. It is easy to operate and gives the same quality of results as the hand-held model, but it has the added advantage of rinsing between each specimen with the push of a lever. However, it does require a larger sample of urine. A small waterbath may be considered if there is a chance the laboratory will expand and deal with more sophisticated tests, but for the routine laboratory, it is an optional piece of equipment.

It may be necessary to have a storage area for volatile reagents. Most regulating agencies require the storage of such material in safety cabinets. If your laboratory is small and will be handling only a small volume, it would be more economical to share storage with another department.

STAFFING A URINALYSIS LABORATORY

As stated earlier, the personnel required to staff adequately the urinalysis laboratory will depend primarily on the numbers and kinds of services the laboratory will provide. It will be necessary, especially if this is a new laboratory, to consult with the medical staff to determine the extent to which they will use the laboratory.

It has been shown that many physicians rely on the results of the urinalysis, while others often overlook significant findings. This leads one to wonder if indeed most urinalysis examinations are not routinely ordered without clinical indications. However, many urine examinations are ordered, and if your laboratory is operating in such a facility, there are several points to consider when hiring the staff:

1. How many specimens will be processed daily?
2. What will be the days and hours of operation?
3. What will be the desired turnaround time for reporting results?
4. How will teaching (if an educational program exists) be handled?

From communications with technologists, it appears that one medical technologist can comfortably handle 50 to 60 specimens per day. If more specimens are tested per day and if frequent teaching is required, one should study the possibility of hiring a technician as an assistant. If the laboratory is required to operate seven days a week, it is imperative to have a well-developed plan for weekend coverage. This is difficult to accomplish with only one or even two persons because they cannot be stretched to cover effectively. Weekend and holiday coverage can best be handled by having another department share the coverage.

The JCAH requires sufficient qualified personnel to perform all technical procedures. As mentioned earlier, the addition of a technician can be an asset to the laboratory. Laws regarding the requirements of a technician vary, but most tend to include a certain amount of education, experience, or both.[21] The only limitation is that the technician must not exercise independent judgment and must at all times work under the direct supervision of a technologist, supervisor, or director.

It is important that the laboratory be certified by JCAH and/or CAP. Currently, if the laboratory is inspected and accredited by CAP, this is equivalent to inspection and accreditation by the federal government be-

cause CAP has stringent standards. The licensed laboratory must also participate in and maintain an acceptable level of performance on surveys and other approved proficiency tests. For this reason, it is important that the staff be aware of the need for proper quality control, the purpose of proficiency testing, and the need for safety at all times. The staff should be well-informed on the proper care and use of equipment and their specific duties as related to providing quality patient care.

COST AND COST EFFECTIVENESS

Laboratories are charged with providing quality patient care and keeping operating costs at a minimum. In dealing with the subject of the cost of performing a urinalysis, one should be aware that the total operating costs can vary.

When trying to get an idea of the cost, short-term planning (one month to one year) should be utilized. One must realize that there are fixed expenses that will occur regardless of the actual number of tests performed. There are also a certain number of costs that will fluctuate with the number of tests that are done. Over a period of time, the total costs versus the number of tests performed can be graphed, and certain trends and patterns associated with the work load may be seen. Before purchasing new equipment or adding new personnel, it is usually necessary to include a graph of this sort to justify the need.

Quality performance by the staff can ultimately help reduce the cost of operation. The more informed the staff members are about the costs of supplies, reagents, and service for equipment, the more helpful they can be in curbing costs.

The cost effectiveness of a test on urine, as with any other laboratory test, includes the consideration of societal benefits in addition to the health benefits to the individual. Societal benefits encompass the contributions of an individual to the pleasure and quality of life of others, e.g., family, professional colleagues, patients, clients, fans, or public. This kind of benefit is the most difficult to analyze, and for this reason it is not included in this discussion of cost effectiveness.

Laboratory scientists have been involved for many years in the calculation of the cost of performing laboratory tests. The analysis of the net health benefit to the patient is a newer approach and is more subject to variation because of the differing uses of the test results by referring physicians, including those who use the same laboratory facility. Baer[22] and others[23] have found that only slightly over one-third of abnormal urinary sediment reports received any detectable attention by the patient's physician.

The components of the health resource cost are direct costs, indirect costs, and induced costs.[24] The items that are included in these categories are listed in Table 8.8. The induced costs of a test are those costs that result from tests or treatments that are added or averted because of the test under study. The difference between the positive and negative aspects of the induced cost items is calculated to give the net effectivenss of the test under study.

In 1979, the direct and indirect costs of a routine urinalysis were calculated to be about $6.00, with a 9 percent increase over that calculated for 1978.[25] The calculation of the net induced cost for a urinalysis has yet to be published. In order to determine this net induced cost, an evaluation of each of the individual tests performed in a routine urinalysis would be necessary. An example of the complexities of the calculation of the net induced cost of a laboratory test is illustrated by Weinstein and Fineberg in their estimation of cost effectiveness for urinary vanillylmandelic acid.[24] Griffith et al have followed two patients from 1967 to 1979 whose nephrolithiasis became a morbid disease.[26] The itemized costs for health service over this 12-year period were calculated for each of these patients to be $43,983 and $70,776. This information was used to support the justification of early diagnosis and treatment of bacteriuria and calculous disease.

TABLE 8.8. HEALTH RESOURCE COSTS: URINALYSIS

Direct Costs
  Capital: microscopes, centrifuges, refractometers
  Labor: medical technologist, laboratory scientist, aides
  Materials: quality control solutions, reagents and reagent strips, microscope slides and coverslips, centrifuge tubes, pipettes, collection vessels, and report forms
Indirect Costs
  Depreciation of capital
  Rental space
  Utilities
  Administrative services
Induced Costs or Effectiveness Factors
  Change in cost due to the performance of a test (+ or −):
    Information obtained from urinalysis—performance of additional tests, alteration of treatment
    Alteration in disease morbidity—improvement of patient's health, leads to treatment of disease
    Side effects of additional tests and treatments—if adverse effects occur from treatment, medication, or additional invasive tests, the cost figures here are negative
    Increased longevity—if the test benefits the patient by prolonging life, other illnesses will occur which will consume health resources

The cost effectivenss of a laboratory test is the ratio of the sum of the direct, indirect, and net induced costs to the net change in the quality (improved function or productivity or pleasure) and years of life.

SUMMARY

Management includes many activities and programs that are not addressed in this chapter, e.g., computerization and data processing. It is hoped that this chapter has introduced the reader to some of the more widely practiced aspects of management as it per-tains to a urinalysis laboratory and encouraged an interest in some other aspects, e.g., cost effectiveness, of this important function of medical technology.

Review Questions

1. Quality control in the urinalysis laboratory depends primarily on:
   A. Performing
   B. Assaying
   C. Monitoring
   D. Planning
   E. Scheduling

2. Major errors committed in the urinalysis laboratory include:
   A. Failure to test a fresh specimen
   B. Inadequate care of reagents
   C. Use of unclean collection containers
   D. Poor technique
   E. Lack of recognition of interfering substances

3. Urine controls that are prepared in the laboratory should meet which of the following criteria?
   A. Should have all values in normal range
   B. Should be very clear
   C. Should be easy to prepare
   D. Should be stable for several months
   E. Should be assayable by routine urinalysis methods

4. Three factors important in the use and storage of lyophilized urine controls are:
   A. Reconstitution with the correct type and volume of diluent
   B. Dating the vial upon receipt and upon opening
   C. Observing storage temperature limits
   D. Selection of the least expensive control
   E. Immediate testing of the control

5. Which of the following situations should prompt the assay of control solutions?
   A. New employee
   B. New reagents
   C. Personnel shift change
   D. Move to a new laboratory
   E. New control solution

6. A medical technologist while performing a Clinitest procedure was called to the telephone. When he returned, the test showed a brown color. Which of the following statements may be correct from the information given here?
   A. The test is positive at a concentration of 1 percent
   B. The test is positive at a concentration of 5 percent
   C. The test is negative
   D. The result is due to interfering substance
   E. The reagent tablet is faulty

7. The glucose oxidase strip test for glucose in a urine specimen is positive, and the Clinitest tablet test is negative. Which of the following explanations is (are) likely:
   A. A false positive glucose oxidase test
   B. The patient is on high doses of vitamin C
   C. The Clinitest tablet is not as sensitive as the glucose oxidase strip test
   D. The Clinitest tablet is more specific for glucose
   E. The Clinitest tablets have been exposed to moisture

8. The three errors that are shared by most tablet and strip tests are:
   A. Improper storage of reagent tablets and strips
   B. Incorrect measurement of urine
   C. Misreading color chart
   D. Incorrect mixing of urine with tablets or strips
   E. Lack of fresh specimen

9. Variation in the report of an examination of urinary sediment is most likely

to occur in which of the following steps?

A. The collection of the specimen
B. The mixing of the specimen prior to centrifugation
C. The removal of the supernatant
D. The speed of centrifugation
E. The counting of elements per microscopic field

10. Two major reasons for participating in a proficiency testing survey program are:
   A. To assure good quality of laboratory results
   B. To receive patient approval
   C. To obtain a comparison of results with those of other laboratories
   D. To meet accreditation standards
   E. To justify a higher charge for the analysis

11. Three steps common to most quality control preventive maintenance programs are:
   A. Monitoring of instrument performance
   B. Evaluation of instruments to be purchased
   C. Maintenance and repair of instruments
   D. Recording the data from the quality control preventive maintenance activities
   E. Sale of outdated instruments

12. In the refractometer function check, the refractometer when filled with 5 percent w/v sodium chloride should give a specific gravity reading of:
   A. 1.000
   B. 1.015
   C. 1.022
   D. 1.030
   E. 1.035

13. A well-planned safety program will do which of the following?
   A. Identify the hazards
   B. Give the procedure to follow to prevent accidents
   C. State the action to be taken following an accident
   D. Provide safety equipment
   E. Have only one person responsible for safety

14. List four areas of biohazard safety control.

15. Disinfection of work areas and equipment is most effectively performed by cleaning with:
   A. 1:10 Sodium hypochlorite
   B. 1:10 Hydrogen peroxide
   C. 1:10 Phenol in alcohol
   D. 1:100 Sodium hypochlorite
   E. 1:100 Phenol in alcohol

16. Match the chemicals in List A with those that are incompatible in List B.

List A
A. Acetic acid
B. Flammable liquids
C. Potassium permanganate
D. Oxalic acid
E. Perchloric acid

List B
1. Hydrogen peroxide
2. Alcohol
3. Silver
4. Nitric acid
5. Ethylene glycol

17. Which one of the following items is to be used continuously in the urinalysis laboratory?
   A. Fire blanket
   B. Fire extinguisher
   C. Laboratory coat
   D. Spill kit
   E. Safety glasses

18. The most important precaution in electrical safety is:
   A. To wear insulated gloves
   B. To establish safety guidelines
   C. To turn off instruments
   D. The presence of ground wire in all cords
   E. Awareness of location of circuit breaker box

19. List four important factors in planning a urinalysis laboratory.

20. What influence can the staff have in the planning phase?

21. A typical sequence for the flow of work in a urinalysis laboratory is:
    A. Receiving, centrifuging, microscopic analysis, processing, confirmation, storage, discard
    B. Receiving, processing, centrifuging, confirmation, microscopic analysis, storage, discard
    C. Receiving, processing, confirmation, centrifuging, microscopic analysis, storage, discard
    D. Receiving, centrifuging, processing, microscopic analysis, confirmation, storage, discard
    E. Receiving, centrifuging, confirmation, processing, microscopic analysis, storage, discard

22. The direct costs of performing a urinalysis include:
    A. Utilities
    B. Capital
    C. Labor
    D. Rental
    E. Materials and supplies

23. The effectiveness factors in the cost-benefit analysis are which of the following?
    A. Alteration in disease morbidity
    B. Information obtained leading to additional tests or alteration of treatment
    C. Side effects of additional tests and treatments
    D. Increased longevity
    E. Inflation

24. The cost effectiveness (CE) of a urinalysis test may be represented by the following formula:

    A. $$CE = \frac{direct + indirect\ costs + net\ induced\ costs}{net\ change\ in\ quality\ and\ years\ of\ life}$$

    B. $$CE = \frac{direct + indirect\ costs}{net\ induced\ costs + net\ change\ in\ quality\ and\ years\ of\ life}$$

    C. $$CE = \frac{net\ change\ in\ quality\ and\ years\ of\ life}{net\ induced\ costs + net\ change\ in\ quality\ and\ years\ of\ life}$$

    D. $$CE = \frac{net\ change\ in\ quality\ and\ years\ of\ life}{direct + indirect\ costs + net\ induced\ costs}$$

    E. $$CE = \frac{direct + indirect\ costs}{net\ induced\ costs}$$

(See Appendix for answers.)

Case Studies

Case Study 1

At the beginning of a day shift, the microbiologist was called to the urinalysis laboratory to identify numerous flagellated microorganisms that appeared on the microscopic slide of a urinary sediment. The microbiologist said it did not look like any organism of medical importance, but he was unsure. Another drop of sediment was examined, and only two such organisms were seen. A senior medical technologist, in passing, saw the congregation at the microscope and joined the crowd. After hearing a recounting of the events, she suggested that an aliquot of the original urine sediment be centrifuged in a clean centrifuge tube and the sediment be transferred to the microscopic slide with a clean pipette. No microorganisms were seen in this preparation. Upon investigation it was found that a pipette that had remained in a small beaker of water was used to transfer the sediment to the slide, and the pipette was flushed with water from this beaker between each sampling. The technologist who was beginning the day's work had not emptied the beaker and cleaned it, nor had she begun with a fresh pipette. A drop of the water from the beaker transferred with the old pipette showed numerous flagellated microorganisms.

Questions
1. What are 3 things that might be done to avoid this problem occurring in the future?
2. What appropriate behavior is noticed in the situation described?

Answers
1. Things that might be done to avoid this problem are:
   a. Establish a well defined laboratory procedure that includes using clean pipets and instruments.
   b. Following established laboratory procedures.
   c. Establish a quality control procedure for urinary sediment analysis.
2. The appropriate behavior is the investigation of any unusual result that is found. The technologist asked for expert consultation when she saw something in the sediment that was unusual.

Case Study 2
   A medical technologist in the urinalysis laboratory of a large hospital had the adhesive tape removed from a sprained ankle. The laboratory worker who helped remove the old tape used ether to remove the sticky adhesive and threw the gauze flats and adhesive tape in the nearest trash can. Approximately 30 minutes later, a medical resident smoking a cigar walked into the urinalysis laboratory to inquire about a report on his patient. During the wait for the report he flicked his cigar in the trash can. An explosion followed. Fortunately, no one was hurt.

Questions
1. What three things could the laboratory personnel have done to prevent this?
2. Are precautions and safety regulations necessary in all parts of the laboratory?

Answers
1. They could have:
   a. Used ether in the laboratory in a more discretionary manner,

   b. Disposed of ether in a proper way, and
   c. Asked nonlaboratory personnel not to smoke or bring lighted smoking material into the laboratory.
2. Yes, ether is not a common chemical in the urinalysis laboratory and yet it was there for an atypical reason. Chemicals and hazards are occasionally in unusual places for unusual reasons. The lack of good safety habits makes these occasions extremely dangerous.

Case Study 3
   A medical technologist at the beginning of the day shift performed a quality control assay on the urinalysis control solution. All chemical tests were within the acceptable ranges, but the specific gravity was 0.003 units outside the acceptable limit.

Questions
1. What should he do next?
2. What should be the first consideration as the cause of the out-of-control assay?

Answers
1. The medical technologist should follow the written procedure that has been established in that laboratory for quality control problems.
2. The use of a 95 percent range for acceptable limits of a test implies that 5 of every 100 assays will be outside these limits for purely statistical reasons.

Case Study 4
   A new urinalysis laboratory has just been occupied. It immediately is found that there are no electrical outlets in the planned microscopy area. There are outlets in all the other walls.

Questions
1. What might have been done to avoid this situation?
2. What can be done to remedy it?

Answers
1. Consideration of the flow of work would have helped, and a scale model

and physical layout (like the one below) with work flow and utilities shown would have helped avoid this problem. The involvement of staff in a review of the layout would have been a good check on the appropriateness of the plans.

2. Add an electrical strip, or, if this is not possible, situate the laboratory instruments to accommodate the same work flow but in a different direction.

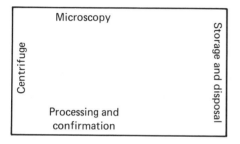

REFERENCES

1. Purvis JJ: Laboratory Planning, Baltimore, Williams & Wilkins, 1973.
2. Bennington JL, Boer GB, Louvac GE, Westlake GG: Management and Cost Control Techniques for the Clinical Laboratory. Baltimore, University Park Press, 1977.
3. Becan-McBride K: Textbook on Clinical Laboratory Supervision. New York, Appleton, 1982.
4. Mac Fate RP: Introduction to the Clinical Laboratory. Chicago, Year Book, 1961, pp. 63–70, 140–143.
5. McLendon WW, Henry JB: Administration of the Clinical Laboratory. In Henry JB (ed): Clinical Diagnosis and Management by Laboratory Methods, 16th ed. Philadelphia, Saunders, 1979, vol 2, pp 1977–2083.
6. Daharan M: Total Quality Control in the Clinical Laboratory. St. Louis, Mo., Mosby, 1977.
7. Surveys 1982, in Pursuit of Excellence, Interlaboratory Comparison Programs. Skokie, Ill., College of American Pathologists, 1982.
8. Steere NV: Safety in the Chemical Laboratory, 2nd ed. Easton, Pa., American Chemical Society, 1980.
9. Manufacturing Chemists Association: Guide for Safety in The Clinical Laboratory, 2nd ed. New York, Van Nostrand, 1971.
10. Free AH, Free HM: Rapid convenience urine tests: their use and misuse. Lab Med 9:10, 1978.
11. Bradley GM, Schumann GB, Ward PCJ: In Henry JB (ed): Clinical Diagnosis and Management by Laboratory Methods, 16th ed. Philadelphia, Saunders, 1979, vol 1, p 565.
12. Peele JD, Gadsden RH, Crews R: Evaluation of Ames Clini-Tek. Clin Chem 23:2338, 1977.
13. Braden M: Evaluation of Kova System. Fountain Valley, California, ICL Scientific Publication.
14. Kurtzman NA, Don Boyd EN: Evaluation of the Kova System of Examination of the Urinary Sediment. Fountain Valley, California, ICL Scientific Publication.
15. University of Texas and Hermann Hospital: Department of Pathology and Laboratory Medicine Laboratory Procedure, Houston, Texas, 1982.
16. College of American Pathologists: Commission of Inspection and Accreditation Inspection Checklist, Section III-A: Urinalysis. Skokie, Ill., College of American Pathologists, March 1982.
17. Linke EG, Henry JB, Statland BE: Theory and practice of laboratory technique. In Henry JB (ed): Clinical Diagnosis and Management by Laboratory Methods, 16th ed. Philadelphia, Saunders, vol 1, p 61.
18. Laboratory Waste and Disposal Manual. Washington, DC, Manufacturing Chemists Association, 1975.
19. Hazardous Chemical Safety. Phillipsburg, N.J., JT Baker Chemical Co, 1977, p. 16.
20. Purvis MJ: Laboratory Planning. Baltimore, Williams & Wilkins, 1973.
21. Halper HR, Foster HS: Laboratory Regulation Manual. Washington, D.C., Aspen, 1976–82, pp 2.3:6, 2.3:18.
22. Baer DM, Berner M: Physicians' responses to abnormal results of routine urinalysis. Canadian Med Assn J 117:1262, 1977.
23. McGuckin MB, Adenbaum AF, Corbin E: Abnormal results are ignored by physicians. Lab World 30:30, 1979.
24. Weinstein MC, Fineberg HV: Cost-effectiveness analysis for medical practices: appropriate laboratory utilization. In Benson ES, Rubin M (eds): Logic and Economics of Clinical Laboratory Use. Amsterdam, Elsevier, 1978, pp 3–32.
25. Kull DJ: Cost containment. the pressures and the impact. Med Lab Observ 12:35, 1980.
26. Griffith DP, Bruce RP, Fishbein WH: Infection(urease)-induced stones in nephrolithiasis. Contemp Issues Nephrol 5:238, 1980.

Ann E. Neely and Kathryn Kilpatrick Cheek

| CHAPTER 9 |

Techniques of Cell Counts and Microscopic Examination of Fluids

Objectives

It is expected that the information presented in this chapter will enable the reader to:

1. Explain methods used for performing cell counts.
2. Compare the advantages and disadvantages of automated vs. manual methods of cell counts.
3. Diagram the various types of hemocytometers including the dimensions of each.
4. Distinguish between RBCs and WBCs on manual hemocytometer counts.
5. Distinguish between mononuclear and polynuclear cells on manual hemocytometer counts.
6. List important techniques to be considered when performing the cell count and differential count on fluid samples.
7. Describe an accepted protocol or methodology for performing manual hemocytometer counts.
8. Calculate the total number of cells present in a fluid specimen.
9. Describe the various concentration techniques.
10. List various stains used on fluid preparations.
11. Identify the staining characteristics of each of the stains described in this chapter.
12. Calculate the final magnification achieved using the light microscope.
13. List the types of microscopy that may be utilized in studying body fluids.
14. Define resolution or resolving power of the light microscope.
15. Describe how greater magnification is achieved using the oil objective of the microscope.
16. Identify the various components that should be incorporated into the final report.

The evaluation of the number of cells present in any fluid provides essential information in the analysis of that fluid. Techniques available for performing cell counts include both manual and automated methods. Current automated methods, however, are not recommended (page 222). Traditionally, due to the low numbers of cells present in body fluids and the problems associated with automated methods, cell counts on body fluids are performed manually. Advantages of the manual method include its simplicity and the low cost of equipment, with the added advantage of easy screening for atypical cell sizes or shapes. Disadvantages include technical variation and the small quantity of sample examined.

MANUAL METHODS

The manual enumeration of cells is accomplished with the use of a hemocytometer. The most commonly used hemocytometers include the Neubauer hemocytometer, the Fuchs-Rosenthal hemocytometer, and the Spears-Levy hemocytometer. Red blood cells and white blood cells in body fluids can be counted by using methods similar to those used for counting them in blood samples. RBCs can be distinguished by their smaller size, uniformity, and smooth homogeneous appearance, while WBCs can be identified by their larger size and granular appearance.

Important Techniques
Techniques that are especially important in regard to cell counts in fluids include:

1. Performing the examination as soon as possible after the fluid is removed from the body cavity, as cellular degeneration occurs rapidly. No fixative is required if the specimen is examined promptly.
2. Adequate mixture of the sample either by placing the sample on an automatic rotator or by slowly tilting the sample back and forth 10 to 15 times.

3. Dilution of the sample is usually not necessary. If, however, on visual examination of the sample the cells are too numerous to count on the loaded chamber, dilutions can be made using either normal saline or a commercially available isotonic solution, such as Isoton.
4. Clean counting chambers, microscope lens, and microscopic slides are essential since any debris may cause inaccurate results.

Hemocytometers
Diagrams of the common hemocytometers are shown in Figure 9.1. It is important to know the dimensions of the chamber used since these dimensions are used in the calculation of the number of cells present in the specimen (Table 9.1).

Accepted Protocol or Methodology
In the literature and at various institutions there are variations in the protocol used for the enumeration of the cells present in a fluid specimen. One recommended protocol follows:

I. Adequately mix the sample.
II. Load one side of a Neubauer hemocytometer with undiluted specimen (referred to as *Side A*).
III. Load the other side of the Neubauer hemocytometer with specimen in which the RBCs have been lysed (referred to as *Side B*). Lysing of the RBCs can be accomplished with any of the WBC-diluting fluids used in manual whole blood WBC counts. WBC-diluting fluid should not, however, be used with synovial fluid since acid will cause protein to precipitate. Since dilution of the sample is usually not necessary, one simple method of lysing the RBCs is to coat the sides of a 44.7γ or 20γ pipette with 1 percent glacial acetic acid. Coating can be accomplished as follows:
A. Fill the pipette with 1 percent glacial

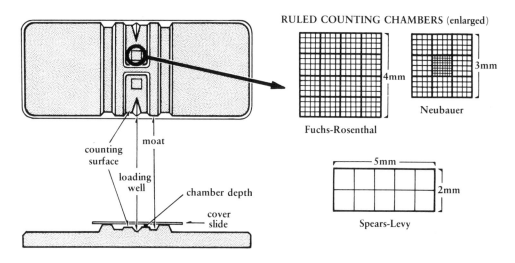

Figure 9.1. Diagrams of hemocytometers.

acetic acid to approximately one-sixth of the tube length.

B. Allow the glacial acetic acid to move from end to end of the pipette several times by rotation of the wrist.

C. Finally, expel the glacial acetic acid out of the pipette with the aid of a piece of lens or tissue paper to facilitate complete removal of the acid.

D. The coated tube is then placed into the body fluid specimen and allowed to fill to approximately one-third of the tube length.

E. Rotate the specimen from end to end of the tube two to three times.

F. The hemocytometer can then be loaded by placing the pipette adjacent to the loading well and allowing the chamber to fill by capillary action.

This method of using a coated glacial acetic acid tube is additionally helpful in that the amount of glacial acetic acid present in the tube is not only sufficient enough to accomplish lysis of the RBCs but also delineates the nuclear material of the WBCs present. This delineation allows one to determine if the WBC is mononuclear or polynuclear (Fig. 9.2).

IV. On *Side A* count the cells in all nine large squares (i.e., count all cells on the counting surface), distinguishing RBCs from WBCs (Fig. 9.3).

V. On *Side B* count the cells present in all nine large squares (i.e., count all the cells on the counting chamber), distin-

TABLE 9.1. DIMENSIONS OF HEMOCYTOMETERS

Hemocytometer	Length	Width	Depth	Counting Surface	Counting Chambers per Counting Surface
Neubauer	3 mm	3 mm	0.1 mm	2	1
Fuchs-Rosenthal	4 mm	4 mm	0.2 mm	2	1
Spears-Levy	5 mm	5 mm	0.2 mm	2	2

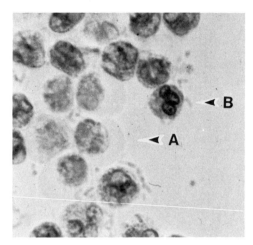

Figure 9.2. A. Mononuclear cell. **B.** Polynuclear cell.

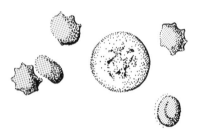

Figure 9.3. Drawing of red (smaller) and white (larger) cells on wet chamber.

guishing mononuclear cells from polynuclear cells (Fig. 9.2).

VI. The number of WBCs counted on *Side A* and *Side B* should be within 10 percent of each other. If they are not within 10 percent, discard the raw RBC and WBC counts and repeat steps I through IV.

VII. Calculate the total number of RBCs, WBCs, mononuclear cells, and polynuclear cells present in the sample as described in the next section.

Calculation of the Total Number of Cells

The International Committee for Standardization in Hematology and other international scientific committees have recommended that all units of volume be reported in liters. The conversion factor for cubic millimeters (mm^3) to microliters (μl) is $1 \; mm^3 = 1.00003 \; \mu l$. However, it is more practical to consider that $1 \; mm^3 = 1 \; \mu l = 1 \times 10^{-6} \; L$. Acceptance and reporting using this recommendation still vary from laboratory to laboratory. For ease in the understanding of how to perform calculations of total cell counts, examples in this book will use mm^3 throughout the problem, with conversion to μl in the final step of the problem.

Calculation of the total number of cells per mm^3 is accomplished by using the following formulae:

$$\frac{\text{Number of cells}}{mm^3} = \text{Number of cells counted} \times \\ \text{dilution correction} \times \\ \text{volume correction}$$

$$[\text{Equation 1}]$$

$$\text{Area} = \text{length} \times \text{width}$$

$$\text{Volume} = \text{depth} \times \text{area}$$

It is important to note that the final value is the number of cells per $1 \; mm^3$. To standardize to $1 \; mm^3$, one must use correction factors for the dilution and volume of fluid from which the raw cell count was actually obtained. These correction factors are the reciprocal of the dilution and of the volume. Therefore, Equation 1 could actually be rewritten as:

$$\frac{\text{Number of cells}}{mm^3} = \text{Number of cells counted} \times \\ \frac{1}{\text{dilution}} \times \frac{1}{\text{volume}}$$

$$[\text{Equation 2}]$$

Example 1. A Neubauer hemocytometer was loaded and counted. All nine 1 mm by 1 mm squares were counted on both *Side A* and *Side B*. On *Side A* 43 RBCs and 24 WBC were counted. On *Side B* 10 mononuclear and 15 polynuclear cells were counted.

$$\text{Dilution correction} = \frac{1}{\text{dilution}}$$

Since the specimen was undiluted, dilution was 1:1. Therefore, the dilution = 1, and dilution correction = 1/1 = 1.

$$\text{Volume correction} = \frac{1}{\text{volume}}$$

$$\text{Volume} = \text{depth} \times \text{area, or}$$

$$\text{Volume} = \text{depth} \times \text{length} \times \text{width}$$

$$\text{Volume} = 0.1 \text{ mm} \times 3 \text{ mm} \times 3 \text{ mm}$$

$$\text{Volume} = 0.9 \text{ mm}^3$$

Volume correction = 1/volume = 1/0.9 mm³

Substituting in Equation 2:

$$\frac{\text{Number of cells}}{\text{mm}^3} = \text{Number of cells counted} \times \frac{1}{\text{dilution}} \times \frac{1}{\text{volume}}$$

$$\frac{\text{Total RBC}}{\text{mm}^3} = 43 \text{ RBC} \times 1 \times \frac{1}{0.9 \text{ mm}^3}$$

$$\frac{\text{Total RBC}}{\text{mm}^3} = \frac{47.7 \text{ RBC}}{\text{mm}^3} = \frac{47.7 \text{ RBC}}{\mu l}$$

Note: Raw WBC counted is obtained by averaging total WBC on *Side A* and *Side B*.

$$\frac{\text{Total WBC}}{\text{mm}^3} = 25 \times 1 \times \frac{1}{0.9 \text{ mm}^3}$$

$$\frac{\text{Total WBC}}{\text{mm}^3} = \frac{27.7 \text{ WBC}}{\text{mm}^3} = \frac{27.7 \text{ WBC}}{\mu l}$$

The number of polynuclear and mononuclear cells is reported as the percentage of the WBC counted. Therefore, using raw counts from *Side B*:

$$\% \text{ mononuclear cells} = \frac{\text{number of mononuclear cells on } \textit{Side B}}{\text{number of WBC on } \textit{Side B}} \times 100$$

$$\% \text{ mononuclear cells} = \frac{10}{25} \times 100$$

$$\% \text{ mononuclear cells} = 40$$

$$\% \text{ polynuclear cells} = \frac{\text{number of polynuclear cells on } \textit{Side B}}{\text{number of WBC on } \textit{Side B}} \times 100$$

$$\% \text{ polynuclear cells} = \frac{15}{25} \times 100$$

$$\% \text{ polynuclear cells} = 60$$

Example 2. A technologist loaded both counting chambers of a Fuchs-Rosenthal hemocytometer with undiluted CSF fluid. On one side she counted 150 RBCs and 40 WBCs, and on the other side she counted 161 RBCs and 36 WBCs.

$$\frac{\text{Total RBC}}{\text{mm}^3} = \text{number of RBCs counted} \times \frac{1}{\text{dilution}} \times \frac{1}{\text{volume}}$$

$$\text{Dilution correction} = \frac{1}{\text{dilution}} = 1$$

$$\text{Volume correction} = \frac{1}{\text{volume}}$$

$$\text{Area of one counting chamber} = \text{length} \times \text{width}$$

$$\text{Area of one counting chamber} = 4 \text{ mm} \times 4 \text{ mm}$$

$$\text{Area of one counting chamber} = 16 \text{ mm}^2$$

However, since the technologist counted both counting chambers:

$$\text{Area of both chambers} = 2 \times 16 \text{ mm}^2 = 32 \text{ mm}^2$$

$$\text{Volume correction} = \frac{1}{0.2 \text{ mm} \times 32 \text{ mm}^2}$$

$$\frac{\text{Total RBC}}{\text{mm}^3} = (150+161) \text{ RBC} \times 1 \times \frac{1}{6.4 \text{ mm}^3}$$

$$\frac{\text{Total RBC}}{\text{mm}^3} = \frac{48.6 \text{ RBC}}{\text{mm}^3} = \frac{48.6 \text{ RBC}}{\mu l}$$

$$\frac{\text{Total WBC}}{\text{mm}^3} = (40 + 36) \times 1 \times \frac{1}{6.4 \text{ mm}^3}$$

$$\frac{\text{Total WBC}}{\text{mm}^3} = \frac{11.9 \text{ WBC}}{\text{mm}^3} = \frac{11.9 \text{ WBC}}{\mu l}$$

Example 3. A technologist loaded all four chambers of a Spears-Levy hemocytometer with undiluted fluid. Upon examination, she realized that the RBCs were too numerous to count and obscured the WBCs. She made a dilution of 1:8 of a portion of the fluid and reloaded two of the counting chambers (chambers 1 and 2). She then took some undiluted sample and lysed the RBCs using a glacial acetic acid coated 44.7γ pipette. She used this pipette to load the other two counting chambers (chambers 3 and 4) of the hemocytometer.

Recording of the raw counts follows:

- Chamber 1: 156 RBCs, 2 WBCs
- Chamber 2: 162 RBCs, 1 WBC
- Chamber 3: 6 mononuclear, 6 polynuclear
- Chamber 4: 8 mononuclear, 5 polynuclear

Dilution for chambers 1 and 2 was 1:8 or 1/8.

$$\text{Dilution correction for chambers 1 and 2} = \frac{1}{\text{dilution}}$$

$$\text{Dilution correction for chambers 1 and 2} = \frac{1}{1/8} = 8$$

Dilution for chambers 3 and 4 was 1:1 or 1.

$$\text{Dilution correction for chambers 3 and 4} = \frac{1}{1} = 1$$

$$\text{Volume correction for each chamber} = \frac{1}{\text{volume of chamber}}$$

$$\text{Volume} = \text{depth} \times \text{length} \times \text{width}$$

$$\text{Volume} = 0.2 \text{ mm} \times 5 \text{ mm} \times 2 \text{ mm}$$

$$\text{Volume} = 2 \text{ mm}^3$$

(Volume of chamber 1 + volume of chamber 2) = $2 \text{ mm}^3 + 2 \text{ mm}^3 = 4 \text{ mm}^3$

$$\text{Volume correction for chambers 1 and 2} = \frac{1}{4 \text{ mm}^3}$$

$$\text{Volume correction for chambers 3 and 4} = \frac{1}{4 \text{ mm}^3}$$

Total RBC = RBC counted in chambers 1 and 2 × dilution correction for chambers 1 and 2 × volume correction for chambers 1 and 2

$$\text{Total RBC} = (156 + 162) \times 8 \times \frac{1}{4 \text{ mm}^3}$$

$$\text{Total RBC} = \frac{636 \text{ RBC}}{\text{mm}^3} = \frac{636 \text{ RBC}}{\mu l}$$

Total WBC = WBC counted in chambers 3 and 4 × dilution correction for chambers 3 and 4 × volume correction for chambers 3 and 4

$$\text{Total WBC} = (12 + 13) \times 1 \times \frac{1}{4 \text{ mm}^3}$$

$$\text{Total WBC} = \frac{6.25 \text{ WBC}}{\text{mm}^3} = \frac{6.25 \text{ WBC}}{\mu l}$$

$$\% \text{ mononuclear WBC} = \frac{\text{number of mononuclear cells in chambers 3 and 4}}{\text{total WBC in chambers 3 and 4}} \times 100$$

$$\% \text{ mononuclear WBC} = \frac{(6 + 8)}{(12 + 13)} \times 100 = 56$$

$$\% \text{ polynuclear WBC} = \frac{\text{number of polynuclear cells in chambers 3 and 4}}{\text{total WBC in chambers 3 and 4}} \times 100$$

$$\% \text{ polynuclear WBC} = \frac{(6 + 5)}{(12 + 13)} \times 100 = 44$$

AUTOMATED METHODS

The practice of using automated whole blood cell counters, such as electronic particle counters and electronic optical counters, is not widely accepted. Advantages include decreased technical time and reduced technical error. Disadvantages result from the fact that these machines are not standardized for the counting of cells suspended in the various body fluids. Several of the problems include the consistency of the body fluids (e.g., increased viscosity of joint fluid), cell size variation (e.g., tumor cells may be two to three times as large as normal WBC), and background debris present in body fluids that may falsely elevate values. For these reasons, it is recommended that body fluid cell counts be performed by manual methods.

MICROSCOPIC EXAMINATION

Direct Chamber Analysis of Mononuclear and Polynuclear Cells

Direct chamber differentiation of mononuclear and polynuclear cells can be performed during the hemocytometer count if glacial acetic acid is used (page 219). Acidified crystal violet may be substituted for the glacial acetic acid. Limitations of this method include the inability to distinguish the exact cell type present (i.e., can only distinguish if the cell is mononuclear or polynuclear, not whether it is a polymorphonuclear leukocyte, lymphocyte, monocyte, eosinophil, and so on). Because of the small sample size, if only a few WBCs are seen in the chamber count, the percentage of cell types present may not accurately reflect the percentage of cell types present in the total volume of fluid.

Concentration Techniques

Various concentration techniques have been described in an attempt to increase the accuracy of the differential count and to facilitate identification of various cell types. Conventional centrifugation or simple sedimentation have both proved unsatisfactory. The most useful techniques described include: (1) the sedimentation technique of Sayk, (2) membrane filter techniques, and (3) cytocentrifugation.

Sedimentation. The sedimentation technique of Sayk utilizes glass or plastic 10 to 14 mm cylinders in which the fluid is placed. The cellular components settle by gravitational forces while the fluid is being removed by the surrounding filter paper. Advantages include excellent preservation of cellular morphology, since the cells remain in a physiologic solution while they are settling onto the slide. Disadvantages include 30 to 80 percent loss of cells onto the filter paper, preparation time of approximately two hours, and difficulty in obtaining equipment resulting in laboratories designing their own sedimentation chambers (Fig. 9.4).

Membrane Filter. Membrane filter techniques utilize suction or pressure to force a volume of fluid through a small-pore filter. The filter is then fixed, stained, and examined. Advantages include good recovery of cells and availability of the cell-free specimen for additional biochemical tests. Disadvantages include some degree of loss of the fine cellular detail and increased technical time and expertise required. (See Fig. 9.5.)

Cytocentrifugation. The cytocentrifugation technique is essentially a slow centrifuge developed by Shandon Scientific Corporation.* The fluid is placed in a specimen cup and is slowly centrifuged between 200 and 1,000 rpm for from 5 to 10 minutes. During this centrifugation, the fluid portion of the specimen is absorbed into filter paper while the cellular portion is concentrated onto a microscopic slide. The cellular portion can then be stained with various cytologic and hematologic stains. A new cytospin machine is now available that incorporates a stainless steel clip as a mechanical advantage. This improvement ensures that optimum pressure is applied to aid in the absorption of fluid and thus decreases the possibility of cell loss. The new machine has a sealed head that can be loaded and unloaded in the safety of a microbiologic cabinet. This assures protection from biohazardous material. Additional safety standards are built in to comply with international safety legislation.

*Shandon Scientific Corporation, 515 Broad Street, Sewickley, Pennsylvania 15143.

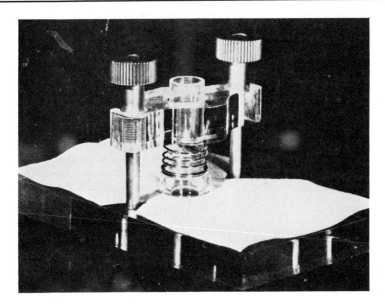

Figure 9.4. Sayk's sedimentation chamber. (From Koelmel HW: Atlas of Cerebrospinal Fluid Cells (2nd ed). New York, Springer Verlag, 1977, p. 4.)

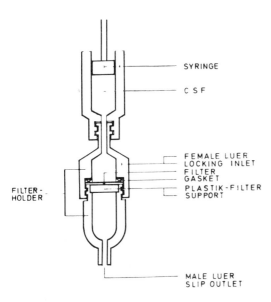

Figure 9.5. Diagram of filter holder. (From Oechmichen M: Cerebrospinal Fluid Cytology: An Introduction and Atlas. Philadelphia, Saunders, 1976, p 5.)

Advantages of the cytocentrifuge method include rapid and easy preparation, good cellular detail, small amounts of sample required, and good recovery of cells. Since the centrifuge head of the Shandon cytospin allows for the preparation of 12 slides simultaneously, the cytospin slides can then be stained by a number of different methods. The major disadvantage of the cytospin is the initial cost of the equipment. (See Fig. 9.6.)

Staining

After microscopic slides have been prepared by the various concentration techniques, a variety of hematologic and cytologic staining procedures may be performed. The Wright, May-Grunwald Giemsa, gram, AFB, Sudan red, and Prussian blue stains can be done with relative ease in most clinical laboratories. The Papanicolaou stain and mucin stain are routine stains used in most cytology laboratories. Most of the stains are available in commercial kits from various manufacturers. Good results have been obtained also using automated staining techniques.

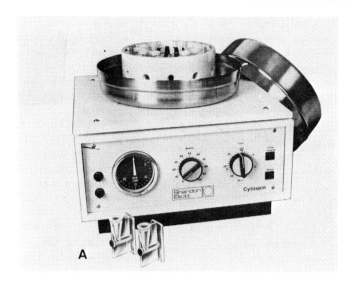

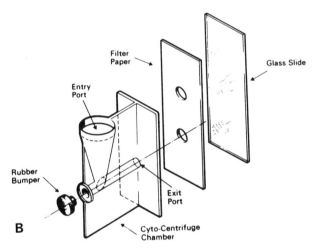

Figure 9.6. A. Cytospin centrifuge. **B.** Cytospin technique. (Courtesy of Shandon Southern Instruments, Inc., Publication No. CYTI, December, 1976.)

Wright's Stain

(Method from Medical College of Georgia, Section of Hematology/Oncology)

Reagents

1. Wright's blood stain crystaline compound, certified by Biological

Stain Commission   9 g

Glycerin, certified, ACS grade   90 ml

Absolute methanol, acetone-free, anhydrous, AR grade   2,910 ml

(a) Mix the glycerin and methanol in a large brown bottle. Add stain powder. Continue mixing powder-glycerin-methanol mixture intermittently for remainder of the day. Stopper bottle tightly overnight. On the next day, loosen the stopper to release any pressure, tighten stopper again, and mix intermittently throughout the day. Repeat this mixing daily through the next 5 to 7 days. Let the stain solution age for another week (or longer) at room temperature.

(b) For daily use, filter a small volume through a number 1 Whatman paper into a dropper bottle.

2. Buffer, pH 6.7

(a) Stock solution

Potassium phosphate, monobasic anhydrous (KH_2PO_4), AR or certified ACS grade   5.13 g

Sodium phosphate, secondary, anhydrous (Na_2HPO_4), AR or certified ACS grade   4.12 g

Distilled water to make 1 L

Check pH with pH paper.

(b) Working buffer

To one volume of the stock buffer, add one volume of distilled water. Mix. Filter through number 40 Whatman paper into a plastic bottle (a wash bottle) or a dropper bottle. Check pH with pH paper.

3. Methanol, absolute (in a dropper bottle), acetone-free, reagent grade.

Technique

1. Place the slides on a support rack so slides are not touching any other slide or object.

2. Cover smear with absolute methanol, then immediately drain off alcohol. This is the primary fixation of blood film.

3. Cover smear and remainder of slide with Wright stain for 1.5 to 2 minutes. Fixation continues with the undiluted stain.

4. Add to the stain an equal volume of working buffer and mix by blowing on the buffered stain until a metallic film begins to appear. Let stain stand for 3.5 to 4 minutes. This is the actual staining period. Mixing is also accomplished by adding the buffer forcefully to the stain in a zigzag fashion from the wash bottle.

5. Wash stain with tap water by flushing stain solution off slide. Immediately place slide in a near vertical position to prevent any wash water remaining on film.

6. Clean back of slide. Allow film to air dry in near vertical position. Label.

Staining Characteristics

- Nuclei: blue
- Cytoplasm: pink to light red
- Bacteria: blue

May-Grunwald Giemsa Stain

(Method from Medical College of Georgia Section of Hematology/Oncology)

Reagents

1. May-Grunwald reagent
May-Grunwald stain (eosin-methylene blue)   2.0 g
Methanol, absolute, acetone-free   500 ml
Mix dye in methanol well and allow to stand two to three days before use. Filter through number 1 Whatman paper before use.

2. Concentrated Giemsa reagent
Giemsa stain (azure-eosin methylene blue)   3.8 g
Glycerin, reagent grade   250 ml
Methanol, absolute, acetone-free   250 ml
Add the Giemsa stain to the glycerin. Mix. Incubate at 55 to 60C (in oven or

elsewhere) for 1.5 to 2 hours. Allow to cool. Mix. With constant stirring, slowly add the 250 ml alcohol. Filter into a reagent bottle. Label Giemsa stock solution. Store in dark.

3. Buffer phosphate
    (a) Stock solutions
        (1) 1/15 molar monopotassium phosphate (9.08 g KH_2PO_4/L) = Buffer A
        (2) 1/15 molar disodium phosphate (11.88 g Na_2HPO_4/L) = Buffer B
    (b) Working buffer, pH 7
        (1) 39.2 ml of stock buffer (A)
        (2) 60.8 ml of stock buffer (B)
        Mix well. Test with pH paper. Filter through number 40 Whatman paper.
4. Giemsa working solution
    Ratio of stain to buffer is 1:4. For two or three cover glasses, 0.5 ml of stain plus 2 ml of buffer is adequate. Mix just before using.

Technique

1. Allow smear to air dry.
2. Place slide on support rack.
3. Flood smear with absolute methanol for 5 minutes for fixing of film.
4. Drain all alcohol off the smear by tilting and touching edge to absorbent material.
5. Add approximately 12 drops of May-Grunwald stain to film for 3 minutes.
6. To the stain, add 9 drops of pH 7 buffer and mix by blowing on stain until a metallic scum/sheen appears. Stain for 3.5 minutes.
7. Wash off stain by adding tap water to one corner of microscopic slide so as to float off metallic scum and then flush off rest of stain with sufficient water. Drain off excess wash water by touching slide to absorbent material.
8. Cover film with diluted Giemsa stain (made just before use) for 5 minutes.

Blow gently on stain to mix residual water on smear with the stain.
9. Wash stain off slide as in Step 7. Clean off back of slide with wet gauze. Air dry smear in vertical position.
10. Label.

Staining Characteristics

- Nuclei: blue
- Cytoplasm: pink to light red
- Bacteria: blue

Gram Stain
(Hucker Modification)

Reagents

1. Solution A: Stock crystal violet solution
    Crystal violet (85 % dye)   20 g
    95 % Ethanol   100 ml
2. Solution B: Stock oxalate solution
    Ammonium oxalate   1 g
    Distilled water   100 ml
3. Working solution
    Mix Solution A 1:10 with distilled water and mix with 4 volumes of Solution B. Store in glass-stoppered bottle.
4. Solution C: Gram iodine solution
    Iodine crystals   1 g
    Potassium iodide   2 g
    Dissolve these in 5 ml of distilled water, then add:
    Distilled water   240 ml
    Sodium bicarbonate,
        5 % aqueous solution   60 ml
    Mix well, store in amber bottle.
5. Solution D: Decolorizer
    95 % Ethanol   250 ml
    Acetone   250 ml
6. Solution E: Safranin counterstain solution
    Safranin O   2.5 g
    95 % Ethanol   100 ml
    Working solution
        Dilute Solution E 1:5 or 1:10 with distilled water, store in glass-stoppered bottle.

Technique

1. Allow specimen to be stained to dry on the slide.
2. Heatfix the material.
3. Cover with crystal violet (gentian violet) for approximately 1 minute.
4. Wash with water.
5. Cover with gram iodine for approximately 1 minute.
6. Wash with water.
7. Decolorize for approximately 10 to 15 seconds with acetone-alcohol.
8. Wash with water.
9. Cover for 10 to 20 seconds with safranin.
10. Wash with water and let dry.

Alternate: In the quick method, the reagents are added in the above sequence but only for 5 to 10 seconds each.

Staining Characteristics

- Gram-positive bacteria: dark blue or violet
- Gram-negative bacteria: red or reddish pink
- WBC: light pink

Prussian Blue Stain
(Method from Medical College of Georgia, Section of Hematology/Oncology)

Reagents

1. Absolute methyl alcohol, acetone-free, reagent grade
2. Potassium ferrocyanide solution, 2% Dissolve 2 g of potassium ferrocyanide in 100 ml of distilled water. Store in a brown bottle. If solution has a color other than a faint tint of yellow-green, discard. Keep only 1 month.
3. Hydrochloric acid solution, 2% Take 2 ml of the stock concentrated HCl and make up to 100 ml volume with distilled water.
4. Neutral red stain, counterstain dye.
   (a) Stock solution, 1 g% (1 g stain dissolved in 100 ml of distilled water.)

(b) Working solution (0.7 ml of stock solution diluted to 10 ml with distilled water. Filter before use.)
5. Staining solution
   Mix just before use.
   - 1 part of 2% potassium ferrocyanide
   - 1 part of 2% hydrochloric acid

Note: All glassware is to be especially cleaned for use in Fe stain procedure.

Technique

1. Allow specimen to air dry on microscopic slide. Include a bone marrow smear known to contain iron for a positive control.
2. Fix control and specimen in absolute methyl alcohol for 10 minutes.
3. Wash smears with distilled or deionized water.
4. Add freshly prepared staining solution to the washed smears for at least 30 minutes.
5. Wash smears with distilled water.
6. Add filtered working counterstain solution to the smears for 1 minute. Rinse with tap water. Air dry.
7. Use Permount coverslip microscope slide preparations.

Staining Characteristics

- Iron: bright blue
- Nuclei: red
- Cytoplasm: light red

Acid-fast Bacteria Stain
(Kinyoun)

Reagents

1. Carbolfuchsin

Basic fuchsin	4 g
Phenol	8 ml
95 % Ethanol	20 ml
Distilled water	100 ml

Dissolve basic fuchsin in 95 % ethanol and add to 8 % aqueous solution of phenol.

2. Acid-Alcohol
   HCl   3 ml
   95 % Ethanol   97 ml
3. Methylene Blue Counterstain
   Methylene blue chloride   0.3 mg
   Distilled water   100 ml

Technique

1. Allow specimen to air dry.
2. Heatfix by quickly passing slide through flame *once*.
3. Stain with Kinyoun's carbolfuchsin for 5 minutes.
   Note: This stain does not require heat.
4. Wash with water.
5. Decolorize with acid-alcohol until red stain stops running.
6. Wash with water.
7. Stain with methylene blue for 1 minute.
8. Air dry.
9. AFB slides to be saved should be sealed with a Permount thin coverslip after oil is removed.

Staining Characteristics

- Acid-fast bacteria: bright red
- Background: light blue

Sudan III

(Method from Medical College of Georgia, Section of Microbiology/Clinical Pathology)

Reagents

1. Sudan III   0.5 g
2. 95 % Ethanol   112.5 ml

Mix Sudan III and 95 % ethanol in a 250 ml Florence flask. Boil gently for 30 minutes. Filter while hot, place in refrigerator, filter while cold. Measure volume and add distilled water to 90 ml. Allow to stand stoppered for 24 hours before using.

Technique

1. Add one drop of stain to one drop of body fluid.

2. Observe under microscope for reddish orange globules.

Staining Characteristics

- Lipids: reddish orange

Microscopy

Light microscopy, phase contrast microscopy, polarized light microscopy, and electron microscopy may all be used to view the various elements in body fluid specimens. Phase contrast microscopy may be useful in viewing living cells, while electron microscopy is used to study the ultrastructure of cells. Both phase contact microscopy and electron microscopy are utilized more as research tools than in the routine clinical laboratory. Polarized light microscopy is utilized in the examination of synovial fluids and is discussed in Chapter 11.

Light microscopy is the usual method of examination of the stained microscopic preparations of the body fluids (Fig. 9.7). Magnification with the compound light microscope is achieved with a series of lens systems. The objective magnifies the specimen initially, and the ocular magnifies the image again as the light travels through the microscope. The total magnification is equal to the product of the ocular magnification and the objective magnification.

$$\text{Final magnification} = \text{ocular magnification} \times \text{objective magnification}$$

The objective magnification is engraved on the side of the objective, and the ocular magnification is marked on either the top or the side of the ocular.

The useful limit of magnification is set by the ability of the optical system of a microscope to distinguish two neighboring points as separate entities. This ability is known as the resolving power or the resolution. Resolving power of the microscope depends on the objective and the wavelength of light according to the formula:

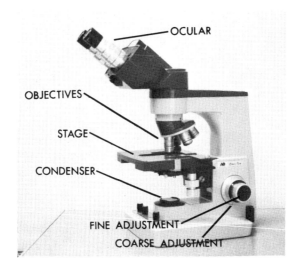

Figure 9.7. Microscope.

$$h = \frac{0.16\lambda}{NA}$$

where h = minimum resolvable distance
    λ = wavelength of light
    NA = numerical aperture

$$NA = N \sin \mu$$

where N = refractive index
    μ = half the angle of the cone of light
       entering that objective

The numerical aperture is given for each of the objectives in Table 9.2.

With the use of the oil objective greater magnification is achieved, since the NA is at its largest value. The refractive index of oil is 1.5, approximately that of optical glass, and this prevents many of the light rays from being refracted, thus increasing the number of light rays that pass through the objective.

Differential Count

The differential count is composed of the percentage of cell types present in the fluid, not including the RBCs. A total of 100 cells are counted. The various types of cells that may be present in the different body fluids are discussed in Chapters 14 and 15. The dif-

ferential count is an important part of the final report.

THE FINAL REPORT

The final report of a fluid specimen should always include the following components:

1. Patient's name and hospital number
2. The time specimen was collected and the time it was received in the laboratory
3. Source of fluid
4. Color and appearance of the fluid
5. Total number of RBC/μl
6. Total number of WBC/μl
7. Differential count of the cellular components (not including normal RBCs)

TABLE 9.2. NUMERICAL APERTURES

Objective	NA
4 ×	.09
10 ×	.25
40 ×	.65
100 ×	1.25

The differential count should include the percentages of the cell types present in the fluid. It is the technologist's task to make observations as to the cell types present and then to report them accurately. The technologist must carefully observe cells for the characteristics described in Chapters 14 and 15. Cells displaying one or more abnormal characteristics should be described in detail and separately from other cells in the same preparation. They should be counted and occupy a unique position in the differential. Preparations containing atypical cells or abnormal cells should always be brought to the pathologist's attention.

It is the pathologist's task to interpret the reported observations because interpretations should be based on careful clinicopathologic correlations that require access to and understanding of all information regarding a case. In view of the potential of its psychologic and social impact, a diagnosis of cancer or malignancy should never be rendered without careful interpretation of all available laboratory diagnostic tools.

Review Questions

Select one best answer.

1. The ability of the optical system of a microscope to distinguish two neighboring points as separate entities is known as the:
   A. Maximal resolvable distance
   B. Numerical aperture
   C. Refractive index
   D. Resolving power
   E. Final magnification

For each of the following problems perform the calculations indicated.

2. A Neubauer hemocytometer was loaded with undiluted CSF and all nine larger squares (1 mm × 1 mm) were counted. On *Side A*, 55 RBCs and 30 WBCs were counted. On *Side B*, 10 mononuclear and 20 polynuclear cells were counted. Calculate total number of WBCs and RBCs. Calculate the percentage of mononuclear and polynuclear cells.

3. A technologist loaded both counting chambers of a Fuchs-Rosenthal hemocytometer with undiluted CSF fluid. On one side, she counted 175 RBCs and 220 WBCs. On the other side, she counted 100 mononuclear cells and 125 polynuclear cells. Calculate the total number of WBCs and RBCs. Calculate the percentage of mononuclear and polynuclear cells.

4. A technologist loaded all four chambers of a Spears-Levy hemocytometer with undiluted fluid. Upon examination, she realized that the RBCs were too numerous to count and obscured the WBCs. She made a dilution of 1:4 of a portion of the fluid and reloaded two of the counting chambers (chambers 1 and 2). She then took some undiluted sample and lysed the RBCs using a glacial acetic acid-coated 44.7λ pipette. She used this pipette to load the other two counting chambers (chambers 3 and 4).

   The recording of her raw counts follows:

   - Chamber 1: 500 RBCs, 4 WBCs
   - Chamber 2: 505 RBCs, 6 WBCs
   - Chamber 3: 15 mononuclear, 4 polynuclear
   - Chamber 4: 14 mononuclear, 6 polynuclear

   Calculate the total number of WBCs and RBCs. Calculate the percentage of mononuclear and polynuclear cells.

For each of the incomplete statements, one or more of the completions given is correct. Select:
   A. If only *1, 2, and 3* are correct.
   B. If only *1 and 3* are correct.
   C. If only *2 and 4* are correct.
   D. If only *4* is correct.
   E. If *all* are correct.

5. Advantages of the manual method for performing cell counts on body fluids include:

1. Technical variation
2. Easy screening for atypical cell sizes
3. The small quantity of sample examined
4. Low cost of equipment

6. Important techniques in regard to fluid examination include:
   1. Performing the examination as soon as possible
   2. Immediate dilution of the sample
   3. Adequate mixture of the sample
   4. Addition of a fixative as soon as fluid is removed from the body cavity

7. The sedimentation technique of Sayk utilizes:
   1. Suction to force fluid through a filter
   2. Glass tube surrounded by filter paper
   3. Slow centrifugation to absorb fluid into filter paper
   4. Gravitational forces to accomplish the formation of a cell concentrate

8. Advantages of cytocentrifugation include:
   1. Rapid and easy preparation
   2. Good cell detail obtained
   3. Good recovery of cell
   4. Availability of the cell-free supernatant for additional biochemical tests

9. Final magnifigation of the light microscope is equal to the product of the:
   1. Numerical aperture
   2. Ocular magnification
   3. Refractive index
   4. Objective magnification

10. Greater magnification is achieved using the oil objective since:
    1. The numerical aperture is at its largest value
    2. Increased numbers of light rays pass through the objective
    3. The refractive index of oil approaches that of optical glass
    4. Light rays are refracted with the use of the oil

11. The final report of a fluid specimen should include:
    1. The time the specimen was collected
    2. Source of the fluid
    3. Differential of the cellular components
    4. Notation of atypical cells when present

Match the labeled cells in the figures below with the correct name in questions 12 through 15.

_____ 12. RBC
_____ 13. WBC
_____ 14. Polynuclear cell
_____ 15. Mononuclear cell

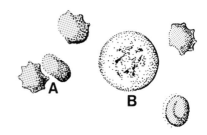

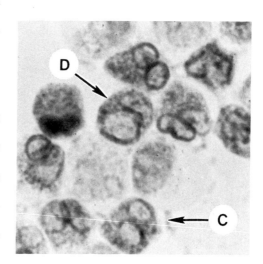

Match the best answer in Column B with the appropriate phrase in Column A. Answers from Column B may be used more than once.

Column A

_____ 16. Wright-stained nuclei
_____ 17. May-Grunwald Giemsa-stained cytoplasm
_____ 18. Sudan red
_____ 19. Gram-positive bacteria
_____ 20. Acid-fast bacteria stain
_____ 21. Prussian blue

Column B

A. Blue
B. Red to light pink
C. Stains iron
D. Stains lipid

Case Study

A 32-year-old female came to the emergency room complaining of headache, earache, and fever. The patient's temperature was recorded at 104F, and nuchal rigidity was noted on physical examination. A spinal tap was performed. Thirty minutes later the preliminary laboratory report was called to the emergency room clerk. It was as follows:

Characteristic	Findings	
Name: B.E. Quick	Hospital No.: 972-861	
Time collected:	7:25 PM	
Time received:	7:30 PM	
Source of fluid:	cerebrospinal fluid	
Color:	colorless	
Appearance:	hazy	
RBC/μl:	12	
WBC/μl:	6,727	
Differential		
Polymorphonuclear leukocytes:		86 %
Lymphocytes:		4 %
Monocytes:		4 %
Macrophages:		5 %
Mesothelial cells:		0
Eosinophils:		1 %

| Basophils: | | 0 |
| Other: | | 0 |

Comments: Intracellular bacteria seen in several of the polymorphonuclear leukocytes.

CSF glucose:	27 mg/dl
Serum glucose:	100 mg/dl
CSF protein:	95 mg/dl

Gram stain: gram-positive diplococci present. Numerous polymorphonuclear leukocytes present. Culture and antibiotic sensitivity performed as requested.

AFB stain: to follow
India ink preparation: to follow
The patient was admitted to the hospital and begun on IV penicillin G therapy.

Question

Abnormal findings in the CSF report include all of the following except:

1. The color
2. The RBC total count
3. The CSF glucose
4. The CSF protein
5. The percentage of macrophages

Answer: 1

Results

The cultures of the CSF were later positive for *Streptococcus pneumoniae* that was sensitive to penicillin. The patient was discharged in good health ten days after admission.

This case illustrates the valuable information that can be obtained from the examination of the various body fluids, such as cerebrospinal fluid.

BIBLIOGRAPHY

Cartwright GE: Diagnostic Laboratory Hematology. New York, Grune & Stratton, 1968.

Finegold SM, Martin WJ, Scott EG: Bailey and Scott's Diagnostic Microbiology. St. Louis, Mosby, 1978.

Henry JB: Clinical Diagnosis and Management by Laboratory Methods, 16th ed. Philadelphia, Saunders, 1979.

Kolmel HW: Atlas of Cerebrospinal Fluid Cells. New York, Springer-Verlag, 1977.

Luna LG: Manual of Histologic Staining Methods of the Armed Forces Institute of Pathology. New York, McGraw-Hill, 1968.

Miale JB: Laboratory Medicine Hematology. St. Louis, Mosby, 1977.

Oehmichen M: Cerebrospinal Fluid Cytology. Philadelphia, Saunders, 1976.

Raphael SS: Lynch's Medical Laboratory Technology. Philadelphia, Saunders, 1976.

Seivard DE: Hematology for Medical Technologist. Philadelphia, Lea & Febiger, 1972.

Spriggs AE, Boddington MM: The Cytology of Effusions and of Cerebrospinal Fluid. London, Heinemann, 1976.

Student's Manual for the Compound Microscope. Rochester, N.Y., Bausch & Lomb, 1975, pp. 33-133.

Williams JW, Beutler E, Erslev AJ, Rundles RW: Hematology. New York, Mc-Graw-Hill, 1977.

Wintrobe MM, Boggs DR, Bithell TC, Athens JW, Foerster J: Clinical Hematology. Philadelphia, Lea & Febiger, 1974.

Ann E. Neely and Kathryn Kilpatrick Cheek

	CHAPTER 10

Cerebrospinal Fluid

Objectives

It is expected that the information presented in this chapter will enable the reader to:

1. Describe the membranous coverings of the brain.
2. Define cerebrospinal fluid, including where it is formed, where it circulates, and where it is reabsorbed.
3. List pathologic states that may cause changes within the cerebrospinal fluid.
4. Describe how cerebrospinal fluid is obtained for laboratory examination.
5. Differentiate between a traumatic and a true hemorrhagic spinal tap.
6. Determine if a cerebrospinal fluid contains increased numbers of white blood cells.
7. Describe the morphologic characteristics, significance and function of ependymal, choroidal, and pia-arachnoid mesothelial cells.
8. List disease states in which various hematologic and nonhematologic cell types may be present.
9. Define melanin, hemosiderin, and hematoidin.
10. Describe the morphologic appearance on Wright-stained preparations of melanin, hemosiderin, and hematoidin and the clinical significance of each.
11. Identify elements that may be present in the cerebrospinal fluid of a patient who has had a recent or old cerebral hemorrhage.
12. Describe the blood-brain barrier.
13. List considerations in determination of cerebrospinal fluid protein level.
14. Identify conditions in which elevated or depressed cerebrospinal fluid total protein values may be found.
15. Utilize the CSF albumin : Plasma albumin ratio to evaluate the integrity of the blood-brain barrier.

16. Utilize the CSF IgG/Plasma IgG ÷ CSF albumin/Plasma albumin ratio to evaluate the integrity of the blood-brain barrier.
17. Identify the cerebrospinal fluid protein electrophoretic patterns that may be present in various disease states.
18. Describe the derivation and importance of cerebrospinal fluid glucose levels.
19. Identify the clinical usefulness of lactate dehydrogenase determination.
20. Describe appropriate techniques for the microbiologic examination of the cerebrospinal fluid.
21. Identify the clinical usefulness and theoretical basis of detection of antigenic microbial substances, gram-negative endotoxin, and microbial antibody.
22. Correlate alterations of cellular content, chemical composition, and microbiologic findings to possible etiologic agents of central nervous system disease.
23. Identify the predominant causative agents of meningitis in various populations of patients.
24. Identify specific laboratory techniques that help make preliminary and definitive diagnosis of aerobic meningitis, anaerobic meningitis, tuberculous meningitis, viral meningitis, fungal meningitis, amebic meningoencephalitis, and CNS infection with spirochetes.

FORMATION AND FUNCTION OF CEREBROSPINAL FLUID

The brain and spinal cord are covered by membranous coverings called the meninges. The meninges are composed of three parts: the pia, the arachnoid, and the dura. The pia is the innermost layer and is intimately attached to the brain and spinal cord. The dura is the tough outermost membranous covering, and the arachnoid lies between the pia and the dura (Fig. 10.1).

Cerebrospinal fluid (CSF) is a modified ultrafiltrate of the blood. It is a clear colorless liquid that is formed in the ventricles of the brain by secretion from the choroid plexus. It is contained within the cerebral ventricles, the neural canal of the spinal cord, and between the pia and arachnoid. This fluid circulates through the ventricles into the spaces between the pia and arachnoid surrounding the brain and spinal cord. It is reabsorbed into the arachnoid granulation of the dural ventricular sinuses and other specialized areas of the dura. Bathing the brain and spinal cord in fluid, the CSF provides a site of metabolic exchange and a site to absorb pressure changes that occur within the central nervous system (CNS) (Fig. 10.1).

ALTERATIONS IN THE CEREBROSPINAL FLUID

Alterations that occur within the CNS may be reflected by changes in the cellular, chemical, and molecular composition of the CSF. Pathologic states that may cause changes in the CSF include meningitis, encephalitis, intracranial abscesses, malignancies, tumors, leukemia, hemorrhage, syphilis, demyelinating diseases, and many other systemic diseases. Specific changes that occur in these various disease states are discussed in the following sections.

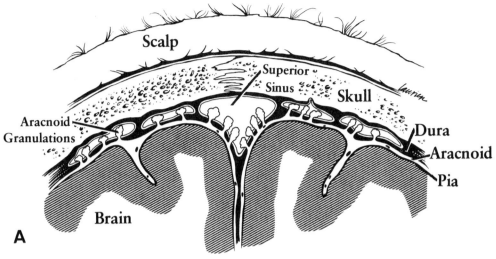

Figure 10.1. **A.** Brain. **B.** Spinal column.

OBTAINING THE CEREBROSPINAL FLUID SPECIMEN

CSF is obtained by the physician through a spinal tap or lumbar puncture. To perform the lumbar puncture, a needle is inserted into the lumbar region of the spinal cord and fluid is withdrawn from the pia-arachnoid space. A manometer is attached to the needle at the beginning and end of the procedure. This facilitates measurement of the opening and closing pressures. Pressure changes are noted in various disease states. For example, elevated pressures are often seen with intracranial tumors and inflammation of the meninges.

CELL COUNTS

Techniques for performing cell counts are discussed in Chapter 9, and characteristic cell counts are shown in Table 10.1. The color and clarity of a CSF specimen should always be noted on both the centrifuged and uncentrifuged specimen. The presence of a pale pink to yellow (xanthrochromia) color after

TABLE 10.1. CSF FINDINGS

Condition	Cell Count (μl)	Protein (mg %)	CSF Glucose / Serum Glucose	Other
Normal	<8	15-45	0.5	—
Bacterial meningitis	↑↑*	↑	↓↓	Gram stain usually positive Polymorphonuclear leukocytes predominant on cell count
Viral meningitis	↑	↑	→	Lymphocytes predominant on cell count
Tuberculous meningitis	↑	↑	↓	Lymphocytes and/or monocytes predominant on cell count
Fungal meningitis	↑	↑	↓	India ink may be positive if *Cryptococcus* is present
Cerebral hemorrhage	↑	↑	→ to ↑	Must distinguish from traumatic tap
Guillain-Barré syndrome	→	↑	→	—
Multiple sclerosis	→ to ↑	→ to ↑	→	—
Syphilis	→ to ↑	→ to ↑	→	May vary depending on stage of disease, serology positive
Leptospirosis	↑	↑	→	Lymphocytes predominant
Encephalitis	↑	→ to ↑	→	Early response is polymorphonuclear lymphocytes, later lymphocytes predominant
Brain abscess	↑	→ to ↑	→	Early response is polymorphonuclear, later lymphocytes predominant
Amebic meningitis	↑	↑	↓	Wet preparation using prewarmed slide to look for motile amebae

* ↑ Increased, ↓ decreased, → normal, ↑↑ markedly increased, ↓↓ markedly decreased.

centrifugation is indicative of previous sub-arachnoid bleeding, while a clear supernatant is expected with a traumatic or bloody tap. A bloody tap and true subarachnoid hemorrhage can be distinguished by performing an RBC count on the first and last tube obtained during the lumbar puncture. If the RBC count decreases significantly from the first to the last tube, a bloody tap is suspected. However, if the RBC count remains within 10 percent in both tubes, a subarachnoid hemorrhage is suspected.

In taps where numerous RBCs are present, a ratio of WBCs to RBCs can be compared to a ratio of WBCs to RBCs present in the patient's peripheral blood to determine if the spinal fluid contains increased numbers of WBCs. Normally the ratio of WBCs to RBCs is 1 to 2 WBCs/1,000 RBCs.

Cell Types Found in the CSF

Cell types that appear in the peripheral blood and in the bone marrow may all appear in the CSF. The characteristic morphology with a representative example of each of the cell types is discussed in Chapter 14.

Cells unique to the CSF include the ependymal, choroidal, and pia-arachnoid meso-thelial (PAM) cells. The cerebral ventricles, neural canal of the spinal cord, and the choroid plexus are lined with epithelial cells of ectodermal origin. The cells of the epithelial lining of the ventricle and neural canal are called ependymal cells, while the epithelial lining cells of the choroid plexus are called choroidal cells. The PAM cells are of mesothelial origin and line the pia and the arachnoid.

There is considerable discussion in the literature as to the exact origin, morphologic characteristics, and function of these cells. There is not universal agreement as to their nomenclature. The ependymal and choroidal cells are difficult to distinguish from each other. Both cells are approximately 25 to 40 μ with a large round to oval nucleus that may lie near the perimeter of the cell. The nucleus occupies approximately one third of the total cell size. Nucleoli may be present in the nucleus, while vacuoles may be present in the cytoplasm. Both cells often appear in large clusters or groups of the same type of cell. Ependymal cells have less distinct cytoplasmic membranes, appear more fragile, and appear in smaller clusters than do the choroidal cells. Both cell types have been reported after the administration of intrathecal drugs and after the removal of ventricular fluid (fluid from the cerebral ventricles) of normal children and hydrocephalic children. The significance of finding these cells in CSF is unknown (Fig. 10.2).

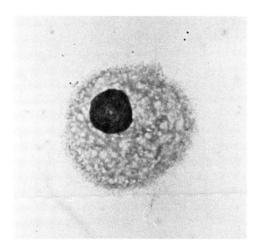

Figure 10.2. Ependymal cell.

The PAM cells are described as young monocytic cells, and it is difficult to distinguish these cells from other cells of the monocytic series. The PAM cells have a round to oval nucleus with loose netted chromatin. The cell size varies from 15 to 25 μ, with the nucleus occupying slightly less than one half of the cytoplasm. The nucleus may have nucleoli, and the cytoplasm may have vacuoles. These cells may appear in clusters. An important characteristic of the PAM cells is that they have the ability to transform into macrophages.

The finding of ependymal, choroidal, or PAM cells occurs rarely. They may be found in the CSF with various other types of hematologic cells. Table 10.2 is a partial list of disease states in which the various cell types may be found.

It is important to remember that cells present in the blood may also be present in the CSF as a result of in vivo bleeding, invasion, or a traumatic tap. Therefore, normal, abnormal, and unusual cells that are seen on peripheral blood films may also be seen in CSF preparations. For example, leukemic blast cells, immature myeloid forms, early erythroid precursors, and immature or abnormal lymphoid cells may all be present in CSF (Fig. 10.3). Leukemic blast cells have very immature homogeneous nuclear material, often containing nucleoli similar to their appearance in peripheral blood films. Lymphoma cells have a nucleus with coarsely clumped chromatin with a very rough appearance. The nucleus of a lymphoma cell may have convolutions or indentations with irregular membranes of the cytoplasm (Fig. 10.4).

A diagnosis of leukemia or lymphoma with or without CNS involvement is made from a review of the total picture of the patient, not just an examination of the blood or the CSF. The important consideration of the technologist is, therefore, to note in the report immature or abnormal cells when they are present in the various concentration preparations.

Additionally, numerous cytoplasmic inclu-

TABLE 10.2. CELL TYPES FOUND IN DISEASE

Cell Type	Disease State
Ependymal and choroidal cells	Ventricular fluid of children in hydrocephalus After intrathecal drugs Pneumoencephalogy
PAM cells	Cerebral hemorrhage Chronic bacterial infection Mixed cellular reaction Chronic infections Multiple sclerosis
Neutrophils	Bacterial meningitis Tuberculous meningitis Early viral meningitis Hemorrhage Fungal meningitis
Lymphocytes	Viral infection of CNS Tuberculous meningitis Fungal meningitis
Monocytes	Viral infection of CNS Tuberculous meningitis Bacterial meningitis
Eosinophils	Allergic reactions Viral meningitis Tuberculous meningitis Parasitic infection of CNS Fungal infection of CNS
Basophils	Chronic granulocytic leukemia Mixed cellular reaction
Plasma cells	Viral infection of CNS Chronic infection Tuberculous meningitis Syphilis Multiple sclerosis
Macrophages	Hemorrhage Bacterial meningitis Tuberculous meningitis Fungal meningitis
Blast cells	Leukemic involvement of CNS
Tumor cells	Primary tumors of CNS Metastatic tumors of CNS

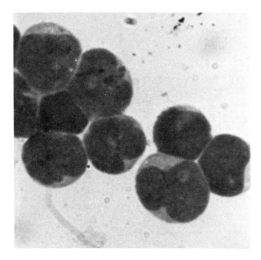

Figure 10.3. Leukemic cells.

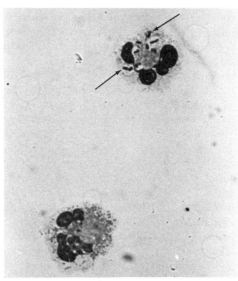

Figure 10.5. Neutrophil containing bacteria (arrows).

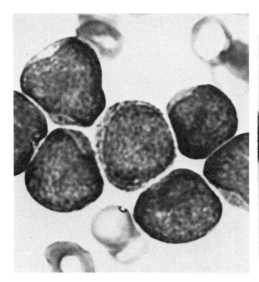

Figure 10.4. Cells from a lymphoma.

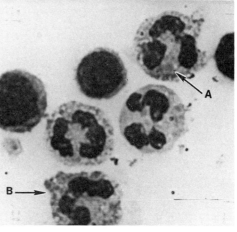

Figure 10.6. Neutrophil containing Döhle body (**A**). **B** indicates toxic granulation.

sions may be seen in the cells present in the CSF. For example, Döhle bodies, toxic granulation, Auer rods, and ingested bacteria may all be seen in neutrophils (Figs. 10.5 and 10.6). Macrophages may be seen containing intact RBCs or with dark pigments in the cytoplasm. The presence of intact RBCs in the macrophage cytoplasm indicates a recent (within three to four days) cerebral hemorrhage. Macrophages whose cytoplasms are filled with dark pigments on the Wright-stained preparations are a result of the cells' phagocytosis of probably melanin, hemoside-rin, or hematoidin (Figs. 10.7 and 10.8). Hemosiderin is an iron-storage molecule and is seen as a dark blue to black inclusion in the macrophage cytoplasm, while hematoidin, which is iron-free, appears as brownish yel-low or red crystals in the cytoplasm (Fig. 10.9). The significance of seeing hemosiderin or hematoidin crystals in CSF is that these may be present after lysis of red cells that has resulted from bleeding in the subarachnoid space. These pigments may be seen within the macrophage from five days to six months after the initial bleeding. Melanin also ap-pears in the cytoplasm as dark blue to black inclusions and is a pigment of skin, hair, eyes, and various tumors. A Prussian blue stain for iron can be done on an additional prepara-tion of the specimen to differentiate between hemosiderin and melanin.

Cells from malignant or benign tumors may be seen in the CSF. These tumor cells

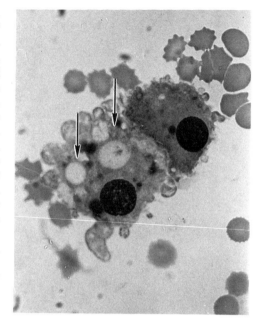

Figure 10.8. Macrophage with ingested red cells.

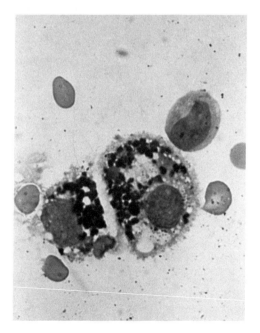

Figure 10.7. Macrophage containing hemo-siderin.

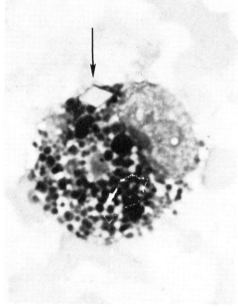

Figure 10.9. Macrophage containing hema-toidin crystal.

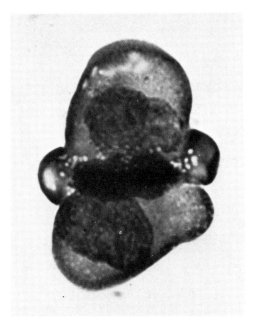

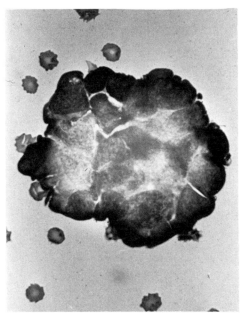

Figure 10.10. Malignant cells in CSF.   **Figure 10.11.** Malignant cells in CSF.

may arise directly from areas of the CNS or may reflect metastatic involvement of the CNS. The criteria for identifying malignant cells are discussed in Chapter 15. Figures 10.10, 10.11, and 10.12 represent examples of malignant cells that may be seen in the CSF.

CHEMICAL EXAMINATION OF THE CSF

CSF is formed in the capillary blood tufts of the choroid plexus. It is felt that the lining cells actively regulate the passage of substances between the CSF and blood, thereby forming a modified ultrafiltrate of the blood plasma. The lining cells of the choroid plexus effectively contribute to the formation of the blood-brain barrier. This barrier and the chemical composition of the CSF may be altered in various disease states.

The chemical examination of CSF routinely includes measurement of the total protein and glucose. Enzyme studies, im-

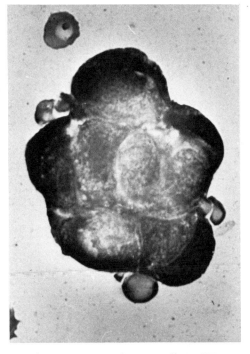

Figure 10.12. Malignant cells in CSF.

munoglobulin levels, and other studies (Na, K, Cl, Ca, bilirubin, creatinine) may occasionally be measured.

Total Protein

CSF total protein can be measured by turbidimetric methods, the Lowry method, ultraviolet light absorption method, gel filtration method, and dye-binding methods. Normal values range from 15 to 45 mg/100 ml, with values up to 70 mg/100 ml in elderly adults and children. Ventricular fluids have lower values than do lumbar fluids. Any CSF specimen for determination of protein should be centrifuged to remove possible RBC and WBC cellular protein contamination. In a traumatic tap, the results of total protein value may be invalid since the value would reflect the protein present in the blood. Even as little as 0.20 ml of blood in a 5 ml specimen can cause a fourfold increase in total protein value. Conditions in which elevated or depressed CSF total protein values may be found are listed in Table 10.3.

To evaluate the integrity of the blood-brain barrier, two ratios are often used. They are the CSF albumin:Plasma albumin ratio and the CSF IgG/Plasma IgG ÷ CSF albumin/Plasma albumin ratio. These ratios can be utilized for this purpose since CSF protein is derived from diffusion of protein from the blood and local secretion of protein. Albumin is not produced in the CNS, and therefore, an elevated CSF albumin/plasma albumin ratio may represent (1) compromise of the blood-brain barrier, (2) impaired reabsorption of CSF protein, or (3) a traumatic tap.

Using the CSF IgG/Plasma IgG ÷ CSF albumin/Plasma albumin ratio an elevated value is indicative of (1) compromise of the blood-brain barrier or (2) increased CSF IgG secretion. The normal ratio is 0.5.

CSF Protein Electrophoresis. Protein electrophoresis may also be performed on CSF. It is advisable to perform simultaneously protein electrophoresis on a serum sample, since abnormal serum patterns may be reflected in the CSF pattern. The CSF protein electrophoresis pattern is composed of a prealbumin, albumin, alpha-globulin, beta$_1$-globulin, beta$_2$-globulin, and gamma globulin bands.

Abnormal CSF electrophoretic patterns include:

1. Elevation in the gamma globulin region reflecting a myeloma protein that is also present in the serum.
2. Elevations in the gamma, alpha, beta$_1$, and albumin regions with depression of the prealbumin and beta$_2$ regions, which may be seen in inflammatory conditions of the meninges, cerebral arterial disease, neoplasms, and Guillain-Barré syndrome.
3. Elevations in the beta$_2$ region, which may be seen in syringomyelia, cerebral atrophy, and cerebral ischemia.
4. Elevations of one or more regions without a corresponding elevation of the same region(s) in the plasma. For example, CSF IgG elevation is seen in multiple sclerosis and CSF IgM elevation is seen in neurosyphilis without the corresponding serum elevation.

CSF Glucose

Glucose obtains entry into the CSF by both active transport and passive diffusion. Changes in the plasma glucose levels are re-

TABLE 10.3. CSF TOTAL PROTEIN LEVELS

Elevated in	Decreased in
Traumatic tap	CSF rhinorrhea (CSF discharged through the nose)
Bacterial meningitis	CSF otorrhea (CSF discharged through the ear)
Viral meningitis	Increased intracranial pressure
Encephalitis	Hyperthyroidism
Obstruction	
Increased synthesis of CNS protein	
Tuberculous meningitis	
Cerebral hemorrhage	
Fungal meningitis	
Neurosyphilis	

flected in the CSF approximately two to four hours after the plasma glucose elevation or depression has occurred. CSF glucose measurements can be performed using the same method utilized for serum glucose measurement. A simultaneous serum glucose measurement should be performed when a CSF glucose is performed. Normal values of CSF glucose are 50 to 75 mg/dl or about 50 to 60 percent of the serum value.

Elevated CSF glucose values reflect an elevation of serum glucose two to four hours prior to the lumbar puncture. Decreased CSF glucose values may be present in a number of conditions, including bacterial meningitis, tuberculous meningitis, hypoglycemia, and leptomeningeal neoplasms. To substantiate a significantly decreased CSF glucose, the CSF glucose/serum glucose ratio is used. A ratio below 0.5 is significant, and the lower the ratio becomes, the more significant the finding.

Enzymes in the CSF

Presently, lactate dehydrogenase (LDH) has proved to be the most clinically useful of the enzymes measured in the CSF. Sources of CSF LDH include diffusion from the blood, brain tissue, WBCs, RBCs, bacteria, and neoplastic cells. Elevated levels may be present in bacterial meningitis, viral meningitis with a poor prognosis, and in any condition associated with CNS tissue destruction.

MICROBIOLOGIC EXAMINATION OF CSF

The microbiologic examination of the CSF is an important part of the overall examination of the CSF. The specimen should be collected aseptically and examined and cultured without delay. Infection within the CNS can result in inflammation of the meninges (meningitis), the brain substance (encephalitis), or localized as intracranial abscess. All of these conditions may cause alterations within the CSF. The infection may be caused by aerobic bacteria, anaerobic bacteria, viruses, fungi, mycobacteria, spirochetes, or protozoa.

Laboratory Techniques

Since there are a variety of agents that may cause infection within the CNS, culture and isolation techniques should include appropriate media and laboratory tests to allow for identification of these agents. Specific considerations for determining the probable and definitive infectious agent are discussed on page 247.

As with any specimen for microbiologic examination, aseptic techniques should be strictly adhered to. The CSF should be transported quickly to the laboratory and should be quickly processed, performing the appropriate stains and inoculation of media. All CSF not utilized for specific stains or culture should be incubated at 37C in 5 percent CO_2 and later reexamined, since CSF itself may serve as a medium for the growth of organisms.

Stains

The importance of the gram stain cannot be overemphasized, since its results are often among the first pieces of information the clinician and the laboratory have as to the etiologic agent responsible for the patient's symptoms. The technique of the gram stain is given in Chapter 9. It should be remembered that as bacteria age they may lose their definitive gram staining characteristics and also decrease in size. Neutrophils should be noted when present. Correlation between the gram stain and the culture isolates should be noted so that infection caused by a multiplicity of organisms will not be overlooked.

Stains for mycobacteria or acid-fast bacteria include the Ziehl-Neelsen, Kinyoun, fluorochrome, and fluorescent antibody stains. A technique for performing the Kinyoun stain is given in Chapter 9. All CSF submitted for culture for mycobacteria should have a portion of the centrifuged sediment stained for AFB.

Cryptococcus neoformans can be tentatively identified by visualization of its capsule with an India ink preparation. This technique is described in the section on fungal meningitis (page 247).

Culture Techniques

Microbiologic culture techniques and biochemical identification are the same as for any other biologic specimen. Care should be taken to include media, biochemical test, and an environment that will allow for the identification of possible causative agents of infection within the CNS.

Gas Chromatography

Gas chromatography has proved most useful in the identification of anaerobes by detection of characteristic short-chain volatile organic acids. However, this method has not been successful for direct identification of organisms from the CSF.

Detection of Antigenic Microbial Substances

Antigenic substances from bacteria can be detected by latex particle agglutination and counterimmunoelectrophoresis techniques. Latex particle techniques employ the coating of latex particles with antibody for detection of antigen present in the CSF by noting the presence of agglutination. Antibody to polysaccharide and to polyribose phosphate-coated latex particles has been used for the identification of *Cryptococcus* and *Haemophilus influenzae*, respectively, for the identification of these organisms in CSF.

Counterimmunoelectrophoresis (CIE) is a process by which antigen is moved by an electric current through a solution of specific antibody. A precipitin line is formed at the site where the antigen-antibody interaction occurs (Fig. 10.13). This technique is more sensitive than the gram stain, and results from CIE can be ready before culture results are available. This technique also offers the advantage of being able to detect antigen present in the CSF when the patient has had prior treatment with antibiotics and the cultures are often negative. CIE has been utilized to identify the following organisms in CSF: *Stretococcus pneumoniae, Neisseria meningitidis, Haemophilus influenzae, Klebsiella pneumoniae, Escherichia coli, Streptococcus* group B, *Cryptococcus neoformans,* and the teichoic acid of *Staphylococcus aureus.*

Limulus Lysate Assay

The limulus lysate assay involves the detection of endotoxin produced in gram-negative meningitis. This is accomplished because endotoxin causes gel formation of an extract (lysate) from horseshoe crabs (*Limulus polyphemus*). Positive findings have been reported in cases of meningitis caused by various gram-negative organisms, including *H. influenzae, E. coli,* and *N. meningitidis.* Although the technique is not specific for the particular gram-negative organism, it does have good sensitivity and specificity for gram-negative meningitis and may prove to be an important technique of the future.

Detection of Microbial Antibody

There are numerous techniques presently employed for the detection of bacterial antibody in serologic or immunologic laboratories. Infection can be established by demonstrating a significant rise or fall in antibody levels (titer) over a 10 to 14 day period. A significant rise or fall means a change of titer level by a factor of $4\times$ or $\frac{1}{4}$, respectively. Demonstration of specific microbial an-

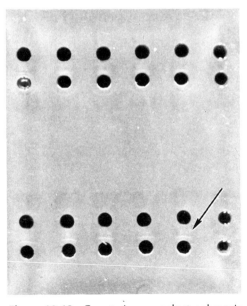

Figure 10.13. Counterimmunoelectrophoresis.

tibodies or specific microbial product antibodies can help establish the diagnosis.

INFECTION WITHIN THE CNS

Characteristic findings of most of the conditions associated with changes in the CSF are found in Table 10.1. The following material deals with specific findings in several of these conditions.

Bacterial Meningitis
Bacterial meningitis may be caused by either aerobic or anaerobic organisms. WBC counts ranging from 50 to 100,000 μl with a CSF glucose/serum glucose ratio of < 0.5 is strongly suggestive of bacterial meningitis. Demonstration of the organism on gram stain helps in making the tentative diagnosis, with bacterial culture confirming the diagnosis.

The most common organisms causing bacterial meningitis are *S. pneumoniae*, *N. meningitidis*, and *H. influenzae*. Many other bacteria may cause meningitis, including the gram-negative bacilli, *Listeria monocytogenes*, group B streptococci, and staphylococci. *E. coli* and group B streptococci predominate as the causative agents in the newborn to 6-month-old patient. *H. influenzae* type B and *S. pneumoniae* infections predominate in patients from 6 months to 3 years and also in patients over 60 years old. *S. pneumoniae* and *N. meningitidis* most commonly cause infections in the patients aged 3 years to 60 years. In patients with altered immune status, staphylococci and the gram-negative bacilli are the common causative agents. There is decreased recovery of the etiologic agent in patients who have received recent antibiotic therapy.

Anaerobic meningitis is not very common and is usually found in association with a brain abscess or other localized intracranial infection. *Fusobacterium*, *Bacteroides*, *Clostridium*, *Actinomyces*, and anaerobic streptococci are among the causative agents. All CSF should be cultured anaerobically as well as aerobically, but often other diagnostic tests, such as CAT scans or arteriography, must be instituted to confirm the diagnosis and the primary focus of the disease.

Tuberculous meningitis results from rupture of a latent tubercle into the CSF or during the hematogenous spread during an early phase of the tuberculosis infection. Tuberculosis skin tests are usually positive in people with tuberculous meningitis. Acid-fast stains, as described in Chapter 9, should be done on the CSF of all patients with possible tuberculous meningitis. Treatment with antituberculosis therapy may have to be instituted without demonstration of the organism on the AFB smear, since AFB smears are often negative in cases of tuberculous meningitis.

Viral Meningitis
Viral meningitis is usually a disease of children and young adults, with mumps, Coxsackie B virus, Echo viruses, and polioviruses among the most common etiologic agents. Lymphocytes usually predominate on the differential count, although polymorphonuclear leukocytes may predominate within the first 24 hours of the onset of symptoms. Definitive diagnosis is established by isolation of the virus or by demonstrating a significant (fourfold) rise or fall in serum titers.

Fungal Meningitis
Fungal meningitis may be caused by *Cryptococcus neoformans*, *Candida albicans*, *Aspergillus*, *Coccidioides immitis*, *Histoplasma capsulatum*, *Blastomyces dermatitidis*, *Mucor*, and other fungi. *Cryptococcus*, *Candida*, *Aspergillus*, and *Mucor* meningitis are most often seen in patients who have a primary malignancy, are immunosuppressed, and/or are receiving corticosteroids. CSF examination should include a wet preparation, India ink preparation, and fungal cultures. An India ink preparation is performed by mixing one drop of centrifuged CSF sediment with one drop of India ink on a slide, covering with a coverslip, and studying under a microscope. The slide should be scanned on 40× with confirmation under oil for the presence of characteristic, budding yeast forms (Fig. 10.14). Diagnosis is made by demonstration of the organism by culture, detection of rising or falling specific

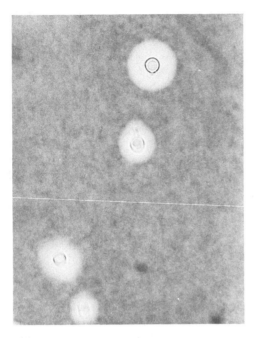

Figure 10.14. *Cryptococcus neoformans* from CSF.

antibody levels, or detection of specific antigen by counterimmunoelectrophoresis.

Amebic Meningoencephalitis

Amebic meningoencephalitis is caused by *Acanthameba* and *Nagleria* species. The amebae are free-living amebae found in fresh water sources. When no bacteria are seen on a gram stain of CSF with an increased cell count, increased protein, and decreased glucose, a wet preparation of the CSF should be made. A wet preparation of CSF should be made on patients with a history of swimming or other exposure to fresh water sources. To perform the wet preparation, one drop of CSF is placed and coversliped on a pre-warmed microscopic slide. The slide is then examined for motile amebae. Tissue cultures may confirm the diagnosis.

CNS Infection with Spirochetes

Two spirochetes are responsible for alterations in the CSF. *Treponema pallidum* is the causative agent for the late (tertiary stage) neurosyphilis that may develop 5 to 35 years

after the primary infection. Establishment of this diagnosis is accomplished by screening the CSF with the nonspecific tests, such as Venereal Disease Research Laboratory (VDRL) or rapid plasma reagin (RPR) test, and confirmation with a specific test, such as the fluorescent treponemal antibody absorption (FTA-ABS) test or microhemagglutination (MHA-TP) test.

Leptospira are the causative agents of a meningitis associated with direct or indirect contact with urine from infected animals. Animals that may be infected include dogs, rodents, cattle, and swine. Confirmation is by serologic techniques that demonstrate a significant rise or fall in antibody titer.

Other Causes of Altered CSF

Many other entities may cause alterations in the CSF and should be considered when an explanation of the changes in the CSF cannot be ascribed to the etiologic agents known to cause CNS infection. Usually, a picture of a slightly increased cell count with a predominance of lymphocytes, normal CSF glucose, and normal to only slightly elevated CSF protein will be seen. Among the entities that may alter the CSF are sinusitis, mastoiditis, vertebral osteomyelitis, intrathecal injections, and neoplastic conditions.

Review Questions

Select the one best answer for each of the following questions.

1. The innermost covering that is intimately attached to the brain and spinal cord is the:
    A. Dura
    B. Pia
    C. Arachnoid
    D. Meninges
2. Cerebrospinal fluid is formed by secretion from the:
    A. Neural canal
    B. Venous sinuses
    C. Arachnoid granulations

D. Choroid plexus

E. Specialized areas of the dura

3. Two CSF specimens were sent to the laboratory. Tube labeled 1 (first tube obtained during the lumbar puncture) had an RBC count of 10,700/μl. Tube labeled 5 (last tube obtained during the lumbar puncture) had an RBC count of 100/μl and a WBC count of 1/μl. The patient's whole blood RBC and WBC counts were within normal limits. These results are indicative of:

A. An infection

B. A traumatic tap

C. A recent subarachnoid hemorrhage

D. Laboratory error

E. An old intracerebral bleeding episode

4. The cell seen in Figure 10.15 was found in the CSF of an 87-year-old male patient on the neurology service.

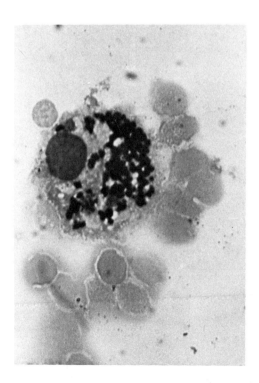

Figure 10.15. Unknown cell on test.

A Prussian blue stain was positive in the same specimen. The dark inclusions seen in this are probably a result of:

A. Recent cerebral hemorrhage

B. Metastatic involvement of the CNS by a malignant melanoma

C. Toxic granulation suggestive of a chronic infection

D. Subarachnoid hemorrhage that occurred four months ago

E. Acute leukemic involvement of the CNS

For each of the incomplete statements, one or more of the completions given is correct. Select:

A. If only *1, 2, and 3* are correct.

B. If only *1 and 3* are correct.

C. If only *2 and 4* are correct.

D. If only *4* is correct.

E. If *all* are correct.

5. In performing a spinal tap, the physician inserts a needle in between which of the following areas to obtain the CSF?

1. Dura

2. Pia

3. Neural canal

4. Arachnoid

6. Which of the following cell types are thought to be epithelial cells of ectodermal origin?

1. Ependymal cells

2. PAM cells

3. Choroidal cells

4. Macrophages

7. Neutrophils may be present in elevated numbers in the CSF of patients with:

1. Bacterial meningitis

2. Fungal meningitis

3. Cerebral hemorrhage

4. Viral meningitis

8. Elevated CSF total protein values may be found in:

1. A traumatic tap

2. Viral meningitis

3. Neurosyphilis

4. Increased intracranial pressure

9. The CSF IgG/Plasma IgG ÷ CSF albumin/Plasma albumin ratio was de-

termined to be 0.7 in a patient with suspected bacterial meningitis. The value may represent:
1. Normal formation of the CSF
2. Compromise of the blood-brain barrier
3. Reabsorption of CSF protein
4. Increased CSF IgG secretion

10. Abnormal CSF electrophoretic pattern may be seen in patients with:
1. Cerebral ischemia
2. Guillain-Barré syndrome
3. Multiple syphilis
4. Multiple myeloma

11. Elevated CSF glucose values may characteristically reflect:
1. Bacterial meningitis
2. Primary CNS tumors
3. Tuberculosis meningitis
4. Elevated serum glucose level 2 hours prior to the special tap

12. Elevated lactate dehydrogenase values may be seen in:
1. Viral meningitis
2. Bacterial meningitis
3. Metastatic involvement of the CNS
4. CNS tissue destruction

13. Definitive diagnosis of fungal meningitis caused by C. neoformans can be made by:
1. Demonstration of the organism by culture
2. A specific antibody titer of 1:2 on the day of the patient's admission to the hospital with a specific antibody titer of 1:4 14 days later

3. Detection of specific antigen by counterimmunoelectrophoresis
4. A positive India ink preparation

Match the best answer in Column B with the appropriate causative agent in Column A. Answers from Column B may be used more than once.

Column A
_____ 14. *Bacteroides*
_____ 15. Staphylococci
_____ 16. Group B streptococci
_____ 17. *H. influenza*
_____ 18. *N. meningitidis*
_____ 19. *Cryptococcus neoformans*

Column B
A. Meningitis in a 2-year-old patient
B. Meningitis in an immunosuppressed patient
C. Meningitis in a 27-year-old patient
D. Meningitis in the newborn
E. Meningitis in a patient with an intracranial abscess

Match the patterns listed in the chart below to the appropriate answers listed in questions 20 through 27. Patterns may be used more than once.
_____ 20. Viral meningitis
_____ 21. Bacterial meningitis
_____ 22. Amebic meningitis
_____ 23. Leptospirosis
_____ 24. Fungal meningitis
_____ 25. Cerebral hemorrhage
_____ 26. Tuberculous meningitis
_____ 27. Encephalitis

Pattern	Cell Count (μl)	CSF Protein (mg %)	CSF glucose / Serum glucose	Comments
A	10,000	50	0.5	Lymphocytes predominate
B	20,000	50	0.4	India ink (positive)
C	47,000	75	0.2	Polymorphonuclear leukocytes predominate
D	5,000	65	0.6	Prussian blue (positive)
E	10,000	60	0.4	Wet preparation (positive)
F	7,500	60	0.4	Monocytes predominate

Case Study

A 27-year-old female had received a 10-dose course of chemotherapy for treatment of acute myelogenous leukemia. On the seventh day of her hospital course, she became confused, with altered awareness of her surroundings. Slight nuchal rigidity was noted on physical examination. A lumbar puncture was performed. The preliminary laboratory report of the CSF follows:

Characteristic	Finding
Time collected:	11:05 AM
Time received:	11:12 AM
Source of fluid:	CSF
Color:	colorless
Appearance:	slightly hazy
RBC/μl:	2
WBC/μl:	997
Differential	
Polymorpho-nuclear leukocytes:	48 %
Lymphocytes:	46 %
Monocytes:	5 %
Macrophages:	1 %
Mesothelial cells:	0
Eosinophils:	0
Basophils:	0
Other:	0
Gram stain:	negative
AFB stain:	negative
India ink preparation:	positive, budding yeast consistent with *Cryptococcus* present
CSF protein:	75 mg %
CSF glucose:	36 mg %
Serum glucose:	94 mg %

The patient was put on intravenous amphotericin B for treatment of *Cryptococcus* meningitis.

Question

The elevated WBC count noted on this CSF report most likely represents:

1. Contamination of the specimen with peripheral blood
2. A defense mechanism of the body to a secondary infection
3. A finding often present in patients receiving chemotherapy
4. The presence of a fungal infection
5. A laboratory error

Answer: 4

Results

Cryptococcus neoformans was isolated from fungal cultures confirming the diagnosis. The patient's mental status returned to normal after several days.

This case illustrates diagnostic information that may be obtained from the evaluation of cerebrospinal fluid.

BIBLIOGRAPHY

Anhalt JP, George EK, Rytel MW: Detection of Microbial Antigens by Counter Immunoelectrophoresis. Washington, D.C., American Society of Microbiology, 1979.

Drewinko B, Sullivan MP, Martin T: Use of the cytocentrifuge in the diagnosis of meningeal leukemia. Cancer 31:1331, 1973.

Esteveg EG, Esteveg BS: Bacteriologic culture of sterile body fluids: assessment of a protocol. Lab Med 11:170, 1980.

Finegold SM, Martin WJ, Scott EG: Bailey and Scott's Diagnostic Microbiology. St. Louis, Mosby, 1978.

Harvey AM, Johns RJ, McKusick VA, Owens AH, Ross RS (eds): The Principles and Practice of Medicine, 20th ed. New York, Appleton, 1980.

Henry JB: Clinical Diagnosis and Management by Laboratory Methods. Philadelphia, Saunders, 1979.

Hoeltge GA, Furlan A, Hoffman GC: Cleve Clin Q 43:237, 1976.

Hoeprich PD, Ward JR: The Fluids of Parenteral Body Cavities. New York, Grune & Stratton, 1959.

Keebler CM, Reagan JD. A Manual of Cytotechnology. Chicago, American Society of Clinical Pathologists, 1977.

Kolmel HW: Atlas of Cerebrospinal Fluid Cells. New York, Springer-Verlag, 1977.

Kent TH, Hart MN, Shires TK: Introduction to Human Disease. New York, Appleton, 1979.

Komp DM: Diagnosis of CNS leukemia. Am J Pediatr Hematol/Oncol 1:31, 1979.

McCormack LJ, Hazard JB, Belovich D, Garner WJ: Identification of neoplastic cells in cerebrospinal fluid by a wet-film method. Cancer 10:1293, 1957.

Oehmichen M: Cerebrospinal Fluid Cytology. Philadelphia, Saunders, 1976.

Spriggs AT, Boddington, MM: The Cytology of Effusions and of Cerebrospinal Fluid. London, Heinemann, 1976.

Tietz NE, Caraway WT, Frier EF, et al.: Fundamentals of Clinical Chemistry. Philadelphia, Saunders, 1976.

Umeo I, Yutaka I: A simple sedimentation chamber adaptable to the laboratory centrifuge. Am J Clin Pathol 58:590, 1972.

Woodruff KH: Cerebrospinal fluid cytomorphology using cytocentrifugation. Am J Clin Pathol 60:621, 1973.

Youmans GP, Paterson PY, Sommers HM: The Biologic and Clinical Basis of Infectious Diseases. Philadelphia, Saunders, 1975.

Ann E. Neely and Kathryn Kilpatrick Cheek

	CHAPTER 11

Synovial Fluid

Objectives

It is expected that the information presented in this chapter will enable the reader to:

1. Define the character, composition, and function of normal synovial fluid.
2. Describe an appropriate method of collection of synovial fluid.
3. Interpret the color and clarity of synovial fluid as to the probable composition of the fluids.
4. Describe how viscosity and mucin clot formation are determined in evaluation of synovial fluids.
5. Utilize synovial glucose, protein, and uric acid levels in relation to serum levels to suggest the possible etiology of a joint fluid accumulation.
6. Define rheumatoid factor.
7. Describe the significance of rheumatoid factor.
8. List appropriate culture media for synovial fluid.
9. Utilize visual appearance, viscosity, mucin clot formation, and cell counts to suggest possible etiology of joint fluid accumulation.
10. Describe dilution techniques of synovial fluid for highly elevated cell counts.
11. Evaluate findings on gram stain and Wright stain of synovial fluids.
12. Define and identify ragocytes (RA cells), LE cells, mast cells, and synovial cells.
13. Describe the appearance under light microscopy, polarized microscopy, and compensated polarized microscopy of monosodium urate crystals, calcium pyrophosphate crystals, corticosteroid crystals, cholesterol crystals, hydroxyapatite crystals, and talcum crystals.
14. Identify birefringence patterns with polarized light and compensated polarized light microscopy of monosodium urate and calcium pyrophosphate crystals.

15. Recognize disease states in which various crystals may be identified in evaluation of synovial fluids.
16. Define the terms positive birefringence, negative birefringence, strongly birefringent, and weakly birefringent.

Synovial fluid is a crystal clear viscous liquid that is found in joint cavities. These joint cavities lack the mesothelial lining found in other body cavities and are called "tissue spaces." The fluid is a protein-containing dialysate of blood plasma. The synovial fluid also contains secretions from the synovium or synovial membrane. The secretions are composed of a high concentration of hyaluronate-protein complex that contains mucin. Hyaluronate is a polymer composed of repeated disaccharide units. Mucin is a mucopolysaccharide or glycoprotein and is the chief constituent of mucus. The presence of mucin in synovial fluid places it intermediate between serous fluid, which is also an ultrafiltrate of plasma, and cerebrospinal fluid, which is a secretion of the choroid plexuses.

Synovial fluid serves the very important functions of moistening and lubricating the joint surfaces, especially those joints subject to heavy weightbearing. It also serves as the mechanism for the movement of nutrient material for the articular cartilage of the joint and for the removal of debris.

The normal amount of synovial fluid is from 1 to 4 ml. It resembles the white of an egg in appearance. The analysis of synovial fluid may furnish diagnostic information, especially when crystal formations and infectious agents are being considered as etiologic agent of a change within the joint. Specific findings must be correlated with the clinical picture by the physician, as frequently two or more disease processes may be occurring at the same time. The removal of the fluid may also relieve a great deal of discomfort to the patient.

COLLECTION OF SPECIMEN

Synovial fluid is extracted aseptically with a 20 gauge or larger needle. If the determination of glucose is of significance, the patient should be fasting at least six hours in order that an equilibrium be obtained between the plasma and synovial fluid glucose. A sterile plastic syringe may be moistened with 25 units of heparin per each ml of fluid withdrawn. An alternate procedure that is recommended is to withdraw the fluid with a dry sterile test tube and have heparin (25 units/ml) in a sterile test tube available to add as desired. Normal synovial fluid contains no fibrinogen, so it does not clot on standing. A portion of the synovial fluid may be placed in a sterile tube and observed for spontaneous clot formation. Spontaneous clotting is seen in the arthritides and is due to the transfer of plasma proteins, including clotting factors, into the fluid. Heparin is recommended as the choice anticoagulant as EDTA and oxalate may contain birefringent crystals. It may be desirable to culture the synovial fluid directly from the needle at the time of aspiration. Cultures may also be done from either the heparinized or unheparinized tube.

EXAMINATION OF SYNOVIAL FLUID

Visual

The color and clarity of the synovial fluid should be examined and recorded. It may be clear, straw-colored, slightly yellow, yellow, orange, green, or bloody in color. The yellow color, or xanthochromia, is the result of a gradual accumulation of blood. Streaks of blood in a fluid are usually due to the aspiration, but a homogeneously bloody specimen is pathologic. Bloody fluid is an indication of a hemorrhage and progresses from dark red to brown as the fluid ages. Clarity may be reported as clear, cloudy, or turbid or may show different amounts of precipitate formation. Clarity may be judged by attempting to read newspaper print through the specimen in a test tube. The degree of cloudiness correlates with either the cells, crystals, or debris present.

Viscosity

Normal synovial fluid shows a high degree of viscosity due to the polymerization of hyaluronic acid. This may be measured satisfactorily by expressing a drop of fluid and letting it drop to a slide. A continuous string of 5 cm before it breaks is normal. A string less than 3 cm means less than normal viscosity. Another method of testing is to place a drop of fluid on the examiner's thumb, which is touched to the forefinger. When the gloved fingers are separated, a continuous string should be 5 cm or more. The hyaluronate concentration is decreased in a variety of inflammatory joint diseases, such as gouty, septic, and rheumatoid arthritis. It is thought that the lysozomal enzymes from the white blood cells break down the hyaluronic acid. The concentration of hyaluronate is also decreased with age.

Mucin Clot

Normal synovial fluid forms a firm clot when the fluid is acidified. The clot formation is dependent on the hyaluronic acid and is produced when 4 ml of 2 percent acetic acid is added to 1 ml of synovial fluid. This should be mixed and allowed to stand one minute.

If a tight, ropy mass is formed surrounded by clear fluid, this is reported as good formation of mucin clot. A softer clot or shredded flakes represent less than normal clot formation, and clot formation is reported as fair or poor. The mucin clot formation and viscosity are usually parallel since both are dependent on the concentration of hyaluronic acid in the synovial fluid. As there is decreased concentration of hyaluronic acid in inflammatory, gouty, and rheumatoid arthritis, it would be anticipated that the mucin clot formation would be poor.

Chemical Examination

The glucose, protein, lactic acid dehydrogenase, and uric acid are measured by the same methods used for serum.

Glucose. Glucose in synovial fluid normally is approximately 90 percent of the blood glucose or about 10 mg/100 less than the blood glucose level. It is suggested that a serum glucose be determined at the same time as the joint fluid glucose level. It is important for optimal interpretation of the values that the patient has fasted for at least six hours. In infections, the glucose of the synovial fluid may be less than 30 mg or may be less than one-half the serum glucose.

Protein. The total protein of synovial fluid ranges from 1 to 3 g/dl, with an average of 2 g. This represents approximately 30 percent of the serum level. The protein is predominantly albumin. The level of protein increases in inflammatory conditions and correlates with the degree of inflammation. A level less than 5 g/dl is considered mildly inflammatory, and a level greater than 5 g/dl correlates with a severe inflammatory state. Septic arthritis may produce a protein level up to 7 g, while the protein level in rheumatoid arthritis may be between 4 and 7 g/dl. The electrophoretic pattern is similar to that found in the serum.

Lactic Acid Dehydrogenase. Lactic acid dehydrogenase is increased in synovial fluid in inflammatory conditions due to the increase in the metabolic activity of the white cells. This may also cause a decrease to less than 7.3 in the pH level. The decreased pH may be associated with a rapid change from aerobic to anaerobic metabolism in the synovial fluid. This determination is not considered a part of the routine examination of synovial fluid.

Uric Acid. The uric acid level is similar to the serum level. The uric acid is increased in gout. The increased serum uric acid in the patient with arthritic symptoms does not establish the diagnosis of gout as this may be secondary to another condition, for example, renal disease or side effects of therapy.

Alkaline phosphatase, acid phosphatase, bilirubin, and numerous enzyme levels have been determined in synovial fluid. These levels appear to be very similar to levels found in the serum.

Rheumatoid Factor (RF)

Rheumatoid factor RF is antibody to immunoglobulins. These antibodies are immunoglobins and may be composed of IgM, IgG, IgA, IgD, or IgE classes. The significance of their presence is not always specific for rheumatoid arthritis, and they may be found in normal and infectious states, hepatitis, and systematic lupus erythematosus. Approximately 90 percent of adult patients with rheumatoid arthritis show the RF, but young patients with rheumatoid arthritis do not show the RF. The titer is lower in synovial fluid than in serum, but it is usually present in both. The gamma globulin is less in synovial fluid, thus accounting for the lower level of RF. However, the synovial fluid may be positive for RF and the serum negative if the RF is being produced by the joint tissues. The test for RF is a slide test using latex particles and is available in commercial kits.

Complement

Measurement of complement may furnish useful information, but it is not a part of the routine examination of synovial fluid. The total hemolytic complement (CH50) and C4 have been measured. The level correlates with the protein and is decreased in more than half of rheumatoid arthritic patients who also show the rheumatoid factor. It may be decreased in negative RF patients as well. Low levels of complement in fluid are found in 60 percent of patients with systemic lupus erythematosus.

Antinuclear Antibody (ANA)

Antinuclear antibodies are found in 60 to 80 percent of patients with systemic lupus erythematosus. A small percentage of patients with rheumatoid arthritis have antinuclear antibodies.

Microbiologic Examination

Any specimen submitted for microbiologic examination should be cultured as soon as possible on the media of choice for aerobic, anaerobic, and acid-fast bacilli, and fungal culture. The recommended media for cultures of all body fluids is found in Chapter 13. A smear is examined with gram stain and acid-fast stain. Although most synovial fluids are sterile, approximately 50 percent of the specimens from septic joint disease show a positive gram stain. Septic arthritis is the most frequently diagnosed problem that produces growth on the culture media. *Neisseria gonorrhoeae*, which causes gonococcal arthritis, is the most common organism grown. Tuberculosis of the joint should be suspected when the causative agent cannot be determined for septic arthritis. Sickle cell anemia patients are especially prone to *Salmonella* infections in the joints.

Cell Counts

The cell count of synovial fluid furnishes a valuable point of reference for the clinician. Rheumatoid diseases have been classified in a number of ways. The white cell count helps the clinician separate the degree of inflammation.

- Group I: normal or noninflammatory
- Group II: mildly inflammatory
- Group III: inflammatory or septic
- Group IV: hemorrhagic

The groupings of synovial fluids is arbitrary. The patient's clinical picture and his immunologic response to challenge are of primary importance. While the grouping may be suggestive of different disease states, it cannot be considered unequivocal. (See Table 11.1.)

TABLE 11.1. CHARACTERISTICS OF SYNOVIAL FLUID

Group	Visual	Viscosity	Mucin	Cell Count	Suggestive of
I	Colorless or straw, clear	High	Good	<200 μl	Normal, trauma degenerative joint diseases
II	Yellow and slightly cloudy	Decreased	Poor	200-2,000 μl	Rheumatoid arthritis, gout, systemic arthritis, lupus erythematosus
III	White, gray, yellow, green, cloudy	Absent	Poor	>100,000 μl	Infectious
IV	Bloody, red, brown	Absent	Poor	RBC and WBC	Trauma, hemophilia, pigmented villo-nodular synovitis

From Rodman G: *Primer on the Rheumatic Diseases*, 7th ed, 1973, p 141. Courtesy of the Arthritis Foundation.

The necessary dilution may be estimated from the visual examination or by preparing a wet preparation by placing a drop on a slide and coversliping it .A specimen with a low count may be put directly on the counting chamber and counted. For higher counts, although the specimen has probably been heparinized, dilution should be made using normal saline as for a manual white blood cell count. This is a 1:20 dilution. If the count is very high, > 50,000, it is more accurate to dilute in a red blood cell pipette with normal saline. Draw saline into the pipette and expel. Draw fluid up to the 1.0 mark of the RBC pipette and fill it to the 101 mark. This gives a dilution of 1:100. The specimen may be diluted with Isoton and lyzed with Zapoglobin. The use of the customary WBC diluting fluid must be avoided as a clot will be formed by the introduction of acid and obviate an accurate count.

Preparation for Staining

A synovial fluid with a normal cell count may be spun down without diluting. A slightly cloudy or hemorrhagic specimen must be diluted 1:1, 1:2, or 1:3 to attain the desirable separation of cells on either a cytospin or a centrifuged specimen and smear made from the centrifuged specimen. The cells in all body fluids tend to group, cluster, and round up. Dilution aids in separating the individual cells.

Gram Stain. The bacteria or fungus will appear as from any other source. Gram stains are positive in approximately 50 percent of joint sepsis samples. The white blood cells are frequently hypersegmented and do not appear to have as firm a cellular membrane as in peripheral blood. This relates to the fluid media and frequently reflects increased activity of the white cells. In inflammatory states, the viscosity will be decreased, and the degree of cloudiness directly correlates with the amount of inflammation (white cell count).

Wright Stain. The synovial fluid slide preparation is stained in the same manner as a peripheral blood film, and various cells will be observed.

Polymorphonuclear leukocytes are seen in the normal state as less than 25 percent of the 100 cell differential. The percentage of polymorphonuclear leukocytes is increased in inflammation and may be as high as 95 percent in septic arthritis. There may also be a shift to the left in extremely high counts. Nonseptic arthritis may show up to 75 percent polymorphonuclear leukocytes. Normal lymphocytes and normal monocytes make up the rest of the 100 cells.

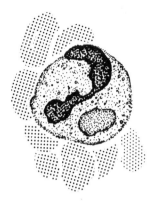

Figure 11.1. Ragocyte.

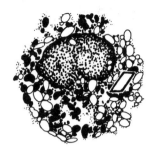

Figure 11.3. Macrophage with hemosiderin.

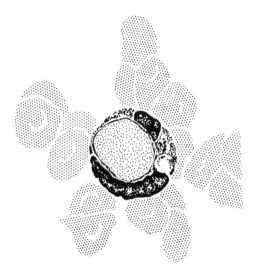

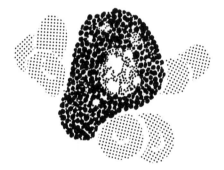

Figure 11.4. Mast cell.

Figure 11.2. Lupus erythematosus cell.

Ragocytes or RA cells (Fig. 11.1) are polymorphonuclear leukocytes that contain round inclusions that stain gray or very dark grayish purple. These inclusions contain immunoglobulins and are seen in rheumatoid arthritis. Ragocytes may be identified using phase microscopy and by immunofluorescent techniques and are shown to consist of immune complexes, IgG, IgM, complement, and rheumatoid factor.

Lupus erythematosus (LE) cells (Fig. 11.2) are polymorphonuclear leukocytes that have phagocytized nuclear material that has lost its basophilia. The nucleus of the phagocytized

polymorphonuclear leukocyte becomes the margin of the cell, encircling a pink, smooth button of nuclear material that occupies most of the cell. The LE cell may appear in synovial fluid.

Macrophages may be seen in synovial fluid. They are large mononuclear cells with a great deal of lacy cytoplasm. Hemosiderin crystals may be seen when bleeding into the joint has occurred (Fig. 11.3). The detailed description and differentiation of crystals found in bleeding problems is found on page 242.

Mast cells (Fig. 11.4) are frequently seen in synovial fluid. The cells are larger than the average basophil. The basophilic granules are dense and encircle a round pink nucleus. The function of the mast cell is not well defined. It has been suggested that the heparin produced by these cells is necessary in the production of hyaluronic acid.

Synovial cells may be seen in some specimens. The synovium is a large tissue space lined with a layer of specialized fibroblasts that differ from the mesothelium that lines other body cavities. These cells may be classified as synovial type A, B, or C (intermediate) cells. They differ greatly ultrastructurally on transmission electron microscopy. The three types of synovial cells also differ in their metabolic function:

1. Synovial cell type A (Fig. 11.5) has prominent Golgi complex, numerous vacuoles and lysozomes, and very little rough endoplasmic reticulum. They are primarily phagocytic scavenger cells. Synovial cell type A is the predominant cell seen.

2. Synovial cell type B (Fig. 11.6) is rich in rough endoplasmic reticulum, has very scant vacuoles, and little Golgi complex. B types may be concerned with production of immunoglobulin, but their true function is unclear.

3. Synovial cell type C has some of the characteristics ultrastructurally of both types A and B.

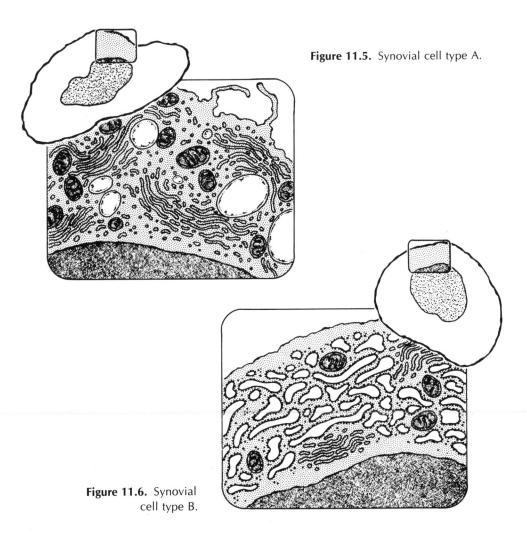

Figure 11.5. Synovial cell type A.

Figure 11.6. Synovial cell type B.

It is established that all three types of synovial cells have cytoplasmic processes. When present in a fluid medium, the cells tend to round up. This gives a much smoother appearance to the surface membrane. It is not possible to separate these cells as synovial cells A, B, or C by light microscopy. The synovial cells are much larger than white blood cells. They vary in size, and the cytoplasm may show a very intense dark blue stain. Nucleoli may be present. These cells may strongly resemble the mesothelial cells seen in pleural fluid.

In the microscopic evaluation of the Wright stain of synovial fluid, some crystal formations may be observed. The appearance of the different crystals is described on page 261.

Other Microscopic Features. The appearance of malignant cells in a synovial fluid examination is extremely rare. One important diagnostic feature of a fluid containing malignant cells is that the fluid is dark and serosanguineous. If other studies or clinical findings have revealed information indicating neoplasm, the specimen should be submitted for sectioned cytologic studies. The most common lesion, pigmented villonodular synovitis, shows a characteristic histologic pattern of dense infiltration with lymphocytes, giant cells, areas of hemorrhage, lipid-laden macrophages, and synovial cell proliferation. Related to villonodular synovitis is a common tendon sheath tumor giant cell or xanthoma. Xanthomas are tumors characterized by collections of foamy histocytes.

Blast cells from leukemic infiltrates and Sézary cells may occasionally be seen.

Wet Preparations for Crystals

For the microscopic examination for the presence of crystals, a drop of well-mixed synovial fluid is placed on a slide, and a coverslip is placed over the drop of fluid. The fluid should barely reach the edge of the coverslip. The coverslip is then rimmed with clear nail polish and allowed to dry. The preparation may be viewed under light microscopy and polarized light microscopy (Table 11.2). Polarized light microscopy is preferred, since the margins of the crystals are much more distinct and the visual characteristics of the crystals are enhanced. The term "birefringence" is used to describe a visual characteristic of crystals. Birefringence is defined as the refraction of light in two slightly different directions to form two rays. The different crystals will show weak or strong birefringence with polarized light and negative or positive birefringence with compensated polarized light.

Polarized microscopy uses an ordinary microscope with two polarizing prisms of filters added. A polarizing filter (the polarizer) is placed between the light source and the condenser. A second filter (the analyzer) is placed between the eyepieces and the objectives. The polarizer causes the light to vibrate in a definite pattern. The analyzer extinguishes the rays of polarized light. The polarizer passes light in only one plane. When the polarizer and the analyzer are at a 90-degree angle to each other, no light passes and the field is dark. When the light passes through the crystal, it will appear white on a black background. If the crystal appears very bright, it is strongly birefringent. If it is dim, it is weakly birefringent.

Compensated polarized light microscopy is accomplished by using a first-order red compensator. The compensator is placed between the polarizer and the analyzer. The compensator may be prepared by placing two pieces of transparent tape lengthwise on a glass slide. The compensator is then placed over the polarizer. The light source provides light consisting of elements having phases of vibration perpendicular to its direction of travel. With the addition of the first-order red compensator the red light is retarded, and the background is red instead of black. The slide is rotated so that the long axis of the crystal is parallel to the axis of slow vibration of the compensator. The slide is placed over the polarizer and rotated until the red color is seen. The crystals in the specimen are lined up to make the axis of the crystal parallel to the transparent tape slide.

TABLE 11.2. CRYSTALS SEEN IN SYNOVIAL FLUID

Type of Crystal	Light Microscopy	Polarized Light	Compensated Polarized Light	Associated with
Monosodium urate	Needlelike 1-20 μ	Strongly birefringent	Yellow, negative birefringence: rotate 90° turns blue	Gout
Calcium pyrophosphate	Rod, rhomboid, or plates	Weakly birefringent	Blue, positive birefringence: rotate 90° turns yellow	Pseudogout or chrondocalcinosis
Corticosteroid	Needle-shaped	Varies according to steroid		Intraarticular injections
Cholesterol	Notched crystals or plates	Strongly birefringent		Chronic effusion, osteo- or rheumatoid arthritis
Apatite	Small chunks or rods	Strongly birefringent		Calcific periarthritis, osteo- or inflammatory arthritis

Both *urate crystals and calcium pyrophosphate crystals* may be seen on light microscopy, but the differentiation of these two crystals is best seen by using the polarizer and the compensator. The urate crystal is seen under dimmed light but is seen clearly as a strongly birefringent needlelike crystal with polarized light. The rhomboid-shaped calcium pyrophosphate crystal is seen more easily on light microscopy than the urate crystal, but with polarized light it is seen less clearly and is considered weakly birefringent. By using the first-order red compensator the crystals may be easily differentiated. When the crystals are lined up so that the axis of the crystal is parallel to the transparent tape, the urate crystal will be yellow. When the red filter is placed perpendicular to the tape, the crystal will be blue. The calcium pyrophosphate will be blue when the axis is parallel and yellow when perpendicular to the compensator. The urate crystals are then described as showing negative birefringence, and the calcium pyrophosphate crystals are positively birefringent. Other birefringent material may be present in synovial fluid. The symmetry of the crystals is an important observation. The extraneous material may be jagged, and sides may not be parallel.

Calcium pyrophosphate crystals (Fig. 11.7) are rod or rhomboid-shaped crystals and may also appear as plates. On light microscopy there appears to be a line running through the middle of the crystal. These crystals are weakly birefringent when viewed under polarized light and positively birefringent under compensated polarized light. In contrast to urate crystals, the calcium pyrophosphate crystals are broader and may be seen up to 25 μ long. Eighty percent of the crystals may be intracellular and may be seen easily on light microscopy using a slightly dimmed light source. These crystals are frequently seen in pseudogout and chrondocalcinosis. The uric acid level of the serum and synovial fluid is normal when calcium pyrophosphate crystals are present.

Monosodium urate monohydrate crystals (Fig. 11.7), commonly called urate crystals, are clear needlelike crystals that may vary from 1 to 20 μ but are usually 8 to 10 μ in length. Urate crystals are water soluble, and if a large amount of anesthetic agent is used with the aspiration of the synovial fluid, the crystals may be dissolved. The crystals may be arranged in small compact clusters. Deposits of the urate crystals in the skin are called tophi. Urate crystals are strongly birefringent

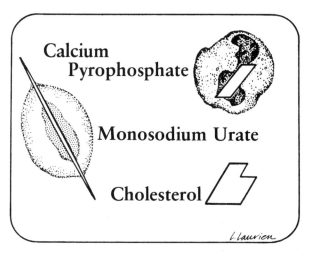

Figure 11.7. Composite of monosodium urate monohydrate, calcium pyrophosphate, and cholesterol crystals.

with polarized light and negatively birefringent with compensated polarized light. In acute attacks of gout, 90 percent of the urate crystals are within the polymorphonuclear leukocytes and macrophages. The report, therefore, should include whether the crystals are intracellular, since acute attacks of gout are unlikely to occur without the presence of intracellular crystals. The number of intracellular crystals decreases as the inflammation decreases.

Cholesterol crystals (Fig. 11.7) appear as notched crystals or plates and are found in turbid, thick, white, or yellow fluids. They are not found intracellularly. These crystals may be seen in synovial fluid from any chronic effusion, osteoarthritis, or rheumatoid arthritis. These are not specific and may be caused by the destructive tissue process or as a result of an infection. Cholesterol crystals are strongly birefringent under polarized light.

Corticosteroid crystals are usually needle-shaped and may be present intracellularly in the leukocytes. Their appearance may vary because they usually result from intraarticular injections of steroid, and the various steroid preparations show different crystal formations. This also causes the birefringent pattern to vary. In order to be specific, it is important to know the patient's drug or treatment history, as the corticosteroid crystal may be confused with urate crystals. The corticosteroid crystals are not a causative agent of the patient's symptoms.

Apatite crystals (hydroxyapatite) may appear with polarized light as small positively birefringent chunks or rods and may be confused with small urate or pyrophosphate crystals. The individual crystals may be as small as 1μ in length. On Wright stain, purple-staining cytoplasmic inclusions or extracellular globules may suggest these crystals. On electron microscopy, these crystals are uniformly dense and may be packed in clumps or individually scattered. They may be seen in the synovial fluid mononuclear cells or in the vacuoles of the neutrophils on electron microscopy. The apatite crystals have been seen in calcific periarthritis, os-

teoarthritis, and acute inflammatory arthritis.

Other Particles. Fragments of cartilage and collagen fibrils may both be present in osteoarthritis. The collagen varies from 2 to 100 μ in length and may resemble urate crystals. The collagen shows no birefringence with polarized light, while the cartilage fragments are strongly birefringent.

Talcum crystals may be seen in synovial fluid specimens as contaminants from gloves worn while obtaining the specimen. With polarized light, the talcum may appear as maltese crosses. Lipid droplets that also appear as maltese crosses may be seen in chronic inflammation or traumatic arthritis.

Review Questions

Select the one best answer for each of the following questions.

1. The laboratory report of a synovial fluid analysis follows:

Character:	white and cloudy
Viscosity:	decreased
Mucin clot formation:	poor
Cell count:	
RBC:	5/mm³
WBC:	57,000/µl
Differential:	
Polymorphonu- clear leukocytes:	79%
Lymphocytes:	16%
Eosinophils:	2%
Basophils:	1%
Macrophages:	2%
LDH (normal 100–200 µ/ml):	220
Protein (normal 1–3 g/100 ml):	5 g/100 ml
Glucose:100 ml):	56 mg/100 ml
Uric acid (normal 4.4–8.8 mg/100 ml):	4.0
Serum glucose:	130 mg/100 ml

These findings would be most consistent with:

A. An infection of the joint
B. Degenerative joint disease
C. Rheumatoid arthritis
D. Gout
E. Lupus erythematosus

2. Dilution of a synovial fluid with an extremely high WBC count may be accomplished using:

A. Normal saline
B. WBC-diluting fluid
C. Hypertonic saline
D. Dilute alkali

3. A crystal described as negatively birefringent would appear as which of the following colors when the axis of the crystal is parallel to the red filter?

A. Red
B. Yellow
C. Blue
D. White

Directions: For each of the incomplete statements, one or more of the completions given is correct. Select:

A. If only 1, 2, and 3 are correct.
B. If only 1 and 3 are correct.
C. If only 2 and 4 are correct.
D. If only 4 is correct.
E. If all are correct.

4. Normal synovial fluid is a crystal clear viscous fluid that contains:

1. Mesothelial cells
2. Hylauronate
3. Crystals
4. Mucin

5. When testing for clot formation of synovial fluid, formation of a tight firm clot is dependent upon:

1. Acidification
2. Reduced viscosity
3. Hyaluronic acid
4. Lysozomal enzymes

6. Rheumatoid factor is:

1. Antigen
2. Antibody
3. Complement
4. Immunoglobulin

7. Rheumatoid factor may be present in:

1. Rheumatoid arthritis
2. Systemic lupus erythematosus
3. Infectious states
4. Normal individuals

8. A clear straw-colored fluid was aspirated from a painful knee joint. Viscosity was high with good mucin clot formation. The total WBC count was 186 μl. These results would be consistent with:

1. Normal joint fluid
2. Degenerative joint disease
3. Trauma
4. Rheumatoid arthritis

Directions: For the following questions, use the key below by answering:

A. If the phrase is associated with *1 only*
B. If the phrase is associated with *2 only*
C. If the phrase is associated with *both 1 and 2*
D. If the phrase is associated with *neither 1 nor 2*

    (1) Strongly birefringent
    (2) Weakly birefringent

_____ 9. Monosodium urate crystals
_____ 10. Corticosteriod crystals
_____ 11. Cholesterol crystals
_____ 12. Calcium pyrophosphate crystals

Directions: Match the one best answer in Column A with the appropriate illustration in Column B (Illustrations at right).

Column A

A. Monosodium urate crystals
B. Calcium pyrophosphate crystals
C. Mast cell
D. LE cell
E. RA cell
F. Cholesterol crystals

Column B

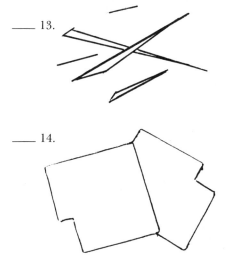

_____ 13.

_____ 14.

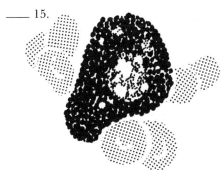

_____ 15.

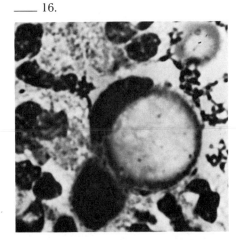

_____ 16.

Directions: Match the one best answer in Column B with the appropriate statement in Column A.

Column A
_____ 17. Chronic effusions
_____ 18. Gout
_____ 19. Pseudogout
_____ 20. Intraarticular injections

Column B
A. Monosodium urate crystals
B. Calcium pyrophosphate crystals
C. Corticosteroid crystals
D. Cholesterol crystals
E. Hydroxyapatite crystals

Case Study

A 28-year-old white male was hospitalized for bilateral knee pain and swelling of three days duration. He had no previous history of arthritis or rheumatic fever. His temperature was 101F. The physical examination revealed a papular rash and a urethral discharge. The complete blood count was as follows:

Characteristic	Finding
WBC:	22,000/mm^3
Hg:	14.5%
Differential:	
Polymorphonu- clear leukocytes:	75%
Bands:	8%
Metamyelocytes:	2%
Lymphocytes:	5%
Monocytes:	10%
Synovial fluid specimen showed	
Visual:	cloudy, slightly yellow
Viscosity:	decreased, less than 2 cm string
Mucin clot formation:	poor
Glucose:	35 mg/100 ml

Characteristic	Finding
Uric acid:	5 mg
Cell count:	125,000/mm³
Differential:	
Polymorphonu-clear leukocytes:	89%
Lymphocytes:	5%
Monocytes:	6%
Gram stain:	numerous WBC with intracellular and extracellular gram-negative diplococci present
Cultures:	aerobic and anaerobic cultures with sensitivity tests were done

Question

Abnormal findings in this report include the:

1. Glucose content
2. Mucin clot formation
3. Cell count
4. Viscosity
5. Differential

Answer: All are correct

Results

This is a typical case of the frequently diagnosed infectious arthritis caused by *Neisseria gonorrhea*.

BIBLIOGRAPHY

Brenenstock H: Arthritis: diagnostic guide. Hosp Med April 1980, pp 27–35.

Hoeprick PD, Ward JR: Synovial fluid. In The Fluids of the Parenteral Body Cavities. New York and London, Grune & Stratton, 1959, Chap 3, pp 31–49.

Germain B: Synovial Fluid Analysis in the Diagnosis of Diseases of the Joints. Upjohn—A Scope Publication, 1976.

Ghadially FN, Submal R: Normal Synovial Membrane. In Ultrastructure of Synovial Joints in Health and Disease. New York, Appleton, 1969, Chap 1.

Phelps P, Steele DA, McCarty DJ Jr: Compensated polarized light microscopy. JAMA 203:166, 1968.

Raphael SS: Collection and examination of specimens. In Lynch's Medical Laboratory Technology, 3rd ed. Philadelphia, Saunders, Chap 17, pp 657–678.

Rippey JH: Synovial fluid analysis. Lab Med 10:140, 1979.

Robbins SL, Cotran RS: Joints and related structures. In Pathologic Basis of Disease, 2nd ed. Philadelphia, WB Saunders, 1979, Chap 30, pp 1513–1517.

Rodman G: Primer on the Rheumatic Diseases, 7th ed. Distributed by the Arthritis Foundation, 475 Riverside Drive, New York, N.Y., 1973, pp 140–141.

Schumacker H, Smolyo AP, Tse RL, Maurer K: Arthritis associated with apatite crystals. Ann Intern Med 87:411, 1977.

Wilkins RW, Lavinsky NG: Joint and connective tissue. Medicine—Essentials of Clinical Practice, 2nd ed. Boston, Little, Brown, 1978, p 598.

Ann E. Neely and Kathryn Kilpatrick Cheek

CHAPTER 12

Analysis of Semen

Objectives

It is expected that the information presented in this chapter will enable the reader to:

1. Identify common reasons for the evaluation of semen.
2. Describe the composition of semen, including the etiology of the various components.
3. Identify hormones which influence the production of semen.
4. Describe the function of Sertoli cells, spermatogenic cells, and Leydig cells.
5. Identify the proper collection and transport techniques for semen.
6. List the major parameters reported in evaluation of semen.
7. Identify the normal values of semen.
8. Utilize reported values of a semen evaluation to assess possibilities of abnormalities that could result in those values.
9. Identify the reason for the initial coagulation with subsequent liquefaction of semen.
10. Describe how to perform a total sperm count.
11. Define azoospermia and oligospermia.
12. Identify causes of azoospermia.
13. Utilize blood hormone levels to differentiate among some of the causes of azoospermia.
14. Explain why it is necessary to perform repeat examinations when an abnormal semen analysis is reported.
15. List situations in which detection of semen may be important.
16. Describe types of specimens that may be submitted for detection of semen.
17. Identify how the detection of semen is accomplished.
18. Identify the usefulness of acid phosphatase levels in detection of semen.

The examination of semen is a laboratory procedure that is usually done in evaluation of infertility, vasectomy procedures, and possible rape victims. Diagnostic evaluation of the male partner in an infertile couple is the most common reason for examination of semen. It has been reported by various authors that up to 25 percent of all marriages produce no children or fewer children than desired, with the male partner being a contributing factor to the couple's infertility in approximately one quarter to one third of these couples. Examination of specimens in alleged rape victims is discussed on page 270.

FORMATION OF SEMEN

Semen is composed of products formed in the various male reproductive organs (Fig. 12.1). The spermatozoa are formed in the testis under the influences of testosterone,

LH, and FSH and stored in the vasa deferentia. The seminiferous tubules account for approximately 75 percent of the total testicular mass and are composed of Sertoli cells and spermatogenic cells. Sertoli cells facilitate the maturation of the spermatozoa. Leydig cells, found in the testis in the connective tissue between the seminiferous tubules, are responsible for production of plasma testosterone. The testis contribute the spermatozoa, which comprise approximately 5 to 7 percent of the total volume of semen.

Over one half of the volume of semen is produced in the seminal vesicles. This fraction provides nutritional components for the spermatozoa. Constituents include fructose, flavins, citric acid, and potassium.

The prostate contributes approximately 20 percent of the total volume of the semen. Its contributions include proteolytic enzymes, citric acid, and acid phosphatase. The epididymis, vasa deferentia, bulbourethral glands,

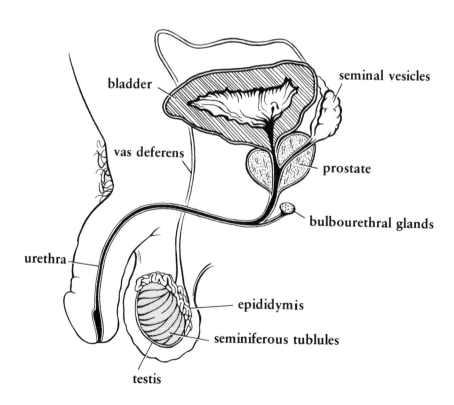

Figure 12.1. Male reproductive system.

and urethral glands contribute only a small portion to the total volume of semen.

SPECIMENS

Ideally, semen should be collected by masturbation after a three-day period of sexual abstinence. The specimen should be collected into a sterile container such as a sputum or urine collection cup. Condoms that contain lubricants or powder and are not sterile are unacceptable. The specimen should be analyzed within 30 minutes to one hour of collection. During transport to the laboratory, it is advisable to keep the specimen as near to body temperature as can be maintained. Avoidance of exposure to temperature extremes is mandatory.

Examination and Interpretation

The major parameters evaluated in the examination of semen are volume, liquefaction, pH, total WBC count, total sperm count, motility, and morphology. Normal values for these parameters are listed in Table 12.1.

The average volume of semen varies from 2 to 5 ml of fluid. Infertility may be associated with both increased and decreased total volume of semen. The pH of semen varies from 7.2 to 8.0, with abnormally low pHs seen in congenital aplasia of the vasa deferentia and seminal vesicles. Normally, no WBCs or an occasional WBC is seen during the performance of the total sperm count. Elevated numbers of WBCs strongly suggest infection within the reproductive tract.

The seminal specimen contains products that cause it to coagulate initially and then to liquefy within 20 minutes after collection. Coagulation results from enzymatic action of a fibrinogen-like precursor formed in the seminal vesicles. Liquefaction occurs as a result of enzymatic action of prostate enzymes. Therefore, coagulation may be abnormal if defects occur within the seminal vesicles, while liquefaction may be abnormal if abnormalities are present in the prostate.

Motility of spermatozoa can be evaluated by placing one drop of semen on a pre-warmed microscopic slide and covering it with a coverslip sealed with petroleum jelly. Examine with the high dry or 40× objective. One should focus, with the fine focus, through the field in order to visualize immobile spermatozoa that may settle to the lower portion of the visual field. Greater than or equal to 80 percent of the spermatozoa should exhibit forward progressive motility.

The morphology of spermatozoa can be evaluated by preparation of smears of semen on microscopic slides, which are then stained using either Papanicolaou stain, Wright-Giesma stain, or hematoxylin stain. Figure 12.2 demonstrates both the normal and abnormal morphology of spermatozoa that may be present. A normal specimen contains 80 to 90 percent normal morphologic forms.

The total sperm count is determined with the use of a Neubauer hemocytometer. A 1:20 dilution of the semen is prepared. Either commercial seminal fluid diluting fluid or a diluting fluid made by mixing 5 g of sodium bicarbonate and 1 ml of neutral formalin in 100 ml of distilled water should be used to make the dilution.

The counting chamber is loaded and allowed to settle for two minutes. The spermatozoa in two of the large 1 mm by 1 mm squares (total of 2 mm^2) are counted. This number is then multiplied by 100,000 to give the number of spermatozoa per milliliter. Normal total sperm counts range from 60 to 150 million/ml. If zero spermatozoa are seen, this is termed "azoospermia." If less than 20 million/ml spermatozoa are seen, this condition is called "oligospermia."

Some of the causes of azoospermia with resulting infertility include hyalinization of

TABLE 12.1. EXAMINATION OF SEMEN

Parameter	Normal Value
Volume	2-5 ml
Liquefaction	Complete in 20 minutes
pH	7.2-8.0
WBC	0-2/μl
Total spermatozoa count	60-150 million/ml
Motility	≥ 80½
Morphology	80-90% normal morphology

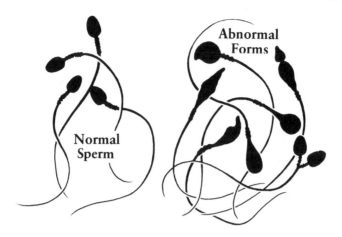

Figure 12.2. Normal and abnormal sperm.

the seminiferous tubules, Sertoli-cell-only syndrome, gonadotropin deficiency, ductal obstruction, maturation arrest, chromosomal disorders, radiation, drugs, renal failure, and pituitary and idiopathic causes. Table 12.2 demonstrates blood hormone levels that may be helpful in differentiating some of these conditions.

It is important that after an abnormal semen evaluation is reported a complete repeat examination of the semen be performed several times before a diagnosis is rendered. One reason for repeat evaluations is that the literature reports a wide variation in spermatozoa total counts even by experienced technologists performing repeat counts on the same specimen.

DETECTING PRESENCE OF SEMEN

Detection of the presence of semen may be important in medicolegal cases of alleged rape or sexual assault. Two types of samples are most helpful. The first of these is a direct smear and/or aspiration with a saline lavage of the contents of the vagina. The second type of specimen, a collection of portions of clothing, skin, or hair, is examined under ultraviolet light, since the flavin present in semen is fluorescent under these conditions. When clothing is obtained as a specimen, it is advantageous to obtain a portion of clothing that is apparently uninvolved with semen. This uninvolved clothing can then be proc-

TABLE 12.2. HORMONE LEVELS IN VARIOUS CAUSES OF AZOOSPERMIA

	Plasma Testosterone	Serum LH	Serum FSH
Hyalinization of seminiferous tubules	↓ to →	↑	↑
Sertoli-cell-only syndrome	→	→	↑
Gonadotropin deficiency	↓	↓	↓
Ductal obstruction or maturation arrest	→	→	→

→ normal, ↑ increased, ↓ decreased.

essed as a negative control. The clothing is usually soaked in isotonic saline for one hour, and the fluid used for soaking can be utilized for additional studies.

The establishment of the presence of semen can be accomplished by (1) demonstration of spermatozoa on Papanicolaou smears made from direct vaginal aspirates or washings from clothings or (2) by demonstrating elevated acid phosphatase on vaginal aspirates or washings from clothing. The use of acid phosphatase levels is more sensitive for the detection of semen than is microscopic identification of the presence of spermatozoa.

Review Questions

Select the one best answer for each of the following questions.

1. Flavins that cause semen to fluoresce under ultraviolet light are thought to be produced in the:
   A. Seminiferous tubules
   B. Testis
   C. Epididymis
   D. Seminal vesicles
   E. Prostate

2. The cell type responsible for the production of plasma testosterone is:
   A. Spermatogenic cells
   B. Leydig cells
   C. Spermatozoa
   D. Sertoli cells

3. A semen analysis appears below. This report would be consistent with:
   A. Normal semen
   B. Azoospermia
   C. Gonadotropin deficiency
   D. Oligospermia
   E. Ductal obstruction

Characteristic	Finding
Total spermatozoa count:	60 million/ml
Total WBC count:	2 WBC/μl
Motility:	80% motility
Morphology:	80% normal morphology
pH:	8.0
Liquefaction:	Complete within 15 minutes
Total volume:	2 ml

4. In azoospermia caused by gonadotropin deficiency, with which of the following hormones would we expect to see an elevated blood level of:
   A. Plasma testosterone
   B. Serum FSH
   C. Serum LH
   D. None of the above

Directions: For each of the incomplete statements, one or more of the completions given is correct. Select:
A. If only 1, 2, and 3 are correct.
B. If only 1 and 3 are correct.
C. If only 2 and 4 are correct.
D. If only 4 is correct.
E. If all are correct.

5. The following male reproductive organs contribute to the formation of semen:
   1. Testis
   2. Prostate
   3. Bulbourethral glands
   4. Seminal vesicles

6. Spermatozoa are formed in the testis under the influence of:
   1. Testosterone
   2. LH
   3. FSH
   4. Growth hormone

7. Semen may be collected for examination in:
   1. An over-the-counter condom
   2. A sterile urine cup
   3. A hand-washed jelly jar
   4. A sputum collection cup

8. Acid phosphatase determination of vaginal fluid and soiled clothing of alleged rape victims are useful because:
   1. Elevated levels are indicative of the presence of semen
   2. Acid phosphatase levels are more sensitive indicators than the microscopic identification of the presence of spermatozoa

3. Acid phosphatase is produced in the prostate
4. Levels may be determined from washings of portions of the victim's clothing

Directions: Match the items in Column A with the appropriate source or location in Column B. Answers from Column B may be used more than once.

Column A

_____ 9. Sertoli cell
_____ 10. Fructose
_____ 11. Testosterone
_____ 12. Acid phosphatase
_____ 13. Fibrinogen-like precursor
_____ 14. Proteolytic enzymes
_____ 15. Liquefaction

Column B

A. Prostate
B. Seminal vesicles
C. Tests

Case Study

A 35-year-old white male submitted a sample of his semen collected after three days of sexual abstinence. The sample in a sterile cup was delivered to the lab within 30 minutes after collection. This man had been married for six years. The couple desired children; however, during their six years of marriage had had none. The wife had one child by a previous marriage. A report of the patient's semen evaluation follows:

Characteristic	Finding
Time collected:	9:10 AM
Time received in laboratory:	9:35 AM
Date:	10-22-81
Total volume:	3.2 ml
pH:	8.0
Total WBC count/μl:	0

Total spermatozoa count:	55,000,000/ml
Motility:	80% motility
Morphology:	95% normal morphology
Liquefaction:	Complete in 15 minutes

Question

In view of the findings of this semen analysis one can say that the male patient:
1. Is probably the reason for this couple's failure to have children
2. Is sterile
3. Deserves a repeat examination
4. And his wife both need repeat physical examinations
5. Is fertile and it is not clear why this couple has failed to have children

Answer: 3

This case illustrates the most common reason that an evaluation of semen is requested which is a case of infertility. In view of this examination a repeat examination was requested in the infertility workup of this couple.

BIBLIOGRAPHY

Freund M, Carol B: Factors affecting haemocytometer counts of sperm concentration in human semen. J Reprod Fertil 8:149, 1964.
Isselbacher KJ, Adams RD, Braunwald E, Petersdorf RG, Wilson J (eds): Harrison's Principles of Internal Medicine, 9th ed. New York, McGraw-Hill, 1980.
Harvey AM, Johns RJ, McKusick VA, Owens AH, Ross RS (eds): The Principles and Practice of Medicine, 20th ed. New York, Appleton, 1980.
Macleod J: The semen examination. Clin Obstet Gynecol 8:115, 1965.
Macleod J, Wang Y: Male fertility potential in terms of semen quality: a review of the past, a study of the present. Fertil Steril 31:103, 1979.
Marmar J, Prass DE, DeBenedictis TJ: An estimate of the fertility potential of the fractions of the split ejaculate in terms of the motile sperm count. Fertil Steril 32:202, 1979.
Schumann GB, Badaway S, Peglon A, Henry JB: Prostatic acid phosphatase. Current assessment in vaginal fluid of alleged rape victims. Am J Clin Pathol 66:944, 1976.

Ann E. Neely and Kathryn Kilpatrick Cheek

CHAPTER 13

Transudates and Exudates

Objectives

It is expected that the information presented in this chapter will enable the reader to:

1. Describe the pericardium, pleura, and peritoneum.
2. Identify three basic processes resulting in effusions of serous cavities.
3. Define effusion, transudate, exudate, edema, anasarca, serous, serosanguineous, ascites, thoracentesis.
4. Differentiate a transudate from an exudate.
5. Identify why careful study of an effusion can be of considerable diagnostic value.
6. Identify disease states that may cause exudates.
7. Identify disease states that may cause transudates.
8. Identify critical considerations in the collection and processing of serous effusions.
9. Recognize synonyms of various body fluids.
10. Determine if a specimen is the result of a traumatic tap or if it represents a hemorrhagic specimen.
11. Use the appropriate terms to describe the appearance of the specimen.
12. Explain the difference between chyle and pseudochyle.
13. Describe the normal appearance of pleural, pericardial, and peritoneal fluid.
14. Correlate total protein, LDH, amylase, cholesterol, and glucose determinations with abnormal states.
15. Describe microbiologic techniques used for identification of bacterial and fungal causative agents of effusions.

The cavities of the human body that contain the heart, lungs, and abdominal organs are lined with a thin layer of connective tissue that forms a sac around the organs. Each sac is lined with cells of mesodermal origin called "mesothelial cells." The sac which contains the heart is the *pericardium*, that which contains the lungs is called the *pleura*, and that which contains the abdominal organs is called the *peritoneum*.

The potential space between the sac and the organ is normally separated by a small amount of fluid, an amount that varies among the cavities. The pericardial cavity normally contains 20 to 50 ml of fluid, which is known as *pericardiocentesis fluid* and fluid from around the heart. The pleural cavity normally contains 30 ml or less of fluid, which is known as *thoracenteseis fluid*, thoracic fluid, and chest fluid. The peritoneal cavity contains less than 100 ml of fluid, which is known as *ascites* and ascitic fluid. Because these fluids resemble serum, they may be referred to as *serous fluid*.

The term *serosanguineous* is frequently used also and refers to a specimen that contains both serum and blood. This term is of pathologic significance. When pathologic conditions cause fluid to accumulate in the potential space between sac and organ, the increased amount of fluid is referred to as an *effusion*.

The accumulation of the fluid is described clinically with specific terms. *Edema* denotes an excessively large amount of fluid in the intercellular tissue spaces of the body, while *anasarca* is used to describe generalized massive edema in all parts of the body. If pus has accumulated in a cavity of the body, it is called *empyema*. This is found often in pleural fluid, when it is called *pyothorax*. In contrast, when air has gained access to the pleural cavity, the term *pneumothorax* is used.

Two similar terms will be used on submitted specimen requests. *Thoracentesis* (thoraco: relationship to chest) is in reference to the surgical puncture of the chest wall for drainage. This is the same as paracentesis when performed on the chest, but the term *paracentesis* is defined as the surgical puncture of any cavity for the aspiration of fluid.

SPECIMEN COLLECTING AND PROCESSING

Fluids from body cavities must be collected in containers that have been cleaned with detergent and further cleaned with alcohol and xylol to remove detergent residue. It is important that an adequate amount of fluid be collected, 300 to 1,000 ml of sample. The more adequate the specimen in relation to volume, the better the sampling for pathologic determinations. For the specimen to be representative, 10 to 15 ml (one or two full test tubes) of well-mixed fluid should be submitted for pathologic determinations. Precautions are taken by the clinician to not take more than 1,200 to 1,500 ml of pleural fluid at one time as vascular collapse and mediastinal shift may occur. Pericardial fluid aspiration requires special precautions to prevent perforation of the heart and pneumothorax. Cardiac arrhythmias, especially venticular fibrillation, are also a possible complication in pericardial fluid aspiration.

Since the fluid may contain a large amount of protein, heparin should be added to prevent clotting. Fluids should be sent immediately to the laboratory to avoid cellular degeneration. If the specimen cannot be examined immediately, it should be refrigerated until it can be processed. Fixatives should not be added to the refrigerated specimen because alcohol hardens cells into a spherical shape, and formalin will cause clumping of nuclear chromatin, obscuring nuclear detail.

BASIC ETIOLOGY OF EFFUSION

The small amount of fluid that is normally present within the body cavities serves to lubricate organ movement. The amount of fluid present is maintained by an equilibrium between the fluid and particulate substances of the capillary blood vessels and the lymphatic vessels. This delicate equilibrium may be compromised by any process which obstructs the flow of fluids, alters the pressure present in the vessels, or alters the constituents present in the vessels.

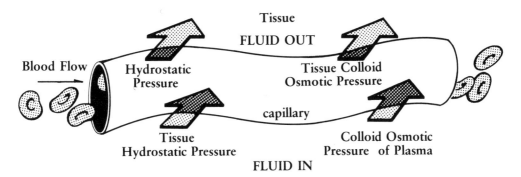

Figure 13.1. Diagram of a capillary.

Figure 13.1 demonstrates the flow of fluid through the walls of a capillary. Blood is flowing through the vessel. Two forces that may contribute to the outward flow of fluid from the capillary are (1) the tissue colloid osmotic pressure resulting from the protein present in the interstitial space and (2) the hydrostatic pressure within the capillary. Forces that contribute to the inward flow into the capillary include the (3) capillary colloid which results from protein present in the blood, (4) osmotic pressure of plasma, and (5) the tissue hydrostatic pressure present within the tissue.

Alterations in the balance of the flow of fluids result in the formation of *effusions.* Processes that alter the forces that control the flow of fluid include inflammation, circulatory disturbances, and neoplasms. An effusion composed of numerous cells (greater than 300/mm³ but usually over 1,000/mm³) and greater than 3 g/100 mm³ protein is called an *exudate.* An effusion composed of fewer than 300 cells/ml and protein less than 3 g/100 ml is referred to as a *transudate.* The white cell count and differential count seen in normal fluids is shown in Table 13.1.

The most frequently encountered causes of a transudate are seen in congestive heart failure, hepatic disease, renal disease, and pulmonary infarction. Exudates may be the result of inflammation, as seen in tuberculosis or bacterial, viral, or parasitic infections. Neoplasms, such as leukemia, lymphoma, metastatic carcinoma, and carcinoma, may also cause formation of exudates. Trauma, rheumatoid arthritis, lupus erythematosus, pancreatis, and asbestosis may exhibit exudates.

MAJOR DIFFERENTIATION OF EXUDATES AND TRANSUDATES

Since the etiology of an effusion determines the effusion's character and composition, careful study of an effusion can be of considerable diagnostic value. Table 13.2 summarizes the major differences between transudates and exudates.

TABLE 13.1. NORMAL CELLULAR CONTENT OF BODY FLUIDS

Type of Fluid	Normal Amount	White Cell Count	Differential
Spinal	—	0-8 /mm³	Lymphocytes, monocytes
Synovial fluid	1-4 ml	200 /mm³	Polymorphonuclear leucocytes < 25%
Pleural fluid	30 ml	300 /mm³	Lymphocytes
Peritoneal fluid	100 ml	300 /mm³	Polymorphonuclear leukocytes < 25%
Pericardial fluid	20-50 ml	300 /mm³	Few macrophages

TABLE 13.2. DIFFERENTIATION OF EXUDATES AND TRANSUDATES

	Exudate	Transudate

Causes	Inflammatory (80-90%)
	Infections; inflammatory or neoplastic
	   processes that cause injury to capillary
	   walls
		Noninflammatory (80-90%)
		↓ in oncotic pressure of
		   plasma
		↑ in hydrostatic pressure in
		   pleural capillaries
		↓ in intrapleural pressure

Condition	Infections Neoplasms	Congestive heart failure Edematous renal disease (retention of salt and water) Cirrhosis of liver Malnutrition
Specific gravity*	> 1.015	< 1.015
Protein	> 3.0 g/100 ml	< 3.0 g/100 ml
WBC	> 1,000/μl	< 300/μl

Differential	> 25% PMN in bacterial inflammations
	Lymphocytes and approximately 5%
	   mesothelial cells predominate in many
	   noninflammatory conditions
	Lymphocytes and very few mesothelial
	   cells with counts > 1000/mm³ in
	   tuberculosis
	PMN, lymphocytes, and numerous
	   mesothelial cells in pulmonary
	   infarction
	Eosinophilia may be nonspecific in
	   chronic process, or from multiple
	   thoracentesis
	Malignant cells
		Lymphocytes and 25% PMN,
		   few macrophages

Fibrinogen†	Enough to cause clotting	None

* May be eliminated if protein determination is available
† Leakage across damaged capillaries

EXAMINATION OF BODY FLUIDS

Visual Examination

Pleural, pericardial, and peritoneal fluids are normally clear, pale, yellow liquids. The clarity or turbidity particularly of the exudates is dependent on the content of the fluid. It is important to remember that in the normal state there is less than 30 ml of pleural fluid, less than 50 ml of pericardial fluid, and less than 100 ml of peritoneal fluid and pathologic changes within the body directly influence the amount, composition, and character of effusions within these cavities.

Sanguineous or *serosanguineous* fluids are hemorrhagic (blood or blood-tinged) speci-mens. When a specimen appears bloody, additional tubes of specimen should be collected. If clearing of blood occurs in the additional samples, a traumatic tap should be suspected. Sixty percent of grossly hemorrhagic specimens that do not clear with subsequent tube collections are due to malignancy. This sanguineous appearance along with an increase in LDH is strong evidence of a malignancy. The diagnosis of tuberculosis must also be considered when the fluid is hemorrhagic.

Purulent is the term used for a thick, white, turbid specimen. This is usually due to a large number of white blood cells present in specimens with an infectious etiology. Bacteria may be present extracellularly in the fluid or within the white blood cells.

A *milky* specimen may be a chylous or pseudochylous specimen. Chylous specimens can be caused by lymphatic obstruction of the thoracic duct caused by a tumor. Chyle is finely emulsified droplets of lipids and some lipoprotein. Effusions that remain in the body cavity for a long period of type may cause destruction of cellular lipids, giving rise to a pseudochylous effusion. Pesudochyle may be seen in effusions caused by tuberculosis and rheumatoid arthritis.

Shimmering is the term used to describe the golden greenish iridescent specimen that contains cholesterol and cholesterol crystals. These specimens have a low lipid content and may also be classified as pseudochylous. This type fluid will frequently contain cellular debris as well as the cholesterol crystals, giving a milky appearance. The color may vary from dark green to a yellowish gold to white depending on the amount of cholesterol crystals.

Fibrinous is the term used to describe a fluid that clots on standing due to increased fibrinogen. Clotting will be seen in exudates because of the passing of fibrinogen across damaged capillary walls.

Transudates have a specific gravity of less than 1.015 and appear very watery or thin. Exudates have a specific gravity greater than 1.015 and are thick. As the specific gravity is dependent on protein content, it is more accurate to separate the transudate and exudate by protein determination.

Chemical Examination

The methodology for the determination of most of the chemical examination in body fluids is the same as for serum. Most specimens will not require a complete chemical examination. The total protein, lactic acid dehydrogenase, and amylase are the most frequent tests requested.

Total Protein. The determination of total protein is the most useful test to separate exudates from transudates. More than 3.0 g/dl of protein is found in exudates, while less than 3.0 g/dl is seen in transudates. It may be necessary to dilute the effusion with isotonic saline if the specimen is thick.

Lactic Acid Dehydrogenase (LDH). The LDH is increased and is higher in body fluids than in serum in rheumatoid diseases, malignant tumor, nonmalignant tumor, and highly cellular fluids. The increase of LDH in cellular fluids may be high due to the release of LDH from the erythrocytes. A normal level is considered as evidence against a malignancy.

Amylase. The amylase level is considerably elevated in pancreatitis. It may be higher than the amylase level in the serum and will remain higher after the level in the serum is lowered. Amylase levels may also be increased in metastatic adenocarcinoma and effusions associated with esophageal perforation.

Glucose. Glucose levels in the various body fluids are normally equal to that of serum glucose. A decreased glucose level of approximately one-half serum level is suggestive of bacterial infection, malignancy, or rheumatoid arthritis. In an inflammatory process, the glucose will be reduced if there are sufficient bacteria present to utilize the glucose. A normal glucose level helps rule out tuberculosis.

Cholesterol. Cholesterol may appear as gold greenish flecks and be found with cellular debris. It is increased in chronic effusions, emphysema, rheumatoid disease, and old hemorrhagic effusions.

Chyle. A Sudanophilia dye (Sudan III) may be used to stain the lipid in the chylous fluids. The drop of fluid and dye are mixed and observed under the microscope for lipid droplets. The lipid droplets appear as maltese crosses under polarized light microscopy. The Sudan III staining method is described in Chapter 9. The creamy consistency in true chylous fluid clears and decreases in volume after extraction with ether and acidification with dilute HCl.

The pH of chylous fluid is alkaline, but the pH of pseudochylous fluid is variable. The cholesterol level of chylous effusions is lower than the serum level but may be higher than the serum level in pseudochylous effusions. Triglycerides may be higher than serum levels in chylous effusions, while in pseudochylous specimens the triglyceride level is lower than serum level. Lipoprotein electrophoresis may also help differentiate chylous from pseudochylous fluids. True chylous fluids show markedly elevated chylomicrons in comparison to normal plasma levels.

pH Determination. The pH of body fluids is usually 7.3 or greater. The pH is determined with a dipstick or any pH meter. The pH of body fluid may be determined after possible esophageal rupture has occurred. The pH would be acid from the contamination of gastric juices. Low values (7.2 or less) may be seen in tuberculosis and malignant effusions.

Chloride. The chloride level will be below blood levels if bacteria and white cells are present to utilize it.

Microbiologic Examination

The body fluid specimens are centrifuged for 10 minutes, and the supernatant fluid is discarded. The sediment is suspended in approximately 0.5 ml of the remaining fluid. If the specimen is purulent and very thick, it is processed without centrifugation. Routinely a gram stain and an acid-fast stain (Kinyoun, Ziehl-Neelsen, or fluorescent stain) are prepared. Cultures of the sediment are aseptically inoculated onto thioglycollate agar, sheep blood agar, MacConkey agar or eosin methylene blue agar, chocolate blood agar, and anaerobic sheep blood agar and incubated at 35C in CO_2.

Frequently, *Mycobacterium tuberculosis* is suspected in body fluids, and the sediment of the fluid is placed on 7 H 11 (Middlebrook) agar medium and Lowenstein-Jensen agar-egg medium and incubated at 37C in CO_2. The mycobacterium cultures are observed for six weeks. For fungal cultures, the sediment is placed on Sabouraud agar and mycosel agar at 25C and 37C and on brain-heart infusion agar with blood at 37C. These are kept for six weeks. Fungal stains and

preparations are done with India ink, potassium hydroxide, Giemsa stain, PAS, and methenamine silver.

Cultures of plate preparations may be discarded after 48 hours. If the patient has received antibiotic therapy, it may be advantageous to view the plate at the end of 72 hours instead of discarding at 48 hours. Broth cultures may be kept up to two weeks. The importance of the smear and culturing for *M. tuberculosis* in effusions cannot be overemphasized.

Infections with multiple organisms may be found. There is a strong correlation with gram stain observations and growth on culture media. A large percentage of body fluids will be sterile.

Microscopic Examination
Methodology for the microscopic examination of body fluids is discussed in Chapter 9. The cellular components of the fluids and characteristics of cells are discussed in Chapter 14.

Repeated examinations of fluids may be necessary before useful data are obtained from the microscopic examination. Varying factors in sampling techniques, freshness of specimen, techniques of preparation, and the mechanism of the cause of the effusion will alter the findings.

PLEURAL FLUID

Pleural fluid usually occurs first at the base of the lungs. The patient will experience a dull aching pain independent of respiration. This is in contrast to the sharp, stabbing sensation seen with the pleuritic pain of pleurisy that is intensified during full respiration. However, pleurisy may occur with a pleural effusion.

The efficiency of lymphatic drainage and the exchange of fluids in the capillary beds are the most important factors in the formation and removal of pleural fluid. When there is an increase in hydrostatic pressure and/or a decrease in oncotic pressure in the pulmonary capillaries, fluid accumulates in the pleural sac. A significant portion of the lymphatic drainage from the abdomen passes by way of the diaphragm, especially on the right. Therefore, a variety of inflammatory conditions within the abdomen or the presence of ascites may be accompanied by pleural fluid accumulating on the right. Pleural effusions are seen in 10 percent of patients with pancreatitis and 5 percent of patients with ascites.

Inflammation within the pleural sac causes an increase in capillary permeability. Cells and protein from the blood as well as fluid may be allowed to escape into the pleural sac. These inflammatory effusions may result from lesions within the mediastinum, diaphragm, or chest wall. Removal of this fluid may be retarded by inflammatory obstruction of the lymphatic channels draining the thorax.

When it is established that an increased amount of fluid, over 30 ml, is present in the pleural, a thoracentesis is performed by the physician. Removal of even a small amount of the fluid may produce marked improvement in symptoms. This not only provides the fluid for examination but the decrease of the effusion permits better radiologic visualization of the lungs. A minimum examination would consist of noting the gross appearance, total protein, lactic dehydrogenase (LDH) content, the determination of total cell count and differential count, and examination of the sediment with Wright stain.

Differentiation between Pleural Transudates and Exudates

To determine the etiology of the pleural effusion, it is necessary to determine if it is a transudate or exudate. In transudates the pleural surfaces are not directly involved by the pathologic process. Exudates are the result of inflammation or other disease processes of the pleural surfaces or from lymphatic obstruction.

In pleural fluid a protein level of 3.0 g/dl classically is used to separate transudates from exudates. About 90 percent of pleural exudates have a total protein greater than 3.0 g/dl, and about 80 percent of pleural transudates have a total protein less than 3.0 g/dl.

An alternative classification has been suggested (Light, 1972) based on these three ratios:

(1) $\dfrac{\text{Pleural fluid LDH}}{\text{Serum LDH}} > 0.6$ suggests exudates

(2) $\dfrac{\text{Pleural fluid protein}}{\text{Serum protein}} > 0.5$ suggests exudates

(3) Pleural fluid LDH > 200 IU suggests exudates

Over 95 percent of pleural exudates show at least one of these changes, while over 95 percent of pleural transudates show none of these findings.

It is possible for a pleural fluid to change from a transudate to an exudate, but the reverse is highly improbable. A congestive heart failure effusion with time and the use of diuretics may develop characteristics of an exudate. There is also a possibility that a new condition has developed.

Visual Examination

The most important observation to be made when examining pleural fluid is if the specimen is bloody or serosanguineous. If a specimen of pleural fluid is grossly bloody and if the patient has had no chest trauma, the chances that the patient has a malignancy are very strong, over 50 percent. If the red cell count is in excess of $100,000/\text{mm}^3$ and trauma and pulmonary infarction are excluded, malignancy is very possible. Other conditions that may show sanguineous pleural fluid are postmyocardial infarction, pulmonary infections, and occasionally tuberculosis. Hemothorax or blood in the pleural space may occur as a sequel to trauma. To distinguish a traumatic tap from a true hemothorax, hematocrit determinations on both the effusion and the capillary blood of the patient should be performed. The hematocrit determinations will be approximately equal in true hemothorax. The specimen may be blood tinged, with a red cell count below $10,000/\text{mm}^3$, in pulmonary embolism and congestive heart failure. This would not be enough blood to call the specimen sanguineous.

Chemical Examination

The *glucose* level in pleural fluid is decreased approximately one to three hours after the serum glucose level is decreased. The pleural fluid glucose levels may be moderately lower than the serum levels in such infections as tuberculosis and in tumors and may be below 12 mg/100 ml in rheumatoid arthritis.

The *LDH* in rheumatoid arthritis will be very high. The LDH will be increased in pleural fluid exudates from malignancies, particularly if malignant cells are found in the specimen.

An increase in *amylase* level may be seen in some malignancies, but the increase in amylase level is marked in pancreatic disease. This is much higher than is the simultaneously drawn serum level of amylase. When the specimen is sanguineous, the amylase level is higher than when the specimen is serous.

PERICARDIAL FLUID

Pericardial fluid is not as frequently removed as are pleural and peritoneal fluid. The diagnosis may be established by other clinical data, and if cardiac function is not impaired, the fluid may not be removed. The relief the patient may obtain is related to physical disorders and the rate at which the fluid has developed. Pericardiocentesis is a relatively dangerous procedure. When an infection or malignant process is suspected, it is necessary to obtain a specimen for culture and cytology.

On visual examination, pericardial fluid may be a clear, straw-colored fluid. The sanguineous pericardial fluid may be due to myocardial rupture following infarction, aortic rupture due to trauma or aneurysm, closed chest trauma, pneumonia, bacterial pericarditis, rheumatoid arthritis, or lupus erythematosus. Anticoagulation and malignancies will also produce bloody pericardial effusions. Hemopericardium may be separated from a traumatic tap by performing a hematocrit determination. The hematocrit results on the effusion and capillary blood will be the same in a hemopericardium. Chylopericardium is rare but is associated with chylothorax caused by a neoplastic process.

In pericardial fluid, the laboratory criteria for transudates are less clearly defined. Most pericardial effusions are caused by damage to mesothelial lining. Pericardial transudates and exudates cannot be reliably separated on the basis of their protein content.

PERITONEAL FLUID

Ascites or accumulation of fluid in the abdomen may be a specific clinical finding, or it may correlate with generalized edema. Chronic liver disease, tumors, nephrosis, congestive heart failure, peritonitis, and pancreatitis are the most frequent conditions in which ascites is present. In chronic liver disease, ascites represents an expansion of the extracellular compartment. A decreased serum albumin is evidence that there is an elevation of portal venous pressure and a decrease in the serum colloidal pressure. This reflects both the impaired protein synthesis by the liver and the dilutional effect of the marked expansion of plasma volume. There are also abnormalities in salt and water metabolism (Harvey et al., 1980, p 713).

Removal of fluid to establish contents of the peritoneal fluid is frequently performed. Hypovolemia and shock may result if a large amount, greater than 1,000 ml, is removed. Body albumin may be further depleted.

On the visual examination of peritoneal fluid, it is expected to be light yellow or straw-colored but may be green or bile stained. These green or bile-stained fluids are found with perforated duodenal ulcer, perforated intestines, perforated gallbladder, cholecystitis, and acute pancreatitis. Sanguineous peritoneal fluids may be seen in peritonitis, ruptured liver, ruptured spleen, tumors, and tuberculosis. Purulent fluids suggest peritonitis due to appendicitis, strangulated intestine, rupture following trauma, or a primary infection. Milky fluids are rare in the peritoneum. They may be obtained in thoracic blockage, tuberculosis, parasitic infections, adhesions, or hepatic cirrhosis.

In the chemical examination of peritoneal fluid, the separation point of transudate and exudate effusions by protein content is not the same as in other fluids. The reference level for peritoneal fluid is 2 g/dl, below 2 g/dl seen in a transudate and greater than 2 g/dl being seen in an exudate. For other fluids the reference point is 3 g/dl of protein. In addition to protein content, the amylase level is frequently requested. The amylase level in peritoneal fluid will be greatly increased in

pancreatitis and bowel necrosis.

Other determinations that are not done routinely are bilirubin determinations, ammonia level, and alkaline phosphatase determination. Bilirubin will be high in the green or amber specimen. The ammonia level will be increased in intestinal necrosis, perforated peptic ulcer, and perforated appendix. Alkaline phosphatase is increased in strangulation or perforation of the small intestine.

Table 13.3 summarizes the findings in peritoneal fluid that are suggestive of various disease states. This is an example of the benefits that may be derived from a complete examination of body fluid.

TABLE 13.3. PERITONEAL FLUID

Examination	Result	Suggested Diagnosis
Visual	Clear, straw-colored	Cirrhosis and nephrosis
	Thick, odoriferous, cloudy	Infection or ruptured viscus
	Milky	Ruptured lympatics, parasitic infections, tuberculosis, hepatic cirrhosis
	Green or bile stained	Perforated duodenal ulcer, perforated intestine, cholecystitis, perforated gallbladder
	Sanguineous	Tumor, tuberculosis, peritonitis, ruptured liver or spleen, pancreatitis
Microscopic Count	< 300 WBC/μl	Noninflammatory transudate, cirrhosis, congestive heart failure
	> 1,000 WBC/μl	Inflammatory
	> 100 RBC/μl	Tumor, traumatic tap, peritonitis, ruptured liver or spleen, tuberculosis
Cells	Bizarre cells, large nuclei	May be reactive mesothelial cells in chronic ascites
	Malignant cells	Tumors
Chemical		
Amylase	↑	Pancreatic ascites and bowel necrosis
Total protein	< 2 g/dl (transudate)	Cirrhosis, nephrosis
	> 2 g/dl (exudate)	Tumor, tuberculosis, infections
Ammonia	Increased	Intestinal necrosis
Alkaline phosphatase	Increased	Strangulation or perforation of small intestine
Microbiologic	Bacteria	Ruptured viscus, peritonitis, tuberculosis

Adapted from Maddrey WC: In Harvey AM, et al.: The Principles and Practice of Medicine, 20th ed. New York, Appleton-Century-Crofts, 1980, p 714.

Review Questions

Select the *one* best answer for each of the following questions.

1. The serous body cavities are lined with
   A. Squamous epithelial cells
   B. Endothelial cells
   C. Transitional cells
   D. Mesothelial cells
   E. White blood cells

2. A hematocrit determination was performed on capillary blood from a patient, and the value was determined to be 30%. A hematocrit test performed on the pleural fluid from the same patient was 29%. The blood in the pleural fluid represents:
   A. A hemothorax
   B. A traumatic tap
   C. A transudate
   D. An infection
   E. An obstructed lymph channel

3. A thick white turbid specimen was received in the laboratory labeled as pericardial fluid. A microscopic examination was performed, and the differential included 90% PMNs. The fluid would be described as:
   A. Serosanguineous
   B. Purulent
   C. Milky
   D. Shimmering
   E. Fibrinous

4. In a pleural effusion caused by *Streptococcus pneumoniae*, the glucose value of the pleural fluid as compared to the serum would probably be:
   A. Increased by 2
   B. Decreased by one half
   C. Increased by one half
   D. Equal
   E. Unpredictable

Directions: For each of the incomplete statements, one or more of the completions given is correct. Select:
A. If only *1, 2, and 3* are correct.
B. If only *1 and 3* are correct.
C. If only *2 and 4* are correct.
D. If only *4* is correct.
E. If *all* are correct.

5. Which of the following may cause a pleural effusion:
   1. Inflammation
   2. Neoplasm
   3. Chronic heart disease
   4. Trauma

6. Careful study of an effusion may be of considerable diagnostic value because:
   1. Inflammatory and noninflammatory conditions give effusions with different characteristics
   2. When fibrinogen is present in a specimen, one would expect the fluid to have a low specific gravity
   3. The etiology of an effusion determines its character and composition
   4. Fluids from infectious processes usually have decreased numbers of PMNs

7. Important considerations in the collection and processing of serous effusions include:
   1. An adequately cleaned container
   2. Immediate examination if possible
   3. Heparin addition if large amounts of protein are present
   4. Addition of formalin for preservation

8. The normal color of peritoneal fluid is:
   1. Green
   2. Pink
   3. Dark amber
   4. Yellow

Directions: Match the one best answer in Column B with the appropriate statement in Column A.

Column A
_____ 9. Fluid accumulation within a cavity
_____ 10. Generalized massive edema
_____ 11. Resembling serum
_____ 12. Fluid accumulation in the abdominal cavity

Column B

A. Effusion
B. Serosanguineous
C. Thoracentesis
D. Empyemia
E. Serous
F. Anasarca
G. Ascites

For questions 13 through 18, use the key below by answering:

A. If the phrase is associated with *1 only*
B. If the phrase is associated with *2 only*
C. If the phrase is associated with *both 1 and 2*
D. If the phrase is associated with *neither 1 nor 2*

　　　　　(1) Transudate
　　　　　(2) Exudate

13. Specific gravity of 1:007
14. An effusion
15. Ratio of pleural fluid protein to serum protein of 0.7
16. Renal failure
17. Tuberculosis
18. Lymphoma

Case Study

A 62-year-old female had weakness, shortness of breath, hemoptysis, and a dull throbbing chest pain beneath her left scapula. Chest x-ray revealed a mass in the upper lobe of her left lung and a left pleural effusion. A thoracentesis was performed, and the laboratory report follows:

Characteristic	Finding
Total number of cells:	155/mm³
Differential	
Polymorphonu- clear leukocytes:	10%

Lymphocytes:	18%
Monocytes:	22%
Macrophages:	10%
Mesothelial cells:	40%

Bronchoscopy revealed inoperable bronchogenic carcinoma. After irradiation of the tumor, the pleural effusion resolved.

A month later on readmission, the patient experienced increased shortness of breath. The chest x-ray showed that the tumor was larger in size and extended to a rib. There were pneumonia and pleural effusion. A thoracentesis was performed, and the laboratory report follows:

Characteristic	Finding
Total number of cells:	3,300/mm³
Differential	
Polymorphonu- clear leukocytes:	4%
Lymphocytes:	20%
Monocytes:	10%
Macrophages:	12%
Mesothelial cells:	44%
Tumor cells:	10%

These two reports illustrate the various characteristics of serous effusions that may result secondarily to the same processes.

Questions
1. What are the two chief differences in the evaluations of the two specimens?
2. What may have caused the first effusion?
3. Why was the second specimen so much more significant?

Answers
1. The cell count is markedly increased and tumor cells are now present in the second specimen.
2. Obstruction.
3. The second report reflects exfoliative cells and probable spread of the tumor.

BIBLIOGRAPHY

Beeson PB, Bass DA: The eosinophil. In Major Problems in Internal Medicine. Philadelphia, Saunders, 1977, Vol 14, pp 238–244.

Dorland's Illustrated Medical Dictionary, 24th ed. Philadelphia, Saunders, 1977.

Estevez, EG, Estevez B: Bacteriologic culture of sterile body fluids: assessment of a protocol. Lab Med 11:170, 1980.

Harvey A, Johns RJ, McKusick VA, Owens AH Jr, Ross R: Congestive heart failure, Chap 19, Pleural effusions, Chap 38, Principle manifestations of liver disease, Chap 64. In The Principles and Practice of Medicine, 20th ed. New York, Appleton, 1980.

Krieg A: Cerebrospinal fluid and other body fluids. In Davidsohn I, Henry JB: Clinical Diagnosis and Management, 14th ed. Philadelphia, Saunders, 1969, Chap 28, pp 1173–1175.

Krieg A: Cerebrospinal Fluid and Other Body Fluids. In Henry JB (ed): Clinical Diagnosis and Management, 16th ed. Philadelphia, Saunders, Chap 18, pp 635–679.

Lennett EH, Spaulding E, Spaulding H, Truent JP:
Manual for Clinical Microbiology, 2nd ed. Washington, D.C., American Society for Microbiology, 1974.

Light RW, Yener SE, Ball WC Jr: Cells in pleural fluid—their value in diagnosis. Arch Intern Med 132:854, 1973.

Light RW, Macgregor MI, Luchsinger PC, Ball WC Jr: Pleural effusions: the diagnostic separations of transudates and exudates. Ann Intern Med 77:507, 1972.

McClement JH: Diseases of the pleura. In Beeson PB, McDermott W (eds): Textbook of Medicine. Philadelphia, Saunders, 1975, pp 873–877.

Rosai J, Ackerman LV: The pathology of tumors. Part II. Diagnostic technique. CA 29:22, 1979.

Shields WF: Transudates, exudates, sweat, vaginal fluid, cystic fluid. In Race GJ (ed): Laboratory Medicine. New York, Harper & Row, 1977, Vol 4, Chap 6, pp 1–4.

Snider GL: Diseases of the pleura. In Wilkins RW, Levensky NG (eds): Medicine—Essentials of Clinical Practice, 2nd ed. Boston, Little Brown, 1978, Chap 21, pp 208–215.

Spieder P: The cytological diagnosis of tuberculosis in pleural effusions. Acta Cytol 23:374, 1979.

Ann E. Neely and Kathryn Kilpatrick Cheek

CHAPTER 14

Cells and Other Fixed Components of Body Fluids

Objectives

It is expected that the information presented in this chapter will enable the reader to:

1. Describe why various cell types present in peripheral blood may also be present in the various body fluids.
2. List considerations that are important in the preparation of the specimen for morphologic examination.
3. Identify the morphologic characteristics of lymphocytes, neutrophils, eosinophils, basophils, monocytes, macrophages, plasma cells, nucleated RBCs, mesothelial cells, atypical lymphocytes, leukemic cells, and lymphoma cells.
4. Differentiate between T and B lymphocytes.
5. Describe the content and function of the neutrophilic granules.
6. List entities in which elevated numbers of eosinophils may be found in pleural fluid.
7. Identify the content of the basophilic granules.
8. Identify functions of the various cell types.
9. List conditions in which both RBCs and nucleated RBCs may be found in fluid specimens.
10. Identify the significance of leukemic and lymphoma cells present in body fluids.
11. Define and identify Döhle bodies, toxic granulation, hemosiderin, and melanin.

Body fluids of normal, reactive, or inflammatory states will contain different types and percentages of cells that correspond with the patient's diagnostic problem. As a result of in vivo bleeding, invasion, or a traumatic tap, it is important to remember that cells present in the blood may also be present in the body fluids. Therefore, it is often possible to see any type of cell that may be seen in the peripheral blood smear in the cytospin preparations of body fluids. The normal white blood cell count in body fluids and the normal differential count are shown in Table 13.1. The characteristic differential findings of various disease states are in the chapters that describe each of the body fluids independently. In the preparation of the specimen for morphologic examination, care must be taken to assure a minimum deposit of debris by using clean slides and pipettes and stain that has been filtered. In making the film deposits with the cytocentrifuge, the speed of the machine should be very slow (500 rpm) so that no distortion of the cells takes place. If the cells are thrown too rapidly onto the slide, the cytoplasmic membrane may be broken or distorted. The morphologic characteristics of the cells will be described as they appear on Wright stain, the routine stain used in the majority of laboratories. The percentage of cells per 100 cells is given as the differential of the cells in making the report. Some laboratories count the malignant cells in excess of the 100 nucleated cells. A standardized method of reporting should be established for each laboratory.

LYMPHOCYTES

Lymphocytes are 9 to 15 μ in diameter and appear very similar to the lymphocytes seen on peripheral blood films. Normal lymphocytes have scant cytoplasm and heavily clumped nuclear chromatin. A few small granules may be seen in the pale cytoplasm. These azurophilic granules stain blue-purple and are peroxidase negative and acid phosphatase positive.

The lymphocyte is involved in two types of immunologic reactions. Approximately 80 percent of the lymphocytes in the peripheral blood are T cells and are concerned with cell-mediated immunity (delayed hypersensitivity graft rejection, graft-vs-host reaction, and the defense against some bacteria, e.g., tubercle bacilli). The B cells account for the other 10 to 20 percent of the lymphocytes in peripheral blood and are concerned with humoral immunity (antibody production). Lymphocytes, particularly the T cell, are thought to be very active in the defense against malignancies.

The lymphocytes are the most predominant cells in body fluids under normal conditions. In general, increased numbers of lymphocytes are present in tuberculosis, tumors, lymphomas, and rheumatoid arthritis. A WBC cell count in pleural fluid over 1,000/mm³, normal lymphocytes, and less than 1 percent mesothelial cells is strongly suggestive of tuberculosis.

NEUTROPHILS

Neutrophils (polymorphonuclear leukocytes, polys, segs) are from 12 to 15 μ in diameter. Neutrophils contain coarse, tightly clumped chromatin in the segmented nucleus. The nucleus contains three or four segments of nuclear material in the normal state. In body fluids, however, it is very common for the neutrophil to exhibit hypersegmentation, showing five to seven lobes. At this time, the cause of this hypersegmentation is not well correlated with peripheral blood counts such that the finding cannot be assumed as evidence of megaloblastic changes. The mature neutrophil shows three different types of granules that vary in staining characteristics. The large primary granules (1.5 μ) are called azurophilic granules. They contain acid hydrylases, neutral proteases, myeloperoxidase, catonic proteins, and lysosomes. The smaller specific granules (0.2 μ) contain alkaline phosphatase, lysosome, and lactoferrin. These smaller granules may vary in shape. The intermediate size are elongated or oval, while the smaller ones are very small and round. The smaller granules take on less dense staining characteristics. The membrane of the neutrophil may not appear as rigid in body fluids as it does in peripheral blood. This may be due to the chemical content of the fluid.

Because the neutrophils' chief function is phagocytosis, they will accumulate in great number under the stimulus of an inflammatory process. Band forms, metamyelocytes, and myelocytes as seen in peripheral blood in inflammatory states are also seen in body fluids (Figs. 14.1 and 14.2).

EOSINOPHILS

Eosinophils are from 12 to 16 μ in diameter, and the nucleus is similar to the neutrophil

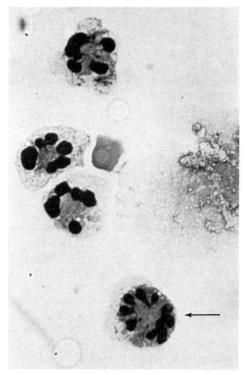

Figure 14.2. Hypersegmented neutrophil.

but is frequently bilobed. The cytoplasm is filled with large red-orange granules that tend to obscure the nucleus. The granules contain various hydrolytic enzymes and are peroxidase positive.

Eosinophils are motile and are active in inflammatory processes. The eosinophil is phagocytic but not as phagocytic as the neutrophil. The exact function of these cells is not fully understood. They are found in effusions when knowledge of the clinical significance of their presence is unknown. The most significant number of eosinophils is found in pleural fluids of all the body fluids, which may indicate the chronicity of many pleural disorders. There is no close relationship between the number of eosinophils in peripheral blood and body fluids. They are very common in exudates but are very uncommon when tuberculosis or malignancies are diag-

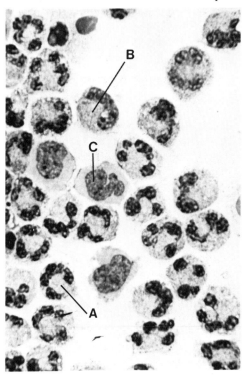

Figure 14.1. Neutrophils (**A**), band forms (**B**), monocytes (**C**).

nosed. Infections (bacterial and parasitic), hypersensitivity states, chest trauma, and hemorrhage into the pleural cavity may be correlated with eosinophilia in body fluids. Repeated tapping, pneumothorax, infarct, and postpneumonic effusions may also show increased eosinophils.

BASOPHILS

Basophils are from 11 to 14 μ in diameter. The nucleus is segmented like a neutrophil, but it may be obscured by the large granules that stain dark blue or dark purple. These granules contain histamine and heparin. The basophil functions in hypersensitivity reactions, such as allergic asthma and contact allergies. The number of basophils found in body fluids is low, and their significance is unknown.

MONOCYTES

Monocytes are quite varied in size, ranging from 15 to 30 μ in diameter (Fig. 14.3). They are usually larger than a neutrophil. The nucleus stains blue-purple and may be round or dented or have superimposed brainlike convolutions. The nuclear chromatin has a tendency to be loose or weblike, giving a coarse linear pattern. The cytoplasm stains dull blue-gray, appears very fragile (less rigid than a neutrophil), and may reveal pseudopods, suggesting its motility. The granules in the cytoplasm are evenly stained and are usually pink in color. The granules may be very fine and resemble dustlike particles. Vacuoles of various size may or may not be present in a normal monocyte.

The monocyte's chief roles are phagocytosis and as an integral part of the immune system. The monocyte is derived from the bone marrow, enters the peripheral circulation, lives from 30 to 100 hours, and becomes fixed in the tissues. At this time it becomes activated and is called a macrophage. This is the mononuclear phagocytic system or reticuloendothelial system.

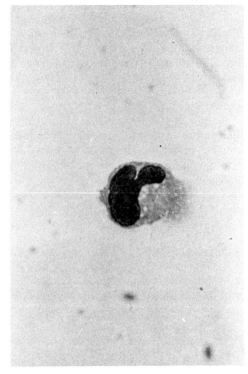

Figure 14.3. Monocyte.

While in the peripheral blood, the monocyte actively phagocytoses bacteria, cellular debris, and red cells. In body fluids, the monocytes are found in active inflammatory processes.

MACROPHAGES

Macrophages vary in size from 30 μ to 150 μ. This is a very broad category of cells and may include monocytes and histocytes. It is thought that most of the macrophages are derived from monocytes. This does not include the reactive mesothelial cells that may also take on properties of macrophages. The macrophage becomes specialized and, according to its location, assumes properties that may alter its appearance slightly, such as the Kupffer's cell of the liver and the alveolar macrophage of the lung.

As a monocyte takes on the properties of the macrophage, the cytoplasm is grossly enlarged, its granules are utilized and disappear, and large numbers of colorless vacuoles appear. The nucleus of the macrophage is round but may be bilobed or many lobed. The many-lobed nuclei in the giant macrophage may become confused with malignant cells. Macrophages may be found in groups frequently. Each macrophage will maintain its separate structure, with each nucleus remaining inside the cytoplasm. This important characteristic of the grouping helps identify nonmalignant cells vs malignant cells and is discussed in detail in Chapter 15. The nucleus contains very open chromatin and may contain dark or blue staining nucleoli.

As the macrophage progresses in its function of phagocytosis, the cytoplasm takes on various colors from gray to pale blue and contains more vacuoles, digested material, iron, and so on. Cells cannot be called macrophages unless they exhibit phagocytosis or evidence of phagocytosis, such as the vacuoles or storage of granules. Macrophages are capable not only of engulfing large particles but also of pinocytosis. Pinocytosis is the minute invagination of the surface of cells in the absorption of liquids to form vacuoles. Macrophages may phagocytize red blood cells, white blood cells, megakaryocyte nuclei, and cellular debris and provide defense against bacteria, viruses, and fungi.

Macrophages also play a very important role in the host defense mechanism (e.g., delayed hypersensitivity). The secretory capability of the macrophage is extremely important in the defense mechanism against foreign cells and tumor cells. They synthesize and secrete several biologically active substances that play the important role of receptors for gamma globulin and for complement. This function of the macrophage is the subject of a great deal of research.

Another function of the macrophage is that it exhibits a regulatory effect in hematopoiesis. The iron from hemoglobin is absorbed by the macrophage and provides nourishment for the red cell precursors (Fig. 14.4).

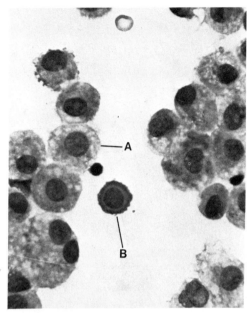

Figure 14.4. Macrophage (**A**) and one mesothelial cell (**B**).

PLASMA CELLS

Plasma cells are from 12 to 16 μ in diameter and are oval in shape (Fig. 14.5). The dense nucleus is eccentrically placed and may be smaller than that of a corresponding lymphocyte. The cytoplasm is intensely dark blue, and there is a clear halo adjacent to the nucleus. The clear zone corresponds to the very large Golgi complex that is seen on electron microscopy.

Plasma cells are involved in antibody production, and the number increases as a result of antigenic stimulation. They may be found in specimens that contain macrophages and lymphocytes. Plasma cells are seen in body fluid specimens that are the result of inflammatory processes.

NUCLEATED ERYTHROCYTES

Nucleated erythrocytes or nucleated red blood cells may be found in body fluid specimens. The orthochromatic normoblast varies

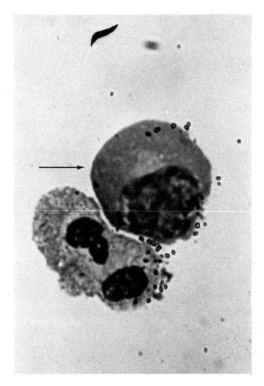

Figure 14.5. Plasma cell.

MESOTHELIAL CELLS

Mesothelial cells are 15 to 45 μ in diameter, and the nonreactive mesothelial cells have a round, coarse, dense, dark nucleus with an occasional nucleoli. The mesothelial cell comes from the simple squamous-celled layer of the epithelium that covers the surface of all true serous membranes, e.g., peritoneum, pleura, and pericardium. The cell has a uniform circular appearance. The cytoplasm is dark blue with a membrane that may contain small vacuoles. Due to the density of the color of the cytoplasm, it may be difficult to determine the separation of the nucleus and the cytoplasm. The nuclear cytoplasmic ratio (1:3) is higher in the mesothelial cell than in the macrophage (Fig. 14.6). The reactive mesothelial cells may contain more than one nucleus and one or more nucleoli (Fig. 14-7).

The nonreactive mesothelial cell, like the monocyte, when confronted with an approp-

from 10 to 13 μ in diameter and is the nucleated RBC most frequently seen. The nucleus is round and stains dark blue-purple. The cytoplasm changes from blue to pink with the maturation of the cell. The cytoplasm completely encircles the nucleus.

The significance of bloody body fluid is dealt with in each of the specific chapters. When the possibility of a bloody tap has been eliminated, in general, the examiner will think strongly of a malignancy being involved in a specimen containing elevated numbers of RBCs. Many of the cells that are malignant or suggestive of malignancy will be found in very bloody or serosanguineous fluids. The appearance of nucleated erythrocytes in a specimen is highly suggestive of a malignant, hemolytic, or abnormal process. This is similar to the situation in a peripheral blood count.

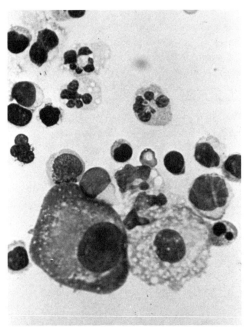

Figure 14.6. Mesothelial cell with macrophage.

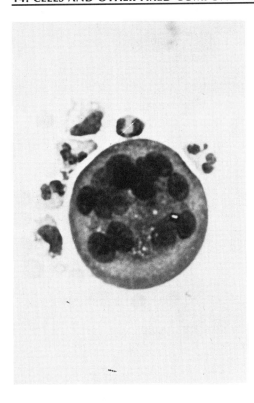

Figure 14.7. Reactive mesothelial cell.

riate stimulus, may transform, becoming a reactive mesothelial cell exhibiting macrophagelike properties.

The designation of a cell as a lymphocyte, monocyte, macrophage, or mesothelial cell (reactive or nonreactive) may pose a problem in terminology, as the role and function of these cells may vary with an individual's concept and training. When a cell fulfils the distinct morphologic characteristics, however, the observer should not hesitate to classify it as a lymphocyte, monocyte, macrophage or mesothelial cell (reactive or nonreactive). When cells do not exhibit all the characteristics of a specific cell type, however, judgments must be made based on experience and interpretation of the characteristics that are present. Often it is most beneficial to use descriptive terms in categorizing cells that do not show all the distinctive characteristics of one or another cell type.

ABNORMAL AND ATYPICAL CELLS

Abnormal and atypical cells that are seen in the peripheral blood may be seen also in body fluids. The most frequent cells of this classification are leukemic blast cells. Any of the leukemias may invade the body cavities, but the leukemic cells are most often seen in the cerebrospinal fluid. The *leukemic cells* (Fig. 14.8) will have the same morphologic characteristics as in peripheral blood, with the exception of the nucleoli being slightly less visible. The nuclei of leukemic cells will appear very immature. The cell count does not have to be increased to contain leukemic cells. If the specimen is from a known leukemic patient, the importance of observing blast cells in spinal fluid is of utmost importance in designing a treatment plan.

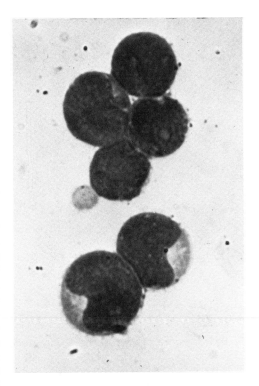

Figure 14.8. Leukemic cell.

ATYPICAL LYMPHOCYTES

Atypical lymphocytes may also be seen in body fluids (Fig. 14.9). The most striking characteristics of atypical lymphocytes are:

1. Increased amount of cytoplasm,
2. Heavy cyanophilic staining, particularly at the periphery of the cytoplasm,
3. Increase in size of the cell,
4. Nucleus may contain nucleoli, and
5. Nucleolar material may be irregularly clumped or disturbed, showing more perichromatin.

It is important in classifying cells in this category to be sure that the cytospin specimen has not been spun too rapidly, since this may distort cellular morphology.

Cells from a *lymphoma* show nuclear material that is more coarse or rough. The nucleus may have convolutions or indentations. Mul-

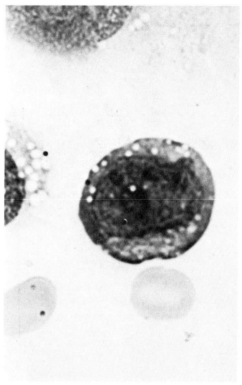

Figure 14.10. Cell from Burkitt's lymphoma.

tiple nucleoli may be present. The increased darkly staining cytoplasm may show irregular plasma membranes. The size of the cell may vary from 10 μ up to 30 μ. The cells from the spinal fluid of a patient with Burkitt's lymphoma may be as large as 30 μ in diameter (Fig. 14.10).

It is important that the examiner note the presence of the immature, atypical, or abnormal cells, such as leukemic or lymphoma cells. The diagnosis of leukemia or lymphoma is made from a review of the total picture of the patient, and the contribution of the observations seen in body fluids gives evidence of the extent of the disease process.

CELLULAR INCLUSIONS

Cellular inclusions that may be seen in body fluids are often the same inclusions as seen in

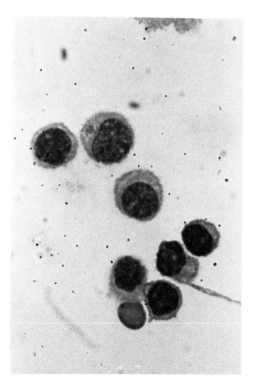

Figure 14.9. Atypical lymphocyte.

peripheral blood cells. *Döhle bodies* are light blue inclusions seen in neutrophils and occasionally in monocytes on Wright stain. They are small amounts of rough endoplasmic reticulum that are retained in the maturation of the cell from the promyelocyte level of maturation. Döhle bodies are seen along with toxic granulation in severe infections and in toxic states. The toxic granules are large azurophilic granules that are peroxidase positive.

Inclusions from the ingestion and degradation of hemoglobin may be seen in cells, particularly macrophages and monocytes. The large deposit of brown to black granules seen in these cells on Wright stain represents hemosiderin (Fig. 14.11). Hemosiderin is a hemogobin-derived deposit that represents stored iron. This is indicative of a large amount of dispersed iron. It can be stained and shows a positive reaction for iron in the Prussian blue stain. Hemosiderin in cells may be evidence of hemorrhage.

Melanin may appear as dark blue to black inclusions and is a pigment of skin, hair, eyes, or various tumors. When melanin is seen in macrophages, it may be evidence of metastatic melanoma. Melanoma cells may also contain melanin pigment, but the morphology of the melanoma cell is quite different from a macrophage. The nucleus:cytoplasm ratio is approximately 3:1 as compared to 1:3 of the macrophage. The membrane of the basophilic cytoplasm of the melanoma cell is fringed with vacuoles. Use of the Prussian blue stain will separate the melanin from hemosiderin.

Bacteria may be seen in polymorphonuclear leukocytes, monocytes, and macrophages and will stain dark purple with Wright stain (Fig. 14.12). The presence of bacteria is distinct, but for further identification a gram stain is necessary.

The appearance of *LE (lupus erythromatosus) cells* in fluids is discussed in Chapter 11, along with the description of RA (ragocyte) cells.

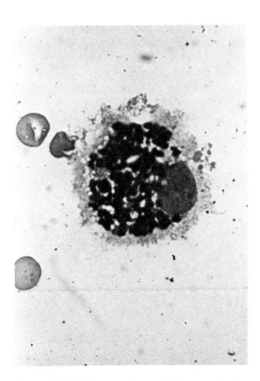

Figure 14.11. Macrophage with hemosiderin.

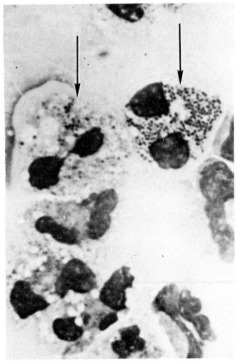

Figure 14.12. Neutrophil with bacteria.

The crystals that are of diagnostic significance and may be seen intracellularly and extracellularly are also discussed in Chapter 11.

SUMMARY

The correct identification of cells seen in body fluids cannot be overemphasized. The differentiation from a normal to a reactive state is frequently difficult to ascertain. A careful consideration of the description of any suspicious cells must be correlated with the rest of the evaluation of a body fluid. Only by incorporating all the available information will the best service for patient care be performed.

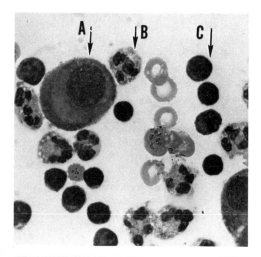

Review Questions

Match the cells in the illustrations at right to the appropriate cell type listed below.

_____ 1. Lymphocytes
_____ 2. Neutrophil
_____ 3. Basophil
_____ 4. Macrophage
_____ 5. Mesothelial cell
_____ 6. Leukemic blast cell

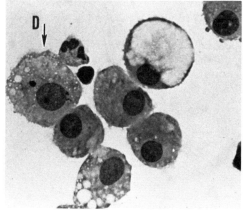

Directions: For each of the incomplete statements, one or more of the completions given is correct. Select:
    A. If *only 1, 2, and 3* are correct.
    B. If *only 1 and 3* are correct.
    C. If *only 2 and 4* are correct.
    D. If *only 4* is correct.
    E. If *all* are correct.
   7. Cell types that are present in a patient's peripheral blood may also be present in a cerebrospinal fluid specimen from that patient as a result of:
    1. A traumatic tap
    2. In vivo bleeding
    3. Local invasion of tumor
    4. Metastatic involvement

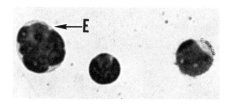

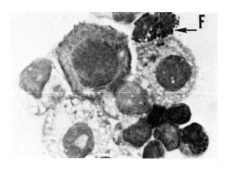

8. Large numbers of eosinophils are often common in exudates resulting from:
   1. Hypersensitivity states
   2. Tuberculosis
   3. Chronic pleural disorders
   4. Malignancies
9. Nucleated RBCs and mature RBCs may be found in various body fluids as a result of:
   1. Underlying hemolytic processes
   2. Malignancies
   3. A traumatic tap
   4. In vivo bleeding

Match the description from Column B to the appropriate entity in Column A.

Column A
_____ 10. Macrophage
_____ 11. Cell-mediated immunity
_____ 12. Contain heparin
_____ 13. Plasma cell
_____ 14. Döhle bodies
_____ 15. Melanin

Column B
A. Iron-containing compound
B. T lymphocytes
C. Skin pigment
D. Eccentric small dense nucleus
E. B lymphocytes
F. Basophils
G. One of its primary functions is phagocytosis
H. Retained rough endoplasmic reticulum
I. Eosinophil

Case Study

A 64-year-old white female was seen in the medicine outpatient clinic. She was very thin, emaciated, and had lost 15 pounds over the past six months. Her chief complaint was a chronic cough and intermittent fever.

On physical examination, her BP was 104/60, temperature 102F, respiration 30/minute. Examination of the chest revealed findings consistent with pleural effusion. There was no lymphadenopathy or splenomegaly.

A thoracentesis was performed, and 300 ml of milky pleural fluid was withdrawn—10 ml of the fluid was sent to the laboratory for examination. The fluid results were:

Characteristic	Finding
Visual examination:	milky
Specific gravity:	1.019
Total protein:	3.8 g/dl
Glucose:	90 mg/dl
LDH:	500 mU/μl
WBC:	1,975/mm^3
RBC:	100/mm^3
Differential:	Lymphocytes 100%
Gram stain:	no bacteria seen
Acid-fast stain:	no acid-fast organism seen
Culture:	pending

The CBC results were:

WBC:	14,000/mm^3
Hg:	10 g%
Hct:	33%
Platelets:	385,000/μl
Differential:	
Polymorphonuclear leukocytes:	30%
Lymphocytes:	54%
Monocytes:	16%

Question
A WBC count of this magnitude may be present as a result of all the following except:
1. A bacterial infection
2. A fungal infection
3. A normal process
4. A malignant process
5. A viral infection

Answer: 3

Comment

With this presentation of history, physical findings, and the abnormal findings on the complete blood count, the physician would list the differential diagnosis as (1) possible fungal infection, (2) tuberculosis, (3) *Mycoplasma* infection, or (4) viral infection.

The differential count on the pleural fluid showed 100% lymphocytes and no mesothelial cells. This is a typical finding of tubercle infections. Subsequently, *Mycobacterium tuberculosis* was reported from the culture.

BIBLIOGRAPHY

Henry JB: Clinical Diagnosis and Management by Laboratory Methods, 16th ed. Philadelphia, Saunders, 1979.

Robbins SL: Pathology, 3rd ed. Philadelphia, Saunders, 1967.

Robbins SL, Cotran RS: Pathologic Basis of Disease, 2nd ed. Philadelphia, Saunders, 1979.

Anne E. Neely and Kathryn Kilpatrick Cheek

CHAPTER 15

Malignant Cells

Objectives

It is expected that the information presented in this chapter will enable the reader to:

1. Define malignancy, cancer, and neoplasm.
2. Identify a situation in which a benign tumor may be life threatening.
3. Differentiate between metastasis and circulating cancer cells.
4. Define adenoma, sarcoma, carcinoma, adenocarcinoma, and in situ tumors.
5. Describe how the appearance of malignant cells as compared to their normal counterparts usually correlates with the classification of the tumor (benign vs malignant).
6. Define anaplasia, pleomorphism, dysplasia, and atypical.
7. Identify morphologic criteria that may cause a cell to be classified as suspicious of malignancy.
8. Utilize morphologic criteria to identify cells that are suspicious of malignancy.

Before undertaking the task of defining the characteristics of malignant cells, it is best to establish the meaning of the word "malignant," since overlapping terms are used in the discussion of cells thought to be malignant. Perhaps specific guidelines can be established for the identification of cells with malignant characteristics, and guidelines can be derived for the reporting of these cells. It is important to remember that there is no one criterion for classifying a cell as malignant. There is no substance, ultrastructurally or biochemical, that is uniquely present in malignant cells and not found in other cells.

Malignancy, cancer, and neoplasm are words that are frequently used interchangeably, and all carry a strong psychologic impact. The term *neoplasm* means literally "new growth" and is an abnormal mass of tissue that may not always be malignant. It may be benign and relatively slowly growing and is not life threatening. A *benign* tumor may become so large or, due to its location, may cause an organ or functional structure of an organ to cease functioning. Only in this manner is the benign tumor life threatening.

In contrast, the word *malignant* means very dangerous and capable of causing death. Malignant tumors have the capacity for rapid growth that can invade contiguous tissue and thereby causes organs to be unable to function. When the extent of malignancy reaches a strategic point, the host will be unable to maintain life and will die. The type of cell causing the invasive process and destruction is not the disease itself. Rather, malignancy is defined in terms of the biologic behavior of these cells, not their appearance. All malignant tumors are cancers and are seldom encapsulated.

There is no single definition of *cancer*. Cancer is a disease of tissue organization and is determined more by the host reaction. The response to the process of cancer is subject to the effects of the ever changing external and internal environment of the host. Most cancers are invasive and are subject to uncontrolled and unregulated growth. Benign tumors may push along the surface wall of an organ, but they do not infiltrate and destroy.

Malignant tumors are capable of infiltration, destruction, and metastasis, and these are the predominant features of cancer.

Metastasis is growth of a cancer separate and distinct from its primary site. Most cancers can metastasize. One factor in the rate of metastasis is that the growth does depend on the vascularity of the cancer's environment. The tumor will not outgrow its blood supply. Circulating cancer cells are not the same as metastasis. If a malignant tumor is manipulated, the number of circulating cancer cells may be increased. There may be an increase in circulating cancer cells following radiation also. However, the rate of metastasic disease is not equated with the number of circulating cells that may be found at any one time. Malignant tumors metastasize through lymphatic, neural, or blood-borne mechanisms depending on the type of cell comprising the tumor.

NOMENCLATURE OF TUMORS

Literally hundreds of types of neoplasms have been defined. For general purposes a word ending in -*oma* means a mass.

Benign
In benign tumor terminology, -*oma* is combined with the cell type in which it is found, e.g., fibroma, lipoma. *Adenoma* is a benign glandular tumor.

Malignant
Sarcomas are tumors arising from mesenchymal origin. The tumors are composed of closely packed cells embedded in a fibrillar or homogeneous substance. *Carcinoma* is the term applied to a malignant growth arising from epithelial cells. It can be derived from any of the three germ layers. *Adenocarcinoma* is the malignant growth of epithelial origin that shows a glandular growth pattern. *In situ tumors* have been retained in the original location and have not spread.

In further differentiating terminology applied to malignancies, one of the most important considerations is the rate and means of growth of the tumor. The rate of growth of a benign tumor is slow and has slight vascularity. In contrast if a malignant tumor is not treated, its growth may be fast, and the tumor shows moderate or marked vascularity. This *usually* correlates with the classification of how closely the malignant cells appear to their normal counterpart. In general, the better differentiated the cell type the slower the tumor grows.

Well-differentiated cells are cells that are present in a specimen that resemble the normal tissue. These tumors are more apt to have well-defined boundaries and contain most normal ultrastructural features. Benign tumors are usually well differentiated. Some tumors even regress spontaneously.

Poorly differentiated cells are cells that bear little resemblance to normal cells in that tissue. The more poorly differentiated the cells, often the more prominent the mitotic figures will be. The mitotic figures will be abnormal. Ultrastructural features are less prominent. There may be a decreased number of mitochondria, decreased endoplasmic reticulum, and decreased number of other recognizable structures.

Anaplasia is a reversal of cells to a very undifferentiated or primitive stage. Anaplasia may be used as a synonym for undifferentiation. There is little or no resemblance to their normal counterpart. Anaplastic cells show a great variation in size, may contain huge nucleoli in very large nuclei, and may have increased and atypical mitotic figures.

Pleomorphism is the assumption of various distinct forms of a cell type. *Dysplasia* refers to an abnormality in the normal organization of cells and tissue. This may precede the development of cancer. *Atypical* denotes a deviation from normal.

MORPHOLOGIC OBSERVATIONS

When an observer encounters a cell that does not qualify as being a normal part of a specific body fluid, a systematic procedure should be followed. The morphologic observations that may suggest the malignancy of a cell are given in Table 15.1. It is important to evaluate the isolated cells as well as the clumps or multiple arrangements of cells. Isolated suspicious cells in a fluid specimen may represent a lack of cohesiveness of malignant cells, as the malignant cells are often easy to separate. This may reflect the fact that malignant cells have less calcium ions and greater electric charges in their cytoplasmic membrane.

The cells should be systematically observed or checked for each of the characteristics listed in Table 15.1. Characteristic findings of malignant cells with examples are described in the remainder of this chapter. Cells displaying one or more of these characteristics should be described in detail and separately from normal cells in the examination of fluid. Preparations containing atypical or abnormal cells should always be discussed with the pathologist or a reliable co-worker. Any preparation that contains malignant cells should be signed out by the pathologist. It is the pathologist's task to confirm the observations, since this frequently requires correlation with other information about the patient. Abnor-

TABLE 15.1. MORPHOLOGIC OBSERVATIONS OF SUSPICIOUS CELLS

   I. Nuclear-cytoplasmic ratio
  II. Nuclear features
       A. Hyperchromasia
       B. Variation in size, shape, number, and appearance
       C. Nucleoli features
       D. Nuclear molding
       E. Intranuclear inclusions
 III. Cytoplasmic features
       A. Well defined
       B. Irregularly defined
       C. Vacuolated
       D. Cyanophilic
       E. Intracytoplasmic inclusions
  IV. Pleomorphism
   V. Size of cells
  VI. Arrangement of cells
       A. Sheetlike
       B. Syncytial
       C. Cell ball
       D. Rosette and glandular
       E. Other forms

malities seen may sometimes be caused by viral infections, fungal infections, megaloblastic changes, or poor preparations as well as by malignancy.

The cells shown in the illustrations in this chapter were made from Wright-stained centrifuged preparations. The morphologic detail is good with this technique, and for this reason various characteristic morphologic changes are readily apparent. It should be remembered, however, that the diagnosis of cancer can rarely be rendered from cytocentrifuged specimens alone.

Morphologic Observations of Suspicious Cells

Nuclear Cytoplasmic Ratio. The nucleus of the normal cell and the cytoplasm are normally found in a 1:4 or 1:6 ratio (Fig. 15.1). The malignant cell appears crowded and the nuclear cytoplasm ratio may be 1:1 (Fig. 15.2). This may be described as having a nuclear area four or five times normal. This nuclear enlargement may be attributed to an increase in DNA content, an increase in the number of chromosomes, or degenerative changes that may be taking place.

Many malignant cells show a marked increase in the number of chromosomes. This may be observed in cells showing very abnormal mitosis. Large spindles may be seen

along with small spindles in the same specimen. The mitotic figures are very important in the classification of malignant tumors, as some malignant tumor cells never show mitosis and other malignant tumors very frequently show bizarre mitosis (Fig. 15.3). The presence of mitosis does not necessarily mean that the cell is malignant.

Nuclear Features. The observations found in the nucleus are the chief factors in suggesting the presence of a malignant condition.

Hyperchromasia. Hyperchromasia is an alteration in the normal chromatin structure. The nucleus contains a large amount of DNA that has an affinity for basic dye. The chromatin may become aggregated in large clumps and irregularly spaced within the nucleus. This is called *heterochromatin,* and when viewed on transmission electron microscopy, it appears as very tight coils that are electron dense. The less dense area between the clumps is called *euchromatin.* The euchromatin is not coiled and is electron lucent on transmission electron microscopy. The aggregates may be so coarsely clumped that the euchromatin is extremely sparse and the background is said to be erased. The large chromatin clumps may be related to the increased functional demands.

The chromatin in the nucleus may have a very jagged appearance (Fig. 15.4). When the

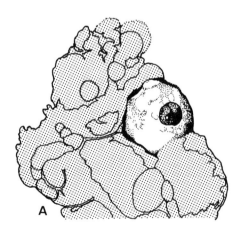
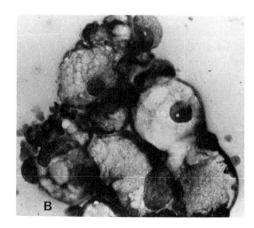

Figure 15.1. Normal nuclear/cytoplasmic ratio 1:3.

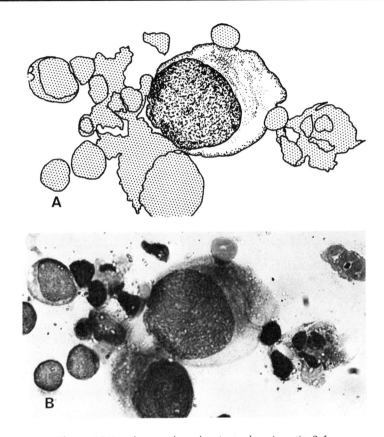

Figure 15.2. Abnormal nuclear/cytoplasmic ratio 2:1.

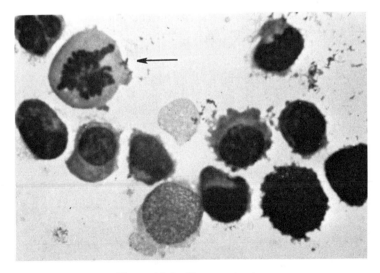

Figure 15.3. Bizarre mitosis.

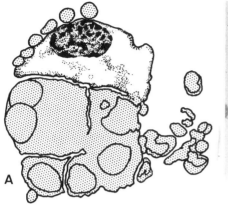 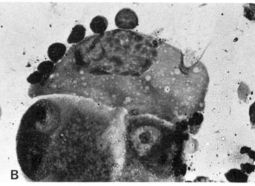

Figure 15.4. Hyperchromatic nucleus.

background is partially cleaned or "erased" the chromatin may be distributed irregularly in deposits along the nuclear membrane. This process is called "nuclear" margination (Fig. 15.5).

Variation in Size, Shape, Number, and Appearance of Nuclei. The nucleus is classically single, round or slightly ovoid, and in the center of the cell. The nuclear chromatin is homogeneously clumped. The normal appearance of the nucleus varies according to the cell type. A cell showing an exaggerated oval nucleus is associated with a high rate of cell division. Whereas the nucleus is centrally placed in most cells, it may be displaced by secretions or cytoplasmic inclusions as one observes in the signet-ring cell (Fig. 15.6).

This displacement is seen frequently in well-differentiated adenocarcinomas that are producing mucin.

Multiple and inconsistently arranged nuclei frequently vary in size and may be bizarre in shape. The nuclei may be lobulated, pyknotic, or may show angular projections (Fig. 15.7). The nuclei may also appear to be notched, or folds or clefts may be present.

The nuclear chromatin may be smooth, fine, and homogeneous, resembling ground glass (Fig. 15.8). In contrast, the chromatin may assume a coarse, heavy, and linear arrangement (Fig. 15.9).

Nucleoli Features. Nucleoli may be prominent and multiple. The nucleolus contains RNA, and the size varies according to the cell

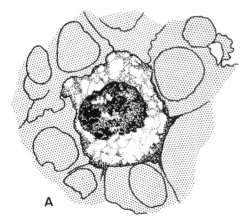 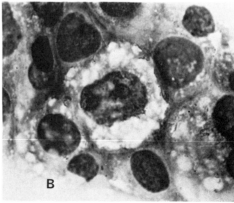

Figure 15.5. Nuclear margination.

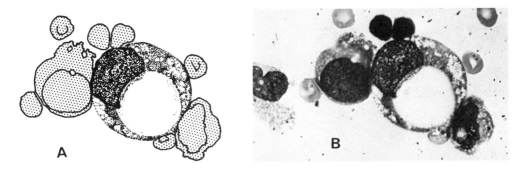

Figure 15.6. Signet-ring form.

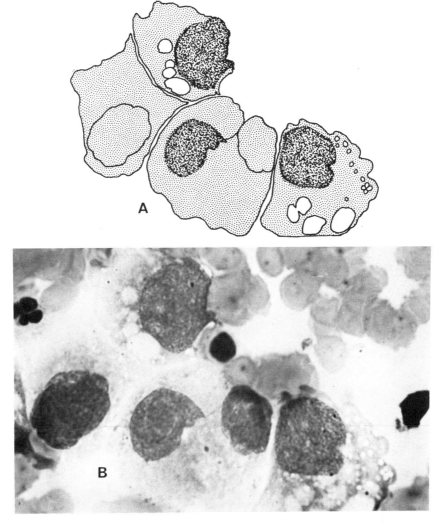

Figure 15.7. Angular projections.

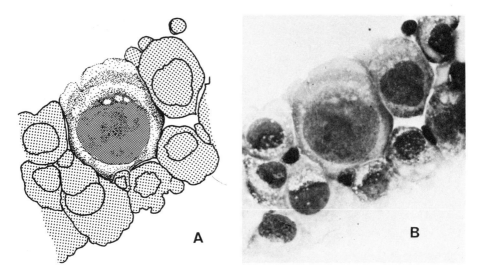

Figure 15.8. Ground glass appearance.

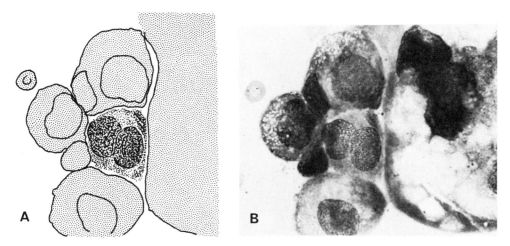

Figure 15.9. Coarse linear chromatin.

involved. Macronucleoli may be present, a reflection of the synthetic activity of these cells. When the nucleolar area is four or five times normal or occupies one third of the nucleus, the cell would be suggestive of an abnormal process. The nucleoli may show irregular configurations with projections or sharp angles (Fig. 15.10).

Nuclear Molding. In groups of abnormal cells, the nuclei may be crowded and molded against one another. Abnormal cells are less subject to contact inhibition. The abnormal cells may be more motile than their normal counterparts so that when they make contact, they continue in an attempt to move. This nuclear molding may occur in a single cell (Fig. 15.11).

Intranuclear Inclusions. Inclusions may be found in both the nuclei and the cytoplasm of cells. They are usually eosinophilic in staining characteristics and may be surrounded by a halo. These may be seen in viral infections, such as cytomegalovirus, as well as in the cells suspicious of malignancy.

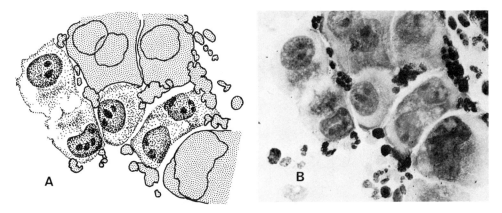

Figure 15.10. Multiple and prominent angular nucleoli.

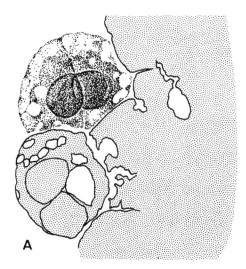

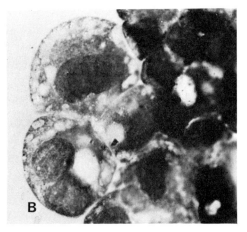

Figure 15.11. Nuclear molding.

Cytoplasmic Features. Observation of the cytoplasmic characteristics is most helpful in identifying the cell type and the rate of proliferation.

Well-defined Cytoplasm. Well-differentiated cells are more likely to have well-defined boundaries (Fig. 15.12). Cells may be seen that show a condensation of staining around the periphery of the membrane. This condensation is called a cytoplasmic matrix and may possibly be related to a secretion on the cell or by the cell.

Irregularly Defined Cytoplasmic Membrane. It is thought that malignant cells with irregular cytoplasmic membranse (Fig. 15.13) may be infiltrative or may spread faster than the better defined cells. The smoother membraned cells are thought to exhibit a tendency to push against tissue in contrast to the irregular edges that invade and infiltrate.

Vacuolated Cytoplasm. The cytoplasm may be very scant, have indistinct boundaries, and be foamy and amorphous. Vacuolated cytoplasm (Fig. 15.14), especially around the periphery of the cell, suggests a glandular origin and may be spoken of as a "string-of-pearls" appearance (Fig. 15.15).

Cyanophilic Cytoplasm. A cyanophilic cytoplasm (dark blue) may be seen in many malignant cells.

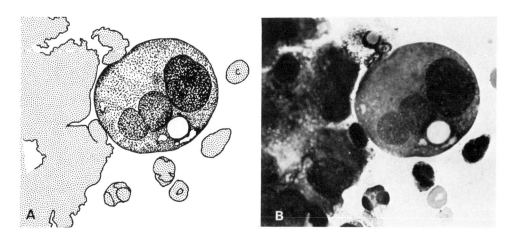

Figure 15.12. Well-defined cytoplasm.

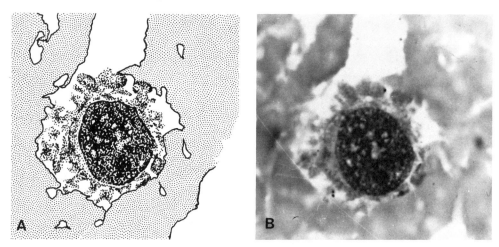

Figure 15.13. Irregular membrane.

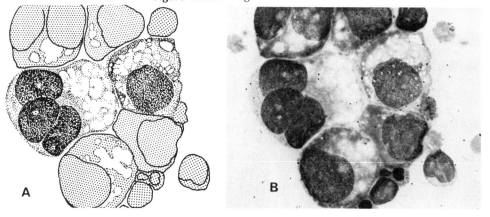

Figure 15.14. Vacuolated cytoplasm.

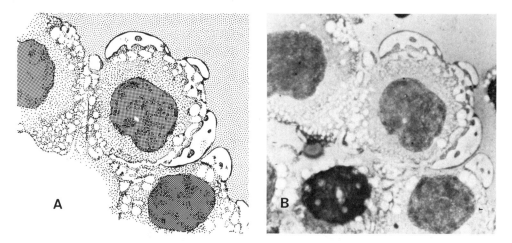

Figure 15.15. String-of-pearls appearance.

Pleomorphism. While some cells may show a marked variation in cell size and shape, other malignancies may be composed of cells of uniform size. Some cells may lose all resemblance to their normal structure and are characterized as poorly differentiated and/or as anaplastic cells. As a general rule, the more malignant the cancerous process, the more pleomorphic the cells (Fig. 15.16).

Size of Cells. The size of a malignant cell may be normal, smaller than normal, or larger than normal, ranging in size up to giant cells.

This lack of uniformity may be an indication of a malignancy. However, it is also possible to have a malignant cell that is smaller than normal and similar in size and shape. Notice the size of the giant cell from a diagnosed malignancy (Fig. 15.17). The cell is approximately 60 to 65 μ in diameter.

Arrangement of Cells. There are several different arrangements or groupings of cells seen in body fluids. In any of the arrangements it is important to observe the individual characteristics of a single cell as well as the

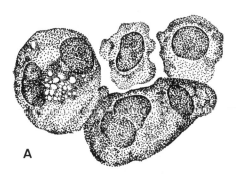

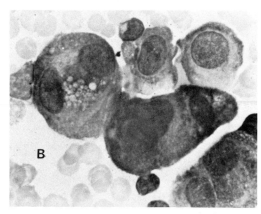

Figure 15.16. Pleomorphism.

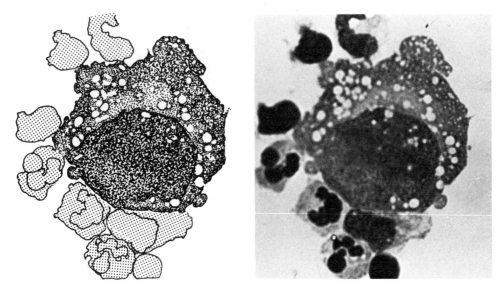

Figure 15.17. Giant cell.

characteristic arrangement of the cells. In evaluating an isolated cell and its frequency, it may suggest a decrease in mutual adhesiveness of the cells. The following are several characteristic arrangements of cells that may appear in body fluids from malignant processes.

Sheetlike Arrangement. Cells are regularly arranged in relationship to one another and have distinct cell boundaries. The individual cells appear normal even though they occur in sheetlike arrangements. They may be growing in a very disorganized manner. Figure 15.18 is a group of nonmalignant cells.

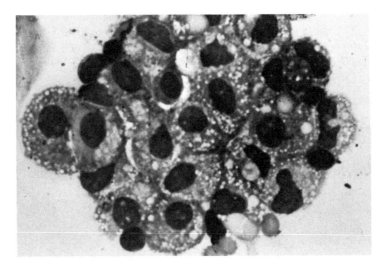

Figure 15.18. Sheetlike arrangement of non-malignant cells.

Syncytial Arrangement. The cells in a syncytial arrangement are irregularly arranged and have poorly defined boundaries (Fig. 15.19). The nuclei may deviate from the normal central position. This is the most important grouping and is very characteristic of malignancies.

Cell Ball. A three-dimensional appearance is seen in a cell ball arrangement (Fig. 15.20). When cells are found in a fluid medium, such as pleural or peritoneal fluid, they tend to grow in spherical aggregates. The cells may appear in wrapped-around groups, in which the cells are crowded and molded against

each other. Mesothelial cells may be seen particularly in pleural fluid in cell ball formation and have a scalloped border.

Rosette and Glandular Formations. Rosette-like arrangements (Fig. 15.21) or side by side groupings may also be found. Cells may form acini (small saclike dilatations), and one may observe hyperdistended secretory vacuoles. These are called "glandular cells" and may suggest adenocarcinoma (Fig. 15.22).

Other Forms. Cells may be seen in several other variations. Mesothelial cells are frequently seen in rows or stacks, resembling an Indian file arrangement sometimes seen in

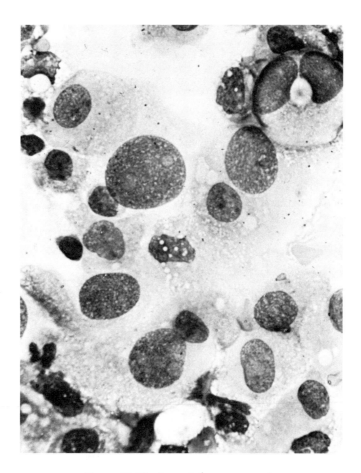

Figure 15.19. Syncytial arrangement.

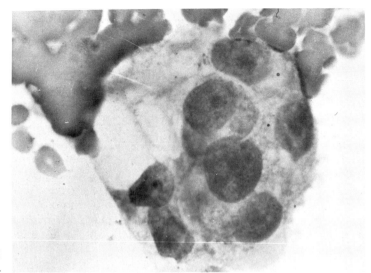

Figure 15.20. Cell ball arrangement.

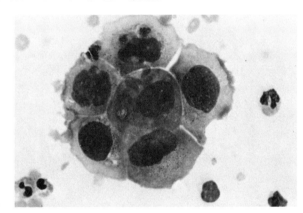

Figure 15.21. Rosette formation.

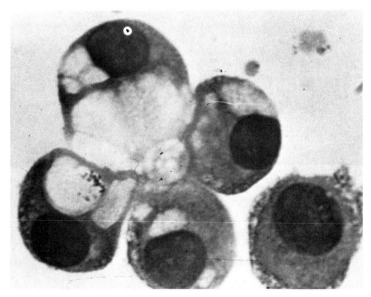

Figure 15.22. Glandular formation.

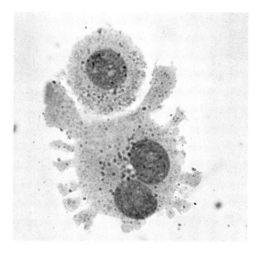

Figure 15.23. Another form of cellular arrangement.

adenocarcinoma. Pyramids and embracing forms may be seen. A cannibalistic activity may be observed in some of the giant cells. Figure 15.23 represents an unclassified cell that appears to exhibit this cannabalistic activity.

SUMMARY

Although a cell may possess one or more of the characteristics to classify it as suspicious or malignant, one must often weigh the overall picture of the cell before a decision is rendered. The more suspicious characteristics a cell displays, the greater the likelihood that the cell represents a malignant process.

Review Questions

Match the word in Column A with its most appropriate definition in Column B.

Column A
___ 1. Malignant
___ 2. Cancer
___ 3. Neoplasm
___ 4. Adenoma
___ 5. Anaplasia
___ 6. Pleomorphism
___ 7. Dysplasia
___ 8. Metastasis

Column B
A. No single definition, a disease of tissue organization
B. A benign glandular forming tumor
C. Tumor arising from mesenchymal origin
D. Abnormal mass representing new growth
E. Assumption of various distinct forms of a cell type
F. Growth of a cancer separate and distinct from its primary site
G. Tumor that has outgrown its blood supply
H. Reversal of cells to a very undifferentiated stage
I. Very dangerous and capable of causing death
J. Abnormality in the normal organization of cells and tissue

Case Studies

Case Study 1

A 68-year-old white female was admitted to the hospital from the emergency room in mild respiratory disease. Past medical history revealed a five-month history of weight loss, anorexia, and chest pain, with recent development of a productive cough. On physical examination a large mass was noted in the right breast. On chest x-ray a large right pleural effusion was seen. A diagnostic tap was performed obtaining 400 ml of bloody pleural fluid.

Cells present on the cytocentrifuge preparation are shown in Figure 1K. Figure 2K demonstrates cells that were present from the fluid sample using a Pappenheim's stain. Figure 3K shows cells on Hematoxylin and Eosin section that were made on axillary lymph node biopsy taken at a later date. A definitive diagnosis of infiltrating ductal carcinoma of the breast was made by breast biopsy several days after admission.

This case illustrates cellular morphology of malignant cells that may be present using various techniques for demonstration of those cells.

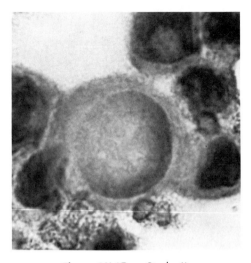

Figure 2K (Case Study 1)

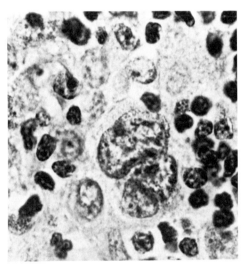

Figure 3K (Case Study 1)

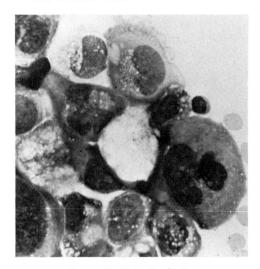

Figure 1K (Case Study 1)

Case Study 2

A pleural fluid was received in the lab at 7:30 PM from a patient admitted through the emergency room. The patient was a 63-year-old white female with a history of alcoholism and malnutrition. The specimen was obtained from a right pleural effusion at approximately 7:00 PM. The following report was developed by the evening technologist:

Characteristic	Finding
Time collected:	7:00 PM
Time received:	7:30 PM
Source of fluid:	right pleural effusion
Color:	orange
Appearance:	cloudy
RBC/mm³:	20,200
WBC/mm³:	4,600
Differential:	
Polymorphonu-	
clear leukocytes:	36%
Lymphocytes:	12%
Monocytes:	20%
Macrophages:	15%
Mesothelial cells (most	
are reactive):	13%
Eosinophils:	2%
Basophils:	2%

Questions

Figure 4K is a view of 63× magnification of one field of the cytospin preparation of this specimen.
1. Identify the cell types present.
2. In your opinion, should the technologist have suspected a malignancy and delayed the final report so that the pathologist could review the slide in the morning?

Answers

1. A. Mesothelial cell (reactive)
   B. Macrophages
   C. Basophil
   D. Lymphocytes
2. No, the cells present do not exhibit any suspicious characteristics.

Case Study 3

A premature 5-day-old infant from a local hospital was transported to the medical center in acute respiratory distress and possible sepsis. Shortly after his arrival, a spinal tap was performed. A specimen was received in the laboratory approximately 20 minutes after the procedure was performed.

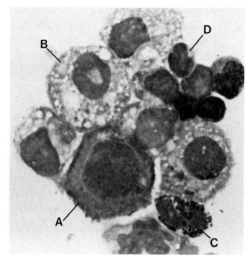

Figure 4K (Case Study 2)

Questions

Figure 5K is a view at 40× magnification of one field of the cytospin preparation of this CSF.
1. Identify the cell types present.
2. Are these cells suspicious for a malignancy?
3. Of what significance are the inclusions in the cytoplasm of some of the macrophages?

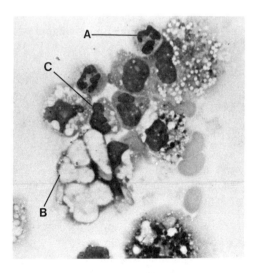

Figure 5K (Case Study 3)

4. What stain(s) might be helpful in identifying the inclusions present in the cytoplasm of some of the macrophages?

Answers
1. A. Neutrophils
   B. Macrophages
   C. Monocytes
2. No.
3. If the inclusions are bacteria, perhaps they are a result of a septic condition present in this child. If the inclusions are hemosiderin or hematoidin, they may indicate a previous bleeding in the area. If they are melanin, they might indicate a tumor.
4. A. Gram stain
   B. Prussian blue stain

Case Study 4

A pleural fluid was received from a 45-year-old black female with a history of recurrent respiratory tract infections. This admission was a result of her most recent recurrence of pneumonia.

Questions
Figure 6K at 40× magnification and Figure 7K at 63× magnification are views of the cytospin preparation from this woman's pleural fluid.
1. How would you report the cell types present in these views?
2. What are some of the predominant features present in the large cells in both of these views?
3. Are these cells suspicious for malignancy?
4. What is the proper procedure for developing the final report on this specimen?

Answers
1. Using descriptive terms.
2. The following characteristics are present:
   Pleomorphism
   Hyperchromatic nucleoli
   Multiple prominent nucleoli
   Irregular cytoplasmic borders
   Vacuoles in the cytoplasm
   Nuclear molding

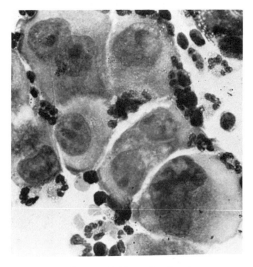

Figure 6K (Case Study 4)

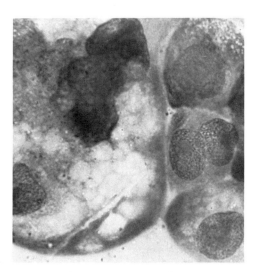

Figure 7K (Case Study 4)

3. Yes.
4. These abnormal cells should occupy a unique position in the differential. They should be categorized using descriptive terms. The slide and technologist's impression should be given to the pathologist so that his impressions may be included in the final report.

Case Study 5

The patient was a 54-year-old white female. Beginning five months prior to admission she developed a productive cough, chest pain, earache, and occasional night sweats. She had been treated twice for pneumonia by her local physician prior to her admission. Figure 8K and Figure 9K represent cells that were seen on the cytocentrifuge preparation of pleural fluid from this patient.

Questions

1. Are these cells suspicious for malignancy? If so, why?
2. Figures 10K and 11K demonstrate cells present in the Hematoxylin and Eosin section of lung from this patient. Figure 12K is a touch preparation (slide touched directly onto section of lung at surgery) of lung tissue from this patient. Do cells present in these preparations demonstrate morphologic

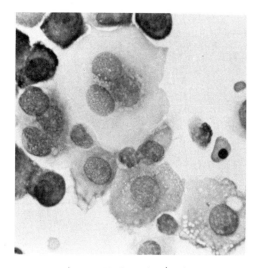

Figure 8K (Case Study 5)

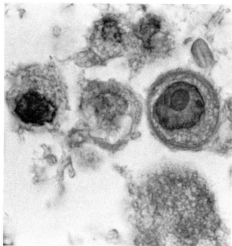

Figure 10K (Case Study 5)

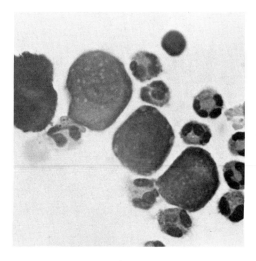

Figure 9K (Case Study 5)

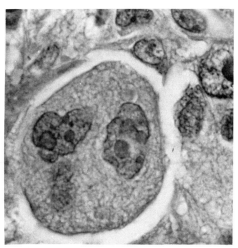

Figure 11K (Case Study 5)

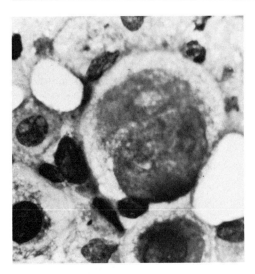

Figure 12K (Case Study 5)

characteristics similar to those seen in Figures 8K and 9K?

Answers

1. Yes. Increased nuclear cytoplasmic ratio, variation in size, shape, number, and appearance of nucleoli, variation in size, shape, number, and appearance

of nucleoli, vacuolated and cyanophilic cytoplasmic pleomorphism.

2. Yes. Patient was diagnosed as having adenocarcinoma of the lung.

BIBLIOGRAPHY

American Society of Clinical Pathologists: A Manual of Cytotechnology, 4th ed. Chicago, 1975.

Bessi M: Living Blood Cells and Their Ultrastructure. New York, Heidelberg, Berlin, Springer-Verlag, 1973.

Henry JB: Clinical Diagnosis and Management by Laboratory Methods, 16th ed. Philadelphia, Saunders, 1979.

Kolmel D, Wolgang H: Atlas of Cerebrospinal Fluid Cells, 2nd ed. Berlin, Heidelberg, New York, Springer-Verlag, 1977.

Oehmichen M: Cerebrospinal Fluid Cytology—An Introduction and Atlas. Philadelphia, Saunders, 1976.

Robbins SL: Pathology, 3rd ed. Philadelphia, Saunders, 1967.

Robbins SL, Cotran RS: Pathologic Basis of Disease, 2nd ed. Philadelphia, Saunders, 1979.

Spriggs AI, Boddington MM: The Cytology of Effusions and Cerebrospinal Fluid, 2nd ed. London, Heinemann Medical Books, Ltd. 1976.

University of Rochester: Clinical Oncology for Medical Students and Physicians, 5th ed. American Cancer Society, Rochester, NY 1978.

Answers to Review Questions

CHAPTER 1

1. A, B, C, D, E
2. C
3. A. 2
   B. 1, 2
   C. 3
   D. 2
   E. 3
   F. 2

4. A
5. A, C, D
6. C, E
7. E
8. A, B

9. A. 4
   B. 5
   C. 3
   D. 1
   E. 2
10. A, B, C, D, E

CHAPTER 2

1. A. 2
   B. 5
   C. 4
   D. 1
   E. 3
   F. 6
2. A. 7
   B. 1
   C. 4
   D. 5
   E. 6
   F. 3
   G. 8

3. A,B,C,D
4. B
5. C,E
6. A,B,E
7. B,C,D
8. D
9. A,B
10. D
11. A
12. A,B,C
13. B
14. B,C
15. A

16. A,D
17. A,B,C
18. A,B,C,E
19. A,E
20. B
21. A,B,C,D
22. A,B,C,D,E
23. A,B,C
24. A
25. E
26. A
27. D
28. x,x,y,x,x,y,y

29. C
30. A,B
31. B
32. A,C,E
33. E
34. A,B,C

CHAPTER 3

1. B
   Blood creatinine: 371.3 μmole/L
      (4.2 mg/dl)
   24-hour urine volume: 840 ml
   Urine creatinine: 2828.8 μmole/L
      (32 mg/dl)
   Height: 132 cm
   Weight: 31.4 kg

   $$C = \frac{UV}{P} \times \frac{1.73}{A}$$

   U = 2828.8 μmole/L

   $$V = \frac{840 \text{ ml}}{24 \text{ hr} \times 60 \text{ min}} = \frac{840 \text{ ml}}{1440 \text{ min}}$$

   $$= 0.58 \text{ ml/min}$$

   P = 371.3 μmole/L

A = body surface area
   log A = (0.425 × log 31.4) + (0.725
      × log 132) − 2.144
   log A = (0.425 × 1.497) + (0.725 ×
      2.121) − 2.144
   log A = (0.636) + (1.538) − 2.144
   log A = 0.03
      A = antilog 0.03 = 1.06 sq m

$$C = \frac{(2828.8)\,(0.58)}{(371.3)} \times \frac{1.73}{1.06}$$

C = 7.2 ml/min

2. A,B,C,D
3. A
4. B
5. B
6. E
7. B
8. C

CHAPTER 4

1. D
2. A
3. B
4. C
5. A
6. A. HCl is dangerous if it comes in contact with skin. It destroys formed elements in the urine and may interfere with specific tests.
   B. Formaldehyde interferes with several tests, including glucose evaluation.
   C. Thymol causes false positive results for protein evaluation by heat and acetic acid.
   D. Toluene is flammable and difficult to separate from the specimen when testing.
7. Twenty-four hour urine collection:
   A. Empty bladder, discard this urine, and note the time on the container.
   B. Collect and refrigerate all voided urine in the next 24 hours.
   C. Remind the patient to include a final voiding at the end of the timing period.
   D. Note the exact time of the final voiding on the specimen container.
8. A. Clean-catch specimen, catheterized specimen
   B. Random or spot specimen
   C. 2-hour afternoon specimen, 24-hour specimen
   D. 24-hour specimen
   E. Three-glass test
   F. Freshly collected random, early morning, or clean-catch specimen; fixative may be added

CHAPTER 5

1. T
2. T
3. F
4. T
5. D
6. F
7. A. 3
   B. 1
   C. 2
8. A. 1,3,6
   B. 2,4,6
9. F
10. F
11. E
12. T
13. C
14. T
15. F

16. A. 3
    B. 4
    C. 1
    D. 2
    E. 5
    F. 7
    G. 6
17. T
18. D
19. A. 1
    B. 3
    C. 3
20. T
21. D
22. F
23. T
24. T
25. T
26. D

27. T
28. B
29. F
30. T
31. C
32. T
33. T
34. F
35. F
36. T
37. F
38. F
39. T
40. D
41. T
42. T
43. A
44. D
45. C

46. F
47. T
48. F
49. T
50. T
51. T
52. D
53. A. 1
    B. 1
    C. 2
    D. 1
    E. 1
54. A. 4
    B. 3
    C. 6
    D. 5
    E. 2
    F. 1
55. T

CHAPTER 6

1. B
2. E
3. C
4. D
5. D
6. A, B, C, D

7. D
8. D
9. A, B, C
10. A, B, C, D
11. B, D
12. D

13. A, C
14. A, B, C, D
15. A, B, C
16. D
17. A, B, C

CHAPTER 7

1. D,E
2. A
3. A
4. A, 2
   B, 4
   C, 3
   D, 1
5. A, B
6. A, B, C, D, E
7. A, 1
   B, 2
   C, 3
   D, 4

8. A, B, D
9. B, C, E
10. A, B, C, D, E
11. C, D, E
12. B, C, D, E
13. A, 2
    B, 5
    C, 4
    D, 3
    E, 1
    F, 2

14. C, D, E
15. A
16. B
17. B
18. A, B, C
19. D
20. B, D
21. C
22. A, 2
    B, 4
    C, 3
    D, 1
    E, 5

23. B, C, D
24. A, B
25. D
26. A, B, C
27. A, B, C

CHAPTER 8

1. C
2. A, B, C, D, E
3. C, D, E
4. A, B, C
5. A, B, C, E
6. A, B
7. C, E
8. A, C, D
9. B, C, D
10. C, D
11. A, C, D
12. C
13. A, B, C, D
14. Disinfection of work area and equipment
    Storage and disposal of biologic specimens and waste
    Precautions in the laboratory
    Identification of hepatitis patients and proper labeling of specimens
15. D
16. A, 4
    B, 1
    C. 5
    D, 3
    E, 2
17. C
18. D
19. Number of tests performed
    Types of tests
    Number of personnel required
    Educational activities
20. The staff can give practical suggestions based upon their familiarity with the performance of the tests and the daily activities of the laboratory. Their acceptance of the final plan is also enhanced.
21. B
22. B, C, E
23. A, B, C, D
24. A

CHAPTER 9

1. D
2. 33 WBC/μl
   61 RBC/μl
   33 % mononuclear
   67 % polynuclear
3. 69 WBC/μl
   55 RBC/μl
   44 % mononuclear
   56 % polynuclear
4. 10 WBC/μl
   1,005 RBC/μl
   74 % mononuclear
   26 % polynuclear
5. C
6. B
7. C
8. A
9. C
10. A
11. E
12. A
13. B
14. D
15. C
16. A
17. B
18. D
19. A
20. B
21. C

CHAPTER 10

1. B
2. D
3. B
4. D
5. C
6. B
7. E
8. A
9. C
10. E
11. D
12. E
13. B
14. E
15. B
16. D
17. A
18. C
19. B
20. A
21. C
22. E
23. A
24. B
25. D
26. F
27. A

CHAPTER 11

1. A	6. C	11. A	16. D
2. A	7. E	12. B	17. D
3. B	8. A	13. A	18. A
4. C	9. A	14. F	19. B
5. B	10. C	15. C	20. C

CHAPTER 12

1. D	5. E	9. C	13. B
2. B	6. A	10. B	14. A
3. A	7. C	11. C	15. A
4. D	8. E	12. A	

CHAPTER 13

1. D	6. B	11. E	16. A
2. A	7. A	12. G	17. B
3. B	8. D	13. A	18. B
4. B	9. A	14. C	
5. E	10. F	15. B	

CHAPTER 14

1. C	5. A	9. E	13. D
2. B	6. E	10. G	14. H
3. F	7. E	11. B	15. C
4. D	8. B	12. F	

CHAPTER 15

1. I	5. H
2. A	6. E
3. D	7. J
4. B	8. F

INDEX

(Page numbers followed by the letters f and t indicate figures and tables, respectively)